D1556924

ATYPICAL DIABETES

Boris Draznin, MD, PhD, Editor

Louis H. Philipson, MD, PhD, Associate Editor
Janet B. McGill, MD, MA, Associate Editor

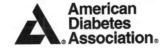

American Diabetes Association®

Associate Publisher, Books, Abe Ogden; *Managing Editor,* Rebekah Renshaw; *Acquisitions Editor,* Victor Van Beuren; *Production Manager,* Melissa Sprott; *Production Services,* Cenveo Publisher Services; *Cover Design,* Design Literate Studio, LLC; *Printer,* Lightning Source®.

1 3 5 7 9 10 8 6 4 2

The suggestions and information contained in this publication are generally consistent with the *Standards of Medical Care in Diabetes* and other policies of the American Diabetes Association, but they do not represent the policy or position of the Association or any of its boards or committees. Reasonable steps have been taken to ensure the accuracy of the information presented. However, the American Diabetes Association cannot ensure the safety or efficacy of any product or service described in this publication. Individuals are advised to consult a physician or other appropriate health care professional before undertaking any diet or exercise program or taking any medication referred to in this publication. Professionals must use and apply their own professional judgment, experience, and training and should not rely solely on the information contained in this publication before prescribing any diet, exercise, or medication. The American Diabetes Association—its officers, directors, employees, volunteers, and members—assumes no responsibility or liability for personal or other injury, loss, or damage that may result from the suggestions or information in this publication.

ADA titles may be purchased for business or promotional use or for special sales. To purchase more than 50 copies of this book at a discount, or for custom editions of this book with your logo, contact the American Diabetes Association at the address below or at booksales@diabetes.org.

American Diabetes Association
2451 Crystal Drive, Suite 900
Arlington, VA 22202

Library of Congress Cataloging-in-Publication Data
Names: Draznin, Boris, editor. | American Diabetes Association, issuing body.
Title: Atypical diabetes : pathophysiology, clinical presentations, and treatment options / [edited by] Boris Draznin.
Other titles: Atypical diabetes (Draznin)
Description: Arlington : American Diabetes Association, [2018]
Identifiers: LCCN 2017017301 | ISBN 9781580406666
Subjects: | MESH: Diabetes Mellitus | Case Reports
Classification: LCC RC660.4 | NLM WK 810 | DDC 616.4/62–dc23
LC record available at https://lccn.loc.gov/2017017301

This book is dedicated to the world's diabetes research community for its effort to solve the diabetes mystery and find a cure for this disease.

Contents

Preface

As a rule, diagnosing diabetes is not that difficult. A constellation of clinical symptoms such as excessive thirst, polyuria, unexplained weight loss, blurry vision, and urinary tract infection, to name a few, immediately brings the diagnosis of diabetes to the top of the list of differential diagnoses in the mind of every physician. Confirmation is then obtained by measuring the level of glucose in blood and hemoglobin A1C (HbA_{1c}). In some patients with mild symptoms or in asymptomatic individuals, laboratory findings may be the only initial manifestations of diabetes.

A more difficult step is to classify diabetes appropriately. Because the term "diabetes" refers to a large group of metabolic disorders characterized by hyperglycemia, it is important to ensure that etiology and pathophysiology of hyperglycemia are identified accurately in every patient. Proper classification of diabetes is not just a theoretical exercise, but also a critically important step in selecting the most appropriate therapy for a given patient.

While type 1 and type 2 diabetes account for up to 90% of all cases of diabetes, the remaining "atypical cases" of diabetes are frequent enough that every practitioner is likely to encounter them in his or her practice. Recognizing these cases and applying appropriate therapy are vitally important for successful treatment of these conditions.

The chapters presented in this volume describe various forms of atypical diabetes and provide insight into their etiology, pathophysiology, clinical picture, and therapeutic options. The cases that follow chapters 1, 4, and 8 illustrate multiple diagnostic and therapeutic challenges and are intended to help practitioners sharpen their clinical skills when encountering similar cases of atypical diabetes.

The authors and the editors are eager to share their knowledge and experience with the readers. We sincerely hope our readers will find the book informative and helpful to their practice.

Boris Draznin, MD, PhD

Introduction

Classification of diabetes includes a long list of common, rare, and not-so-rare conditions characterized by hyperglycemia of variable degrees. Whereas the majority of patients with diabetes are easily classified as having type 1 or type 2 diabetes, the other forms of diabetes, in aggregate, account for approximately 10% of diabetes cases. These cases may be grouped under the umbrella of rare forms of diabetes or "atypical diabetes." Even though individually rare, these atypical types of diabetes are frequent enough that every practitioner is likely to encounter such cases in his or her practice. The challenge is in recognizing them.

Cases of atypical diabetes are not only challenging from the diagnostic perspective, but more often than not, they demand distinct therapeutic approaches, emphasizing that "one size does not fit all" in clinical medicine.

This book groups cases of atypical diabetes into three broad categories:

Part I, edited by Dr. Louis H. Philipson, illustrates the difficulties in making a diagnosis and the importance of obtaining genetic analysis in cases of monogenic diabetes, which together account for 2–3% of all cases of diabetes before ages 25–35. In some cases, the impact of proper diagnosis can be immediate and profound, such as in the use of sulfonylureas in neonatal diabetes caused by mutations in *KCNJ11* and *ABCC8*, or in diabetes caused by HNF1A mutations (MODY3) presenting in young adults that is also highly responsive to sulfonylureas. Where there might not be a change in treatment, there can be a change in how other organs are potentially impacted, such as the great vessels in *GATA6*, thyroid abnormalities with *GLIS3*, bone abnormalities with *EIF2AK3*, or variably presenting multi-organ involvement with mitochondrial diabetes (MELAS, MIDD, etc.).

The detailed discussion of the genetic and clinical presentations of monogenic diabetes is followed by 22 cases that illustrate the most important examples of monogenic diabetes.

Part II, edited by Dr. Boris Draznin, presents important examples of diabetes arising as a consequence of insulin resistance, genetic defects in insulin action, and diseases of exocrine pancreas. The 21 cases in this part of the text clearly demonstrate challenges both in diagnosis and therapy of these conditions.

Genetic syndromes of insulin resistance are rare, but when encountered, they present challenging diagnostic and therapeutic dilemmas. Cases of lipodystrophy occur with somewhat greater frequency than genetic syndromes of severe insulin resistance, but are equally challenging, particularly in aspects of therapy. Pancreatogenic diabetes follows the destruction of exocrine and endocrine pancreas by disease processes usually initiated in the exocrine part of this important organ or after surgical removal of the pancreas due to either pancreatitis or cancer. Diabetes also develops in many patients with cystic fibrosis who have much improved life expectancy. Patients with hemochromatosis and liver diseases may develop diabetes as do those treated with certain medications that interfere with either insulin secretion or insulin action, thus promoting hyperglycemia.

Part III, edited by Dr. Janet B. McGill, highlights the clinical presentation of diabetes in patients with endocrinopathies, immune-mediated pathogenesis of diabetes, diabetes of unknown cause, and diabetes arising in patients with other genetic diseases. The discussion includes the frequent development of diabetes in patients with other endocrine diseases, such as acromegaly, Cushing's syndrome, pheochromocytoma, and glucagonoma. Successful therapy of the underlying disease in these cases usually dramatically improves or completely normalizes glycemic control.

Patients with Latent Autoimmune Diabetes of Adults (LADA)* are often initially mistakenly diagnosed as having type 2 diabetes. Once an appropriate diagnosis is made, insulin therapy is instituted and these patients are managed similarly to those with type 1 diabetes. Other examples of immune-mediated diabetes include Type B insulin resistance, polyglandular failure, and stiff person syndrome.

An unusual entity of ketosis-prone diabetes is also discussed in detail in this part of the text. This form of diabetes is not as rare as was originally thought, and many diabetologists see these atypical cases of diabetes in their practices. Finally, there are other genetic syndromes associated with diabetes and Part III of this volume offers an in-depth discussion of these conditions as well.

In summary, the growing recognition of these atypical cases underscores the importance of considering and diagnosing rare forms of diabetes accurately and expeditiously in a cost-effective manner. We hope this compilation of cases and didactic chapters will help physicians encountering similar cases in their practice understand pathophysiology of these conditions and will guide them in their effort to diagnose and treat these atypical forms of diabetes. Finally, the text offers an extensive list of references to aid practitioners to navigate the literature about atypical cases of diabetes they will certainly encounter in their offices.

Boris Draznin, MD, PhD
Louis H. Philipson, MD, PhD
Janet B. McGill, MD, MA

---

*The American Diabetes Association does not recognize Latent Autoimmune Diabetes of Adults (LADA) as a distinct form of diabetes. ADA categorizes any diabetes that is due to an autoimmune β-cell destruction as a form of type 1 diabetes. A person with LADA with evidence of autoimmune dysfunction would be said to have type 1 diabetes, otherwise the person has either type 2 diabetes or a specific type due to other causes, such as monogenic diabetes syndromes. Content about LADA provided in this book is not consistent with the information in the ADA *Standards of Medical Care in Diabetes*.

PART I:
Monogenic Diabetes: Genetic Defects of β-Cell Development and Function

1
Monogenic Diabetes: Maturity-Onset Diabetes of the Young (MODY) and Neonatal Diabetes

Rochelle N. Naylor, MD;[1] Siri Atma W. Greeley, MD, PhD;[1] David Carmody, MD;[2] Jessica L. Hwang, MD;[3] May Sanyoura, PhD;[1] Lisa R. Letourneau, MPH, RD;[1] Graeme I. Bell, PhD;[2] and Louis H. Philipson, MD, PhD[1]

Introduction

M onogenic diabetes is a heterogeneous group of uncommon but important causes of diabetes, accounting for 1–2% of all diabetes worldwide. Monogenic diabetes can be distinguished from other forms through genetic testing. Accurate diagnosis of monogenic forms of diabetes is one of the most compelling clinical examples of personalized genetic medicine for affected individuals and their families. In the majority of cases, diagnosis of monogenic diabetes via genetic testing leads to improved diabetes control through therapy selection based on the genetic cause of diabetes. Less expensive and less burdensome therapy makes genetic testing for monogenic diabetes in appropriately

[1]Departments of Medicine and Pediatrics, Section of Adult and Pediatric Endocrinology, Diabetes, and Metabolism, The University of Chicago, Chicago, IL
[2]Singapore General Hospital, Singapore
[3]Cook County Hospital, Chicago, IL

DOI: 10.2337/9781580406666.01

selected patients a cost-effective practice. Diagnosis of monogenic diabetes also has important implications for surveillance for associated extra-pancreatic features and complications and for identifying at-risk family members for diagnostic and predictive genetic testing.[1,2] However, the possibility of an underlying monogenic diagnosis is rarely considered. Data from numerous studies suggest that more than 80% of monogenic diabetes cases are missed, emphasizing the need to address barriers to identifying patients with monogenic diabetes and acquiring genetic testing.

Here we present case reviews that illustrate the clinical features, family history, and validated biomarkers, including absence of markers of autoimmunity and high-sensitivity C-reactive protein (hs-CRP) that can aid in identifying individuals highly likely to have monogenic diabetes. We review the first-line therapies and appropriate management for the most common monogenic diabetes subtypes.

Nomenclature

The various forms of monogenic diabetes are due to sporadic or dominantly or recessively inherited highly penetrant single gene mutations or chromosomal abnormalities that are sufficient to cause diabetes. Most of the causative genes are critical for β-cell development, function, or regulation, or involve the insulin gene itself.[3,4] The nomenclature used to describe monogenic forms of diabetes can be confusing as many of the terms were established before the advent of molecular genetic testing. Phenotypically, monogenic diabetes can be divided into three overlapping categories: maturity-onset diabetes of the young (MODY), neonatal diabetes (ND), and syndromic forms with a variety of features in addition to diabetes (Table 1.1).

Dominantly inherited young-onset diabetes was described by Tattersall in 1998,[6] later termed MODY. MODY is the predominant form of monogenic diabetes. Reported estimates of MODY prevalence vary by country, by pediatric versus adult populations, and by method of ascertainment, but MODY is thought to represent at least 1% of all diabetes cases.[7-10] Neonatal diabetes is traditionally defined as persistent hyperglycemia in the first 6 months of life requiring treatment.[11-15] Since many cases are diagnosed after the neonatal period, the term "congenital diabetes" might be more appropriate; however, ND has been used most consistently in the literature. Although later presentations have been described, nearly all cases of

Table 1.1—Highly Penetrant Gene Causes of Monogenic Diabetes Characterized by β-Cell Dysfunction

Gene	Inheritance	Clinical Features
Genetic disorder of glucose metabolism		
GCK	AD	**MODY 2:** Stable, nonprogressive elevated fasting blood glucose; typically does not require treatment; microvascular complications are rare; small rise in 2-hour glucose level on OGTT (<54 mg/dL; <3 mmol/L)
Genetic disorders of gene expression		
HNF1A	AD	**MODY 3:** Progressive insulin secretory defect with presentation in adolescence or early adulthood; lowered renal threshold for glucosuria; large rise in 2-hour glucose level on OGTT (>90 mg/dL; >5 mmol/L); sensitive to sulfonylureas
HNF4A	AD	**MODY 1:** Progressive insulin secretory defect with presentation in adolescence or early adulthood; may have large birth weight and transient neonatal hypoglycemia; sensitive to sulfonylureas
HNF1B	AD	**MODY 5:** Developmental renal disease (typically cystic); genitourinary abnormalities; atrophy of the pancreas; hyperuricemia; gout
PDX1	AD / AR	**MODY 4:** Rare; diabetes appears to be mild / **ND:** SGA; diarrhea; malnutrition; parents have PDX1-MODY (MODY4)
NEUROD1	AD / AR	**MODY 6:** Rare / **ND:** Cerebellar hypoplasia; deafness
GATA6	AD	**ND:** Pancreatic hypoplasia; gastrointestinal and cardiac malformations
GLIS3	AR	**ND:** Congenital hypothyroidism; glaucoma; kidney cysts; hepatic fibrosis
PAX4	AD	**MODY 9:** Rare
PAX6	AR	**ND:** Brain malformations; microcephaly; microphthalmia; panhypopituitarism
NEUROG3	AR	**ND:** SGA; severe intractable congenital diarrhea
PTF1A	AR	**ND:** Pancreatic hypoplasia; cerebellar hypoplasia
RFX6	AR	**ND:** SGA, intestinal atresias; gallbladder hypoplasia/aplasia; diarrhea
KLF11	AD	**MODY 7:** Rare
BLK	AD	**MODY 11:** Rare
NKX2.2	AR	**ND:** Rare
MNX1	AR	**ND:** Rare; pancreatic hypoplasia
Genetic disorder of ion channels		
ABCC8	AD	**ND:** IUGR; responsive to sulfonylureas
KCNJ11	AD	**ND:** IUGR; possible developmental delay and seizures; responsive to sulfonylureas

(Continued)

Table 1.1 — (*Continued*)

Gene	Inheritance	Clinical Features
Genetic disorder of insulin synthesis		
INS	AD	**ND:** IUGR **MODY 10:** Rare
Genetic disorders of ER stress/cell death		
EIF2AK3	AR	**ND:** Wolcott-Rallison Syndrome; epiphyseal dysplasia; exocrine pancreatic insufficiency
WFS1	AR	**Variable age of diabetes diagnosis (3 weeks to 14 years):** Rare; optic atrophy; deafness; diabetes insipidus
IER3IP1	AR	**ND:** Rare; Microcephaly with simplified gyral pattern; infantile epileptic encephalopathy
TRMT10A	AR	**MODY:** Rare; short stature; microcephaly
Epigenetic disorders of the β-cell		
6q24 (PLAGL1, HYMA1)	AD for paternal duplications	**Transient ND:** IUGR; macroglossia; umbilical hernia; mechanisms include UPD6, paternal duplication or maternal methylation defect
ZFP57	AR	**Transient ND:** Rare; IUGR; macroglossia
Genetic disorder of glucose transport		
SLC2A2	AR	**ND:** Rare; hepatomegaly; proximal tubular nephropathy
Primary genetic disorder of auto-immunity		
FOXP3	X-linked	**ND:** IPEX syndrome; autoimmune diabetes; autoimmune thyroid disease; exfoliative dermatitis
Genetic disorder of insulin secretion		
SLC19A2	AR	**ND:** Rare; thiamine-responsive megaloblastic anemia; deafness
Disease of the exocrine pancreas		
CFTR	AR	**Variable age of diabetes diagnosis:** Pulmonary disease; exocrine pancreatic dysfunction; decreased insulin production; insulin resistance
CEL	AD	**MODY 8:** Rare; atrophy of the pancreas; exocrine pancreatic dysfunction
Mitochondrial disorders		
MT-TL1, MT-TK, MT-TE	Maternally inherited	**MIDD:** Maternally inherited diabetes and deafness
Iron deposition within β-cells		
HFE	AR	**Variable age of diabetes diagnosis:** Hepatic disease; skin pigmentation; arthropathy; hypogonadism in males; cardiomegaly

AD, autosomal dominant; AR, autosomal recessive; IUGR, intrauterine growth restriction; ND, neonatal diabetes; MODY, maturity-onset diabetes of the young; SGA, small for gestational age. Shaded rows indicate gene causes that should be routinely tested in most MODY or ND cases. Unshaded causes are typically considered when suggestive features are present or other testing was negative. Rare syndromic monogenic diseases associated with variable diabetes penetrance were not included.
Source: Modified from Carmody D et al.[5]

diabetes diagnosed before 6 months of age will be monogenic, rather than autoimmune, in origin.[16,17] High-risk HLA haplotypes that are overrepresented in people with type 1 diabetes are rarely found in this group, and pancreatic autoantibody production is markedly rare.[18,19] An exception is immunodysregulation polyendocrinopathy enteropathy X-linked (IPEX) syndrome, an X-linked syndromic cause of autoimmune-mediated neonatal diabetes due to mutations in FOXP3.[1,2,20]

Over the last 20 years, the molecular underpinnings of monogenic diabetes have been elucidated, and genetic testing is now widely available on a commercial or research basis. Testing allows the replacement of a broad clinical classification, which can be confusing, inaccurate, and misleading, with a specific molecular genetic diagnosis. We advocate the use of terms that include the gene/locus that has been mutated.

Maturity-Onset Diabetes of the Young (MODY)
Pathophysiology

MODY is the most common subset of monogenic diabetes and accounts for 1–2% of all diabetes cases.[3,4,21] The identified genes that lead to MODY encode transcription factors important for β-cell function and regulation and an enzyme that allows the β-cell to respond to changes in glycemia.[3,6,22] Linkage studies identified loci on chromosomes 7p, 20q, and 12q as causes of MODY. The glucokinase (GCK) gene was the first gene to be subsequently identified in 1992, shortly followed by discovery of HNF1A and HNF4A in 1996.[7-10,23-25] These three genes along with HNF1B account for more than 90% of all MODY with a known genetic diagnosis.[7,11-15] Altogether, there are at least 13 MODY genes that affect insulin secretion in five major ways:

1. encode transcription factors that are critical for β-cell development, function, or regulation
2. an enzyme (GCK) that allows the β-cell (and liver) to respond to changes in glycemia
3. involve the insulin gene
4. lead to endoplasmic reticulum (ER) stress and damage the β-cell
5. part of complex genetic syndromes

Several genes involved overlap with neonatal forms of monogenic diabetes or have mutations that can cause both forms.[3,16,17,22]

Clinical Presentation and Diagnosis

MODY is classically defined as autosomal dominant, nonketotic, non–insulin dependent diabetes with onset typically before 25 years of age with 2–3 consecutively affected generations.[18,19,26] Patients typically lack significant obesity or metabolic features and pancreatic autoantibodies. However, studies show that less than 50% of individuals with a genetic diagnosis of MODY fit the classic description of onset before 25 years with positive family history.[7,27] Studies using widened testing criteria have identified MODY in 10–25% of the tested population.[28]

There is significant clinical overlap between MODY and type 1 and type 2 diabetes, leading to frequent misdiagnosis. Studies from the U.K. suggest that more than 80% of MODY goes unrecognized.[7,10] Misdiagnosis may be more prevalent in racial and ethnic minorities. Efforts to assess diagnosis of MODY in Asians in the U.K. showed that the study prevalence and clinical features of MODY did not differ between Asians and Caucasians. However, while Asians represented 4% of the country's population, only 0.5% of referrals for MODY testing were for Asians.[29] SEARCH for Diabetes in Youth reported on 586 U.S. participants who were sequenced for MODY. Mutations were found in 8% of the tested individuals, estimating a MODY prevalence of at least 1.2% in the pediatric diabetes population. In this study, 64% of those originally misdiagnosed and subsequently determined to have MODY were ethnic minorities, mainly African American and Hispanic.[30]

There can be significant clinical overlap between MODY and type 1 or type 2 diabetes (Table 1.2). Difficulty in identifying people likely to have MODY is a major barrier to diagnostic genetic testing and subsequent appropriate clinical management.

Because MODY lacks a singular phenotype that would capture all affected patients, a combination of clinical features, history, biomarkers, and clinical tools must be used to identify those most likely to benefit from genetic testing (Table 1.3).[31] Measuring pancreatic autoantibodies, C-peptide, urine C-peptide creatinine ratio (UCPCR), and/or hs-CRP can provide further evidence of a likely underlying monogenic etiology of diabetes. In the case of differentiating MODY from type 1 diabetes, lack of pancreatic autoantibodies at diabetes diagnosis should raise suspicion for MODY, particularly with familial diabetes. Measurement of C-peptide or UCPCR three years or more after diabetes onset is helpful to identify individuals with continued significant endogenous insulin production, as occurs in MODY. Both C-peptide and UCPCR are higher in HNF1A-MODY and HNF4A-MODY compared to type 1 diabetes.[32–34] Type

Table 1.2—Clinical Comparison of Type 1 Diabetes, Type 2 Diabetes, and Maturity-Onset Diabetes of the Young (MODY)

	MODY	Type 1 Diabetes	Type 2 Diabetes
Prevalence	1–5% of diabetes cases	5–10% of diabetes cases	90% of diabetes cases
Age at onset	Typical presentation in adolescence or early adulthood (<35 years)	Typical presentation in childhood	Typical presentation in later adulthood. Pediatric cases occur postpuberty.
Family history	2–3 consecutive unilineal generations	Affected parent is rare	Often 1 or both parents have a history of obesity and/or type 2 diabetes
Obesity or metabolic features	Classically absent, though impact of current obesity epidemic is unclear	Classically absent, though impact of current obesity epidemic is unclear	Frequent
Clinical presentation	Typically without significant ketosis or acidosis	Usually with ketosis and varying degree of acidosis	Insidious onset. Typically without ketosis or acidosis though exceptions occur.

1 and 2 diabetes are associated with inflammation, making elevated hs-CRP a useful biomarker. Conversely, levels of hs-CRP are low in HNF1A-MODY and can be used to distinguish HNF1A-MODY from type 1 and type 2 diabetes.[35–37]

Genetic testing for MODY can be accomplished through standard Sanger sequencing or via next generation sequencing and is commercially available in Clinical Laboratory Improvement Amendments–certified laboratories. Medical insurance coverage varies and prior authorization should be sought before ordering testing. Several considerations must be made with regard to diagnostic diabetes genetic testing, including appropriate patient selection and genetic counseling, recognition of the possibility of false negative results, correct interpretation of genetic testing results, correct handling of variants of uncertain significance, and appropriate treatment following confirmed genetic diagnosis of monogenic diabetes.[42,43] All clinicians should have a low threshold for consulting with experts in monogenic diabetes for interpretation of genetic testing results prior to implementing therapy and management changes (Tables 1.4, 1.5).

Table 1.3—Laboratory Tests to Aid in Identifying MODY

Laboratory Test	Clinical Utility	Interpretation
Pancreatic autoantibodies (GAD65, islet cell antibodies, insulin,* ZnT8)	All MODY types	Present in only 1% of MODY
C-peptide after 3–5 years diabetes duration	All MODY types	Random or glucagon-stimulated C-peptide ≥0.2 nmol/L can distinguish MODY from type 1 diabetes
Urine C-peptide creatinine ratio (UCPCR)	HNF1A-MODY, HNF4A-MODY	UCPCR >/= 0.2 nmol/mmol distinguishes HNF1A-MODY and HNF4A-MODY from type 1 diabetes with 97% sensitivity and 96% specificity
High-sensitivity C-reactive protein (hs-CRP)	HNF1A-MODY	hs-CRP <0.75 mg/L shows 79% sensitivity and 67% specificity to distinguish HNF1A-MODY from type 1 diabetes hs-CRP <0.75 mg/L shows 79% sensitivity and 70% specificity to distinguish HNF1A-MODY from type 2 diabetes
HbA$_{1c}$	GCK-MODY	Values very stable with little intra-patient variation HbA$_{1c}$ typically ranges from 5.6–7.3% (38–56 mmol/mol) at ages ≤40 years; 5.9–7.6% (41–60 mmol/mol) at ages >40 years

*Should only be tested in insulin-naive patients.
Source: Ludvigsson J et al.,[32] Besser REJ et al.,[33] Owen KR et al.,[35] McDonald TJ et al.,[36] Thanabalasingham G et al.,[37] McDonald TJ et al.,[38] Urbanová J et al.,[39] Thomas NJ et al.,[40] and Steele AM et al.[41]

Table 1.4—Clinical Tools and Genetic Testing Approaches to Aid in MODY Diagnosis

Clinical Tools and Resources	Description
Centre for Molecular Genetics at the University of Exeter (http://www.diabetesgenes.org) and MODY Probability Calculator (diabetesgenes.org/content/mody-probability-calculator)	For use in estimating the likelihood of a MODY diagnosis in patients with diabetes onset before age 35 years. This tool provides a post-test probability of MODY based on the clinical features of the patient.
Calculator proposed by Bellanné-Chantelot	For use in estimating the likelihood of HNF1A-MODY versus early-onset type 2 diabetes
US Monogenic Diabetes Registry (http://monogenicdiabetes.uchicago.edu)	Experienced team available for advice regarding genetic testing and interpretation

Table 1.4 — (*Continued*)

Clinical Tools and Resources	Description
Genetic testing considerations	
Sanger sequencing	Analytical sensitivity is nearly 100% for mutations in coding regions, flanking intronic regions; Analytical specificity is nearly 100%
Multiplex Ligation-dependent Probe Amplification (MLPA)	Analytical sensitivity is nearly 100% for detection of partial and whole-gene deletions; analytical specificity is nearly 100%
False positives	Can occur in MLPA due to SNPs preventing probe binding and ligation; benign sequence variants can be reported as pathogenic or interpreted by clinicians as pathogenic
False negatives	SNPs within PCR primer-binding sites can result in false negatives; deep intronic splice site mutations and mutations in other regulatory sites will be missed
Next-generation sequencing (NGS) panels	Allow for testing many genes at once and are usually designed very specifically to identify all known mutations in any gene included
Whole exome or genome sequencing	Should be used with caution by experienced clinical genetics teams, usually only after other testing of known causes has been negative; some genes and/or intronic regions may not be well covered and without appropriate testing strategies and filtering these approaches are likely to result in many variants of uncertain significance

Source: Bellanné-Chantelot C et al.,[27] and Colclough K et al.[44]

Table 1.5 — Clinical Features and Treatment of the Common Subtypes of MODY

Monogenic Diabetes Phenotype and Clinical Features	First-line Therapy
HNF1A-MODY (MODY 3) Progressive insulin secretory defect with presentation in adolescence or early adulthood; lowered renal threshold for glucosuria; large rise in 2-hour glucose level on OGTT (>90 mg/dL; >5 mmol/L)	Sulfonylureas (frequently low doses) GLP-1 agonists may be considered for adjunctive therapy

(*Continued*)

Table 1.5—(Continued)

Monogenic Diabetes Phenotype and Clinical Features	First-line Therapy
HNF4A-MODY (MODY 1) Progressive insulin secretory defect with presentation in adolescence or early adulthood; may have large birth weight and transient neonatal hypoglycemia	Sulfonylureas (frequently low doses)
HNF1B-MODY (MODY 5) Developmental renal disease (typically cystic); genitourinary abnormalities; hypoplasia, atrophy of the pancreas; hyperuricemia; gout; HNF1B mutations often cause renal disease without diabetes	Variable Type 1 diabetes (around 30%)
GCK-MODY (MODY 2) Lifelong stable, elevated fasting blood glucose with minimal age-related progression	Treatment is not needed for isolated GCK-MODY except during pregnancy with an unaffected fetus

Sequence information is based on GenBank reference sequences. OGTT, oral glucose tolerance test; HbA_{1c}, hemoglobin A1C.
Source: Carmody D et al.[5]

GCK-MODY (previously referred to as MODY 2)

Glucokinase is an enzyme that catalyzes the conversion of glucose to glucose-6-phosphate, which is the first step in glycogen storage and glycolysis. Glucokinase acts as the body's glucose sensor, linking increased glucose levels to the secretion of insulin and hepatic glucose production. Heterozygous inactivating GCK mutations increase the serum glucose level that triggers insulin release, resulting in persistent, mild hyperglycemia.

GCK-MODY has a prevalence of 1 per 1,000, is the second most commonly identified cause of MODY, and is more common than HNF1A-MODY as a cause of incidental hyperglycemia in pediatric populations.[45] GCK-MODY is characterized by persistent, mild hyperglycemia with fasting serum glucose typically ranging from 99–144 mg/dL (5.5–8.0 mmol/L).[46] Hemoglobin A1C (HbA_{1c}) is generally just above the upper limit of normal, ranging from 5.6–7.6% (38–60 mmol/mol).[41] The metabolite profile in GCK-MODY is similar to healthy controls, with free fatty acid levels lower than controls.[47]

GCK mutations cause mild, regulated nonprogressive hyperglycemia, so treatment is not needed. Studies have shown that discontinuation of therapy in GCK-related hyperglycemia does not alter HbA_{1c}.[48] Most individuals with GCK mutations do not require care under a diabetes specialist or frequent medical evaluation.[21,49] Exceptions to this include co-occurrence of other diabetes types and pregnancy, when women with GCK mutations are frequently treated with insulin in an effort to avoid fetal macrosomia in fetuses who do not carry the GCK mutation.[50] Once a GCK mutation is identified in a proband, fasting serum glucose or HbA_{1c} identifies family members who also should be tested.

There is very minimal deterioration of glucose tolerance over the long term. This minimal deterioration is due to the same mechanism of age-related increases in insulin resistance that is seen in healthy people without diabetes.[51] At this level of glycemic control, diabetes-related complications are exceedingly rare. In a recent study of GCK-MODY, overall rates of microvascular complications were very low and not significantly different from controls without diabetes. Rates of retinopathy were increased above controls (30% versus 14%). However, this was due to background retinopathy with 81% having minimal disease and none requiring laser therapy. Rates of persistent microalbuminuria did not differ from controls. Neuropathy was rare (2% in GCK versus 0% controls) and macrovascular disease was less prevalent in GCK mutation carriers versus controls (4% versus 11%).[52]

HNF1A-MODY (previously referred to as MODY 3)

Mutations in the transcription factors HNF1A lead to a progressive insulin secretory defect. Evidence of impaired β-cell function has been demonstrated even in asymptomatic mutation carriers before development of overt diabetes.[53,54] There is deterioration in glycemic control over time and progression from subtle abnormalities in glucose tolerance to overt diabetes symptoms.

Worldwide, HNF1A-MODY is the most commonly identified form of MODY, particularly in adult cohorts and regions such as the United Kingdom and Norway. There is a progressive insulin secretory defect, and fasting blood glucose values may remain normal while postprandial values are in the diabetic range. HNF1A mutations result in a low renal threshold for glucose, so glucosuria can be found at relatively normal blood glucose values. Increased HDL values are also commonly seen in affected individuals but are not cardioprotective.[55] Liver adenomatosis may occur in HNF1A-MODY due to somatic inactivation of the wild-type allele.

HNF1A-MODY often exhibits a marked sensitivity to sulfonylurea agents, which is the established first-line therapy resulting in equal or improved control as compared to insulin therapy.[56,57] Starting doses should be one-fourth of typical doses. Studies have demonstrated a mean decrease in HbA_{1c} ranging from 0.8–1.5% in a majority of patients transferring from insulin to sulfonylureas even after decades of insulin therapy.[29,58] The durability of sulfonylurea effect is not necessarily lifelong. However, individual cases have shown successful glycemic control with sulfonylurea therapy for decades.[59] Other insulin secretagogues, such as nateglinide, have been successfully used in HNF1A-MODY and may result in less hypoglycemia as compared to sulfonylureas. The best second-line therapy for waning efficacy or failure of sulfonylureas is not fully established. However, improved glycemic control with incretin-based therapies has been demonstrated in HNF1A-MODY, including a randomized crossover trial showing adequate glycemic control with glucagon-like peptide-1 agonists with fewer hypoglycemic events compared to sulfonylureas.[60]

Due to increased cardiovascular risk in HNF1A-MODY, statin therapy should be initiated by 40 years of age.[18] Additionally, screening liver ultrasonography can be considered for detection of liver adenomatosis, although clinical guidelines for evaluation, surveillance, and management do not exist.

Microvascular complications are common in HNF1A-MODY tied to level of glycemic control.[61] Additionally, despite elevated levels of HDL cholesterol in patients with HNF1A-MODY, their risk for cardiovascular disease is higher than in unaffected relatives.[55] Coronary heart disease is more prevalent in HNF1A-MODY as compared to type 1 diabetes despite a similar prevalence of hypertension. However, it is lower than in type 2 diabetes (16 % versus 33% in one cohort).[62]

HNF4A-MODY (previously referred to as MODY 1)

HNF4A-MODY is also characterized by a progressive insulin secretory defect with deterioration in glycemic control over time. HNF4A-MODY accounts for about 10% of MODY cases and mutations in HNF4A cause diabetes that is nearly indistinguishable from HNF1A-MODY. A personal or family history of neonatal macrosomia and/or neonatal hypoglycemia may be found in HNF4A-MODY.

HNF4A-MODY may also respond to sulfonylurea agents or other insulin secretagogues. However, descriptions of the clinical course of HNF4A-MODY are lacking due to lower frequency, with the exception of a well-characterized pedigree.[9]

Similar to HNF1A-MODY, microvascular complications are tied to glycemic control in HNF4A-MODY.[61]

HNF1B-MODY (previously referred to as MODY 5)

In HNF1B-MODY, due to haploinsufficiency of HNF1B, diabetes is due to both β-cell dysfunction and insulin resistance, with some studies suggesting that insulin suppression of endogenous glucose production is impaired while peripheral insulin sensitivity remains intact.[63] There is often overlap with a form of renal cystic disease, so that the term RCAD applies to "renal cysts and diabetes" due to HNF1B mutations (mostly deletions).

Heterozygous mutations in HNF1B cause several different phenotypes of disease and account for up to 5% of MODY.[7] Mutations in HNF1B more commonly present with diabetes associated with renal cysts than diabetes in isolation and may present solely with developmental kidney disease. Genotype-phenotype variation occurs.

Despite homology between the HNF1A and HNF1B transcription factors, HNF1B-MODY does not exhibit the same sulfonylurea-responsiveness as HNF1A-MODY, and insulin therapy is often required.[63,64] Individuals with HNF1B-MODY should be evaluated and treated for accompanying development of renal disease and genitourinary malformations.

Neonatal Diabetes

ND occurs in 1:90,000–260,000 live births and is traditionally defined as persistent hyperglycemia requiring treatment.[11,12] Although later presentations have been described, nearly all cases of diabetes diagnosed before 6 months of age will be monogenic, rather than autoimmune, in origin.[16,17] Indeed, high-risk HLA haplotypes that are overrepresented in people with type 1 diabetes are rarely found in this group, and pancreatic autoantibody production is markedly rare.[18,19] An exception is IPEX syndrome, an X-linked syndromic cause of neonatal diabetes.[20,65]

Pathophysiology

ND can be transient or permanent, each accounting for approximately 50% of cases.[4] The majority of cases of transient ND are due to an overexpression of the imprinted chromosome 6q24 genes PLAGL1 and HYMAI.[66] Since 2004, it has become clear that the most common causes of permanent ND are heterozygous activating mutations in the genes *KCNJ11* and *ABCC8*, encoding respectively the Kir6.2 and SUR1 subunits of the ATP-sensitive potassium (K_{ATP}) channel regulating insulin secretion from β-cells. These two genes also account for nearly all remaining cases of transient ND.[67,68] Linkage studies by Støy et al. [69] in a family with ND without mutations in either *KCNJ11* or *ABCC8* led to identification of INS gene mutations as the second most common cause of permanent ND and an infrequent cause of transient ND.[69,70]

Although sporadic heterozygous mutations in these few genes account for the majority of ND cases, more than 20 different genes have now been described as causing many rare forms of neonatal monogenic diabetes that are most often due to recessively inherited homozygous or compound hetero-zygous mutations (Table 1.1).[71-73] With the common dominantly inherited causes, occasional parental germline mosaicism not detectable in blood or saliva can lead to unexpected recurrence in future offspring due to inheritance of the mutation from an unaffected parent.[74]

Clinical Presentation and Diagnosis

Most neonates with ND have intrauterine growth restriction and are born small for gestational age, reflecting the role of insulin as a growth factor *in utero*. Transient ND typically presents in the first several days to weeks of life and remits, on average, by 12 weeks of age. Interestingly, an uncertain but large pro-portion of cases will redevelop diabetes later in life, most often as adolescents or young adults.[66] Average onset of diabetes in permanent ND is at 5 weeks of life (range birth to 26 weeks).

Diabetes onset before 6 months of age should prompt genetic testing. As these infants are typically hospitalized, genetic testing is most often sent in the hospital directed by the medical team and with consultation of experienced geneticists and pediatric endocrinologists. Imaging studies to assess for hypoplasia or aplasia of the pancreas can help to direct selection of genes to test and identify patients who will definitively require lifelong insulin therapy (Table 1.1). Genetic testing should also be considered for diagnoses between 6 and 12 months of age in the absence of islet cell autoantibodies or in the presence of any family history or extrapancreatic fea-tures suggestive of a monogenic diabetes syndrome.

6q24-Related Transient Neonatal Diabetes

6q24-related diabetes accounts for approximately 70% of transient ND.[66] Affected individuals have intrauterine growth restriction and may additionally have macroglossia and/or an umbilical hernia. Overexpression of maternally imprinted genes PLAGL1 and HYMAI at the 6q24 locus can occur via paternal uniparental isodisomy of chromosome 6, paternally inherited duplication of 6q24, or maternal methylation defects. Paternal uniparental isodisomy and methylation defects cause sporadic cases, with negligible recurrence risk to offspring. However, individuals carrying a duplication of 6q24 have a 50% chance of passing on the duplication to their offspring.[75] If the duplication is paternally inherited, children will develop transient ND; if it is maternally inherited, affected offspring will be carriers and male children will subsequently have a 50% chance of transmission to their children.

The best therapy in relapsed 6q24-related ND is unclear; however, case reports and studies utilizing dynamic stimulation testing of a few patients suggest that treatment with sulfonylureas and incretin-based therapies may result in lower doses or discontinuation of insulin injections.[76]

KCNJ11- and ABCC8-Related Diabetes

Activating mutations in *KCNJ11* and *ABCC8* render the K_{ATP} channel less sensitive to ATP, with failure of channel closure resulting in insufficient insulin secretion from the β-cell. Since K_{ATP} channels are widely expressed in the brain, patients with ND due to *KCNJ11* and more rarely *ABCC8* mutations may have a spectrum of neurologic features that are highly correlated with specific mutations causing different degrees of impairment of ATP inhibition of K_{ATP} channels. Rare cases with the most severe developmental delay, epilepsy, and neonatal diabetes (DEND) syndrome have profound global developmental delay and may exhibit mildly dysmorphic features, including bilateral ptosis, downturned mouth, and a prominent metopic suture.[67,77] More common is a less severe phenotype characterized by moderate developmental delay and intellectual impairment that is termed intermediate DEND and usually lacks seizures. Impairments seen in intermediate DEND include mild dystonia, learning difficulties, and/or ADHD-like behaviors.[16,68]

The majority of patients with ND due to K_{ATP} channel mutations are able to transition from insulin to oral sulfonylureas due to closure of the K_{ATP} channel by sulfonylureas in an ATP-independent manner. Transition to sulfonylureas almost always leads to better control of diabetes characterized by improved HbA_{1c} along with decreased episodes of hypoglycemia and decreased needed frequency of self–blood glucose monitoring. The typical effective doses for treatment of ND due to K_{ATP} channel mutations are notably higher than for type 2 diabetes relative to body weight. Thus far, serious adverse effects of high doses of sulfonylureas have not been reported in monogenic neonatal diabetes, but long-term follow-up is needed.[16,78–80]

Several case reports of improvement in neurodevelopmental features, such as immediate gains in motor function, support the notion that sulfonylureas may also restore K_{ATP} channel function in the brain.[81] However, the degree to which neurodevelopmental impairments may be ameliorated remains unclear. Our study of children with KCNJ11-related ND showed that those with DEND associated mutations had lower performance on a standardized test of visual-motor integration (VMI).[82] That the age of sulfonylurea initiation was inversely correlated with VMI scores in this group raises the possibility that such problems may be at least partially prevented by early initiation of sulfonylurea treatment. There is also growing evidence that transition from insulin attempted at older ages may be more difficult, with requirements for higher sulfonylurea doses and/or other agents.[16] There are now reports of affected infants who are trialed on sulfonylurea therapy immediately without use of insulin.[83] However, sulfonylureas are established therapy only for neonatal diabetes due to K_{ATP} channel mutations and will cause further deterioration of glycemia and clinical status in other causes of neonatal diabetes. Patients with K_{ATP} channel mutations who do not respond to sulfonylureas and those with other forms of neonatal diabetes must continue on insulin therapy, though case reports of relapsed 6q24-related ND suggest that treatment with sulfonylureas and other noninsulin therapies may result in lower doses or discontinuation of insulin therapy.[84] Pearson et al.[85] provide a detailed approach for transition from insulin to sulfonylureas.

INS

Mutations in the insulin gene (INS) are the second most common cause of permanent neonatal diabetes.[69,86–89] Heterozygous dominantly acting missense mutations impair folding of the protein and lead to dysfunction and death of β-cells as a result of increased ER stress.[90–94] As a consequence, the early-onset diabetes in these patients involves progressive insulin-deficiency that is clinically similar to type 1 diabetes. Similar to other forms of ND, INS-related ND is associated with mildly reduced birth weight, but no other consistent clinical features other than diabetes. Although most patients are diagnosed with diabetes before 6 months of age, many others have been diagnosed between 6–12 months of age or even later. Approximately 7–10% of patients with a type 1 diabetes phenotype but negative autoantibody testing may carry INS mutations (especially when diagnosed at younger ages), and other INS mutations appear to be a very rare cause of MODY.[95-99] While most mutations are exonic missense mutations, some patients have intronic mutations that affect splicing and appear to cause similar pathology,[100] and still other rare recessive cases with biallelic deletions, mutations affecting gene expression,[70,101] or deep intronic mutations affecting mRNA stability.[102] For all patients with INS gene mutations, insulin is the mainstay of treatment and since young infants require such small doses of insulin, continuous subcutaneous insulin infusion is a logical approach and can be augmented with continuous glucose monitoring when feasible. Future treatment modalities to be considered could include therapies that mitigate ER stress, or potentially cell-replacement strategies.

EIF2AK3

Wolcott-Rallison syndrome (WRS) is the most common recessive form of neonatal diabetes. It is a rare syndromic disorder caused by mutations in EIF2AK3, located on chromosome 2p12. It encodes the pancreatic eukaryotic initiation factor-2 alpha kinase protein (PEK or PERK) highly expressed in pancreatic islet cells.[103] PEK/PERK resides in the ER protein and is critically involved in the response to an increase in misfolded proteins. When it is expressed, it inactivates the alpha subunit of EIF2 (eukaryotic translation-initiation factor 2) via phosphorylation, resulting in a general downregulation of protein synthesis. PEK/PERK is also involved in the cell cycle during the G1 growth arrest first phase.

WRS is typically seen in consanguineous families and presents as ND combined with bone pathologies: multiple epiphyseal dysplasias, a short trunk-to-armspan ratio, osteopenia, and bone demineralization.[104] Other clinical findings may include developmental delay, mental retardation, hepatic or renal dysfunction, cardiac abnormalities, exocrine pancreatic dysfunction, and neutropenia resulting in frequent infections.[105] Hepatic dysfunction manifests as recurrent acute episodes of cytolysis, with or without cholestasis. These episodes usually remit spontaneously, but their severity is variable and they have been associated with multi-organ failure and death. Liver function should be closely monitored in all those with EIF2AK3-related diabetes. The appearance and severity of these additional clinical findings is highly variable even among patients with the same mutation or within the same kindred.[106] This suggests that the clinical features of *EIF2AK3* mutations are susceptible to environmental factors and/or modifier genes. Diabetes may appear first before the bone or other abnormalities so that WRS should be considered in all cases of ND with or without parental related-ness. Treatment of WRS diabetes is based on insulin administration.

GATA6

GATA6 is a highly conserved transcription factor (GATA-binding fac-tor 6) located on chromosome 18q11.2 that plays an important role during the development of several organs, most notably the pancreas and heart. The *GATA6* protein encodes a 449-amino acid protein with two zinc finger/basic domains.[107] Heterozygous mutations in *GATA6* have been described as a rare cause of neonatal diabetes, usually characterized by pancreatic agenesis in association with other features including major cardiac defects.[72] Atrial and ventricular septal defects are common. All those diagnosed with pathologic *GATA6* mutations have insulin-requiring ND in the first week of life. Pancre-atic agenesis or hypoplasia has been consistently noted. Other gastrointesti-nal abnormalities are common such as intestinal malrotation and gallbladder agenesis. Lifelong replacement therapy of exocrine and endocrine pancreas is required in most cases. Those with significant cardiac/intestinal disease often require surgery (or multiple surgeries) and may have delayed developmen-tal milestones. With limited published data, the full phenotypic spectrum is incompletely understood, particularly in regard to whether neurodevelopment is impaired. However, neurocognitive and neurodevelopmental delay is not a universal feature later in childhood despite protracted neonatal hospitalization. Treatment is complex but at a minimum involves insulin treatment and exo-crine pancreatic enzyme replacement as well as surgical management.

WFS1

Wolfram syndrome (WS) is a complex autosomal recessive syndromic genetic disorder that includes diabetes. It is characterized by a complex of variable expression of diabetes insipidus, diabetes, optical atrophy, deafness, and brain atrophy. Death usually results in middle adulthood, typically due to brainstem atrophy–induced respiratory failure.[108–110] Mutations in two genes have been implicated, with most of them in WFS1, and several reports describe a similar syndrome in the WFS2 gene. WFS1 is located on chromosome 4 and encodes wolframin, an intracellular transmembrane protein of 890 amino acids. It has been implicated in playing a role modulating ER stress, cytosolic Ca^{2+} disturbances, impaired mitochondrial dynamics, and abnormalities in certain neurons and pancreatic β-cells.[111] In addition to the syndromic form, several cases have been reported with juvenile onset diabetes as the initial manifestation with homozygous or compound heterozygous mutations.[112] Other reported forms include an autosomal dominant expression, autosomal dominant deafness only, and an association with type 2 diabetes and neuropsychiatric illness. The severe prognostic implications underlie the importance of considering WS in autoimmune-negative young-onset diabetes. Treatment is supportive and will usually include insulin management of diabetes.

Mitochondrial Diabetes

Mitochondrial diabetes refers to syndromes that include diabetes that arise from alterations in mitochondrial DNA.[113] Inheritance is maternal, since the vast majority of mitochondria are contributed to the fetus from the ovum. Diabetes is usually not present in isolation but is part of a syndrome caused by the variable numbers of defective mitochondria in any given tissue, a process known as heteroplasmy. This simply refers to the number of mitochondrial genomes per cell or tissue that can vary. While most are normal, some are not. The distribution of normal versus abnormal mitochondria in any given tissue can be different in the same kindred, meaning that the exact manifestations of tissue damage secondary to defective mitochondria can be different. The most common manifestation of mitochondrial diabetes is the maternally inherited diabetes and deafness (MIDD) syndrome. This syndrome also overlaps with a related syndrome with mitochondrial encephalomyopathy, lactic acidosis, and stroke-like episodes (MELAS) that arises from the same mitochondrial DNA mutation; in fact there is a continuum of symptoms for these and related entities such as Leigh syndrome.[113] The prevalence estimations have ranged from 1% of all cases of diabetes,[113] to about 0.9% in a population under 30,[114] to a recent study that suggests a much lower prevalence of 0.02% in people with a diabetes diagnosis under age 30, with Kearns Sayre, MELAS, and Pearson syndromes being the most frequent causes.[115] The syndrome results from an A to G substitution at position 3243 (m.3243A>G) of the mitochondrial DNA encoding the gene for tRNALeu.[116-118] This defect leads to an impairment of energy generation by the defective mitochondrion, giving rise to defects first in the most energetically demanding tissues, such as the cochlea and insulin-producing cells, as well as many other neurons, cardiac myocytes, retina, and kidney cells. The hearing loss is sensorineural. Diabetes can present with DKA but is most often anti-islet antibody negative. Therefore, it can be mistaken for either type 1 or type 2 diabetes. Retinal disease, psychiatric disease, strokes, short stature, and heart failure (sometimes in pregnancy, where the miscarriage rate is also high) can also be part of the syndrome. Diagnosis is best done with urine or mouth samples that tend to have a higher degree of heteroplasmy than white blood cells.[119,120] Treatment may include CoQ10, but mitochondrial toxins should be avoided, including metformin, as well as any agent that has been associated with lactic acidosis.[113] The cornerstone of the treatment of blood glucose in MIDD remains insulin. Follow-up of maternal relatives is critical, as a significant proportion may be asymptomatic yet carry the mutation,[121] and genetic counseling is strongly recommended.

Summary and Recommendations for Clinical Guidelines and Practice

Monogenic diabetes represents an important category of heritable disorders for which an accurate genetic diagnosis affects clinical care, including use of genetically targeted therapies and disease surveillance. Over the last 20 years, the molecular underpinnings of monogenic diabetes have been elucidated, and genetic testing is now available on a commercial or research basis for the common and rare causes of monogenic diabetes. However, monogenic diabetes is almost always misdiagnosed and patients are frequently improperly treated. While most studies are cross-sectional in design, misdiagnosis of monogenic diabetes has been convincingly shown across numerous studies. Glycemic control has been shown to improve after sulfonylurea transfer in many forms of monogenic diabetes, which could feasibly decrease long-term diabetes complications. However, formal studies on impact of quality of life are lacking and are an area for future research. Additionally, transition off therapy or to sulfonylureas in monogenic forms of diabetes is cost-saving on an individual basis. Cost-effectiveness analyses of genetic testing for neonatal diabetes and MODY have shown that genetic testing can be cost-effective but additional formal economic evaluations are needed.[122,123]

Currently, there are clinical guidelines for diagnosing monogenic diabetes in children and adults (Table 1.6). These guidelines advocate for clinical features and family history of diabetes to guide patient selection for genetic testing. For suspected MODY cases, they also cite the use of biomarkers whose efficacy has been established in several studies. All guidelines advocate for testing for monogenic causes where clinical management will be impacted. While studies show that selection for genetic testing by clinical features may miss as much as 50% of affected patients with MODY, this is a reasonable approach

Table 1.6—Clinical Guidelines-Criteria for MODY Genetic Testing

American Diabetes Association: classification and diagnosis of diabetes-MODY
1. Diagnosis in childhood or early adulthood
2. Diabetes without typical features of type 1 diabetes (negative diabetes-associated autoantibodies) or type 2 diabetes (nonobese, lacking other metabolic features)
3. Strong family history of diabetes in successive generations, suggesting an autosomal dominant pattern of inheritance

European Molecular Genetics Quality Network MODY group
4. Mild fasting hyperglycemia (testing for GCK)
5. Gestational diabetes (testing for GCK)
6. Children and young adults with diabetes and a strong family history of diabetes (testing for HNF1A, HNF4A)
   a. Young onset
   b. Non–insulin-dependent beyond 3 years
   c. Two generations of familial diabetes
   d. Absence of pancreatic autoantibodies
   e. Sensitivity to sulfonylureas
   f. No marked obesity; insulin resistance, or acanthosis nigricans; ethnic background with low prevalence of type

ISPAD clinical practice consensus guidelines for diagnosis and management of monogenic diabetes in children and adolescents
7. Family history of diabetes in one parent and first-degree relatives of that parent who lack characteristics of type 1 and type 2 diabetes
8. Mild stable fasting hyperglycemia
9. Renal development disease or renal cysts
10. Ethnic background with a low prevalence of type 2 diabetes

Recommendations for treatment
11. Sulfonylureas for HNF1A-MODY and HNF4A-MODY
12. No treatment for GCK-MODY

Source: Stride A et al.,[48] Shepherd M et al.,[58] Fajans SS and Brown MB,[59] Rubio-Cabezas et al.,[124] American Diabetes Association,[126] Ellard S et al.[127]

until genetic testing is more affordable and universally covered by medical insurance. Current guidelines also include race/ethnicity as a relevant factor when considering MODY.[124,125] However, studies by Porter and Pihoker et al.[29,30] suggest that minorities are underrepresented in studies of MODY prevalence and those with MODY are likely to be misdiagnosed. Thus, inclusion of race/ethnicity in guidelines may exacerbate underdiagnosis of MODY in minority ethnic groups.

Diagnosing monogenic diabetes in one patient also identifies affected and at-risk family members who may benefit from targeted diagnostic and predictive genetic testing, respectively. Genetic testing of at-risk family members leads to earlier diagnosis and potentially improved outcomes. Predictive genetic testing in asymptomatic first-degree relatives can be undertaken. In such cases, guidelines endorse referral to specialty centers.[124]

Universal diabetes genetic testing incorporated at diabetes diagnosis for correct classification would ensure cases of monogenic diabetes are not missed, but current costs of genetic testing prohibit this approach. However, next-generation sequencing platforms and monogenic diabetes panels hold promise to increase efficiency of genetic testing at lower costs through simultaneous sequencing of multiple relevant genes in a single test.[128–130] Formal economic studies that account for these cost-saving technologic advances will be needed to inform future practice guidelines as well as insurance coverage for genetic testing for correct diabetes classification. Large, multicenter, and randomized control trials assessing long-term treatment outcomes, including potential adverse effects of therapy and quality-of-life effects are also needed to increase recognition and diagnosis of this less common but important cause of diabetes.

References

1. Shepherd M, Hattersley AT, Sparkes AC. Predictive genetic testing in diabetes: a case study of multiple perspectives. *Qual Health Res* 2000;10:242–259

2. Shepherd M, Ellis I, Ahmad AM, et al. Predictive genetic testing in maturity-onset diabetes of the young (MODY). *Diabet Med* 2001;18:417–421

3. Fajans SS, Bell GI, Polonsky KS. Molecular mechanisms and clinical pathophysiology of maturity-onset diabetes of the young. *N Engl J Med* 2001;345:971–980

4. Edghill EL, Hattersley AT. Genetic disorders of the pancreatic beta cell and diabetes (permanent neonatal diabetes and maturity-onset diabetes of the young).

In *Pancreatic Beta Cell in Health and Disease.* Seino S, Bell GI, Eds. New York, Springer, 2008, p. 399–430

5. Carmody D, Støy J, Greeley SAW, Bell GI, Philipson LH. A clinical guide to monogenic diabetes. In *Genetic Diagnosis of Endocrine Disorders.* 2nd ed. Weiss RE, Refetoff S, Eds. United Kingdom, Academic Press, 2016, p. 21–30

6. Tattersall R. Maturity-onset diabetes of the young: a clinical history. *Diabet Med* 1998;15:11–14

7. Shields BM, Hicks S, Shepherd MH, Colclough K, Hattersley AT, Ellard S. Maturity-onset diabetes of the young (MODY): how many cases are we missing? *Diabetologia* 2010;53:2504–2508

8. Kropff J, Selwood MP, McCarthy MI, Farmer AJ, Owen KR. Prevalence of monogenic diabetes in young adults: a community-based, cross-sectional study in Oxfordshire, UK. *Diabetologia* 2011;54:1261–1263

9. Fendler W, Borowiec M, Baranowska-Jazwiecka A, et al. Prevalence of monogenic diabetes amongst Polish children after a nationwide genetic screening campaign. *Diabetologia* 2012;55:2631–2635

10. Irgens HU, Molnes J, Johansson BB, et al. Prevalence of monogenic diabetes in the population-based Norwegian Childhood Diabetes Registry. *Diabetologia* 2013;56:1512–1519

11. Iafusco D, Massa O, Pasquino B, et al. Minimal incidence of neonatal/infancy onset diabetes in Italy is 1:90,000 live births. *Acta Diabetol* 2012;49:405–408

12. Wiedemann B, Schober E, Waldhoer T, et al. Incidence of neonatal diabetes in Austria-calculation based on the Austrian Diabetes Register. *Pediatr Diabetes* 2010;11:18–23

13. Grulich-Henn J, Wagner V, Thon A, et al. Entities and frequency of neonatal diabetes: data from the diabetes documentation and quality management system (DPV). *Diabet Med* 2010;27:709–712

14. Slingerland AS, Shields BM, Flanagan SE, et al. Referral rates for diagnostic testing support an incidence of permanent neonatal diabetes in three European countries of at least 1 in 260,000 live births. *Diabetologia* 2009;52:1683–1685

15. Shankar RK, Pihoker C, Dolan LM, et al. Permanent neonatal diabetes mellitus: prevalence and genetic diagnosis in the SEARCH for Diabetes in Youth Study. *Pediatr Diabetes* 2013;14:174–180

16. Støy J, Greeley SAW, Paz VP, et al. Diagnosis and treatment of neonatal diabetes: a United States experience. *Pediatr Diabetes* 2008;9:450–459

17. Greeley SAW, Tucker SE, Naylor RN, Bell GI, Philipson LH. Neonatal diabetes mellitus: a model for personalized medicine. *Trends Endocrinol Metab* 2010;21:464–472

18. Shield JP, Gardner RJ, Wadsworth EJ, et al. Aetiopathology and genetic basis of neonatal diabetes. *Arch Dis Child Fetal Neonatal Ed* 1997;76:39–42

19. Edghill EL, Dix RJ, Flanagan SE, et al. HLA genotyping supports a nonautoimmune etiology in patients diagnosed with diabetes under the age of 6 months. *Diabetes* 2006;55:1895–1898

20. Rubio-Cabezas O, Minton JAL, Caswell R, et al. Clinical heterogeneity in patients with FOXP3 mutations presenting with permanent neonatal diabetes. *Diabetes Care* 2009;32:111–116

21. Murphy R, Ellard S, Hattersley AT. Clinical implications of a molecular genetic classification of monogenic beta-cell diabetes. *Nat Clin Pract Endocrinol Metab* 2008;4:200–213

22. Frayling TM, Evans JC, Bulman MP, et al. Beta-cell genes and diabetes: molecular and clinical characterization of mutations in transcription factors. *Diabetes* 2001;50(Suppl. 1):S94–S100

23. Vionnet N, Stoffel M, Takeda J, et al. Nonsense mutation in the glucokinase gene causes early-onset non-insulin-dependent diabetes mellitus. *Nature* 1992; 356:721–722

24. Yamagata K, Oda N, Kaisaki PJ, et al. Mutations in the hepatocyte nuclear factor-1alpha gene in maturity-onset diabetes of the young (MODY3). *Nature* 1996;384:455–458

25. Yamagata K, Furuta H, Oda N, et al. Mutations in the hepatocyte nuclear factor-4alpha gene in maturity-onset diabetes of the young (MODY1). *Nature.* 1996;384:458–460

26. Tattersall RB, Fajans SS. A difference between the inheritance of classical juvenile-onset and maturity-onset type diabetes of young people. *Diabetes* 1975;24:44–53

27. Bellanné-Chantelot C, Lévy DJ, Carette C, et al. Clinical characteristics and diagnostic criteria of maturity-onset diabetes of the young (MODY) due to molecular anomalies of the HNF1A gene. *J Clin Endocrinol Metab* 2011;96:E1346–E1351

28. Thanabalasingham G, Pal A, Selwood MP, et al. Systematic assessment of etiology in adults with a clinical diagnosis of young-onset type 2 diabetes is a successful

strategy for identifying maturity-onset diabetes of the young. *Diabetes Care* 2012;35:1206–1212

29. Porter JR, Rangasami JJ, Ellard S, et al. Asian MODY: are we missing an important diagnosis? *Diabet Med* 2006;23:1257–1260

30. Pihoker C, Gilliam LK, Ellard S, et al. Prevalence, characteristics and clinical diagnosis of maturity onset diabetes of the young due to mutations in HNF1A, HNF4A, and glucokinase: results from the SEARCH for Diabetes in Youth. *J Clin Endocrinol Metab* 2013;98:4055–4062

31. Shields BM, McDonald TJ, Ellard S, Campbell MJ, Hyde C, Hattersley AT. The development and validation of a clinical prediction model to determine the probability of MODY in patients with young-onset diabetes. *Diabetologia* 2012;55:1265–1272

32. Ludvigsson J, Carlsson A, Forsander G, et al. C-peptide in the classification of diabetes in children and adolescents. *Pediatr Diabetes* 2012;13:45–50

33. Besser REJ, Shepherd MH, McDonald TJ, et al. Urinary C-peptide creatinine ratio is a practical outpatient tool for identifying hepatocyte nuclear factor 1-{alpha}/hepatocyte nuclear factor 4-{alpha} maturity-onset diabetes of the young from long-duration type 1 diabetes. *Diabetes Care* 2011;34:286–291

34. Besser REJ, Shields BM, Hammersley SE, et al. Home urine C-peptide creatinine ratio (UCPCR) testing can identify type 2 and MODY in pediatric diabetes. *Pediatr Diabetes* 2013;14:181–188

35. Owen KR, Thanabalasingham G, James TJ, et al. Assessment of high-sensitivity C-reactive protein levels as diagnostic discriminator of maturity-onset diabetes of the young due to HNF1A mutations. *Diabetes Care* 2010;33:1919–1924

36. McDonald TJ, Shields BM, Lawry J, et al. High-sensitivity CRP discriminates HNF1A-MODY from other subtypes of diabetes. *Diabetes Care* 2011;34:1860–1862

37. Thanabalasingham G, Shah N, Vaxillaire M, et al. A large multi-centre European study validates high-sensitivity C-reactive protein (hsCRP) as a clinical biomarker for the diagnosis of diabetes subtypes. *Diabetologia* 2011;54:2801–2810

38. McDonald TJ, Colclough K, Brown R, et al. Islet autoantibodies can discriminate maturity-onset diabetes of the young (MODY) from type 1 diabetes. *Diabet Med* 2011;28:1028–1033

39. Urbanová J, Rypáčková B, Kučera P, Anděl M, Heneberg P. Should the negativity for islet cell autoantibodies be used in a prescreening for genetic testing in

maturity-onset diabetes of the young? The case of autoimmunity-associated destruction of pancreatic β-cells in a family of HNF1A-MODY subjects. *Int Arch Allergy Immunol* 2013;161:279–284

40. Thomas NJ, Shields BM, Besser RE, et al. The impact of gender on urine C-peptide creatinine ratio interpretation. *Ann Clin Biochem* 2012;49:363–368

41. Steele AM, Wensley KJ, Ellard S, et al. Use of HbA_{1c} in the identification of patients with hyperglycaemia caused by a glucokinase mutation: observational case control studies. *PLoS One* 2013;8:e65326

42. Rubio-Cabezas O. Diagnosing monogenic diabetes: common misinterpretations of genetic findings. *Pediatr Diabetes* 2009;10:497–499

43. Stein SA, Maloney KL, Pollin TI. Genetic counseling for diabetes mellitus. *Curr Genet Med Rep* 2014;2:56–67

44. Colclough K, Saint-Martin C, Timsit J, Ellard S, Bellanné-Chantelot C. Clinical utility gene card for: maturity-onset diabetes of the young. *Eur J Hum Genet* 2014;22

45. Chakera AJ, Spyer G, Vincent N, Ellard S, Hattersley AT, Dunne FP. The 0.1% of the population with glucokinase monogenic diabetes can be recognized by clinical characteristics in pregnancy: the Atlantic Diabetes in Pregnancy cohort. *Diabetes Care* 2014;37:1230–1236

46. Osbak KK, Colclough K, Saint-Martin C, et al. Update on mutations in glucokinase (GCK), which cause maturity-onset diabetes of the young, permanent neonatal diabetes, and hyperinsulinemic hypoglycemia. *Hum Mutat* 2009;30:1512–1526

47. Spégel P, Ekholm E, Tuomi T, Groop L, Mulder H, Filipsson K. Metabolite profiling reveals normal metabolic control in carriers of mutations in the glucokinase gene (MODY2). *Diabetes* 2013;62:653–661

48. Stride A, Shields B, Gill-Carey O, et al. Cross-sectional and longitudinal studies suggest pharmacological treatment used in patients with glucokinase mutations does not alter glycaemia. *Diabetologia* 2014;57:54–56

49. Schnyder S, Mullis PE, Ellard S, Hattersley AT, Flück CE. Genetic testing for glucokinase mutations in clinically selected patients with MODY: a worthwhile investment. *Swiss Med Wkly* 2005;135:352–356

50. Colom CC, Corcoy RR. Maturity onset diabetes of the young and pregnancy. *Best Pract Res Clin Endocrinol Metab* 2010;24:605–615

51. Martin D, Bellanné-Chantelot C, Deschamps I, Froguel P, Robert JJ, Velho G. Long-term follow-up of oral glucose tolerance test-derived glucose tolerance and insulin secretion and insulin sensitivity indexes in subjects with glucokinase mutations (MODY2). *Diabetes Care* 2008;31:1321–1323

52. Steele AM, Shields BM, Wensley KJ, Colclough K, Ellard S, Hattersley AT. Prevalence of vascular complications among patients with glucokinase mutations and prolonged, mild hyperglycemia. *JAMA* 2014;311:279–286

53. Herman WH, Fajans SS, Ortiz FJ, et al. Abnormal insulin secretion, not insulin resistance, is the genetic or primary defect of MODY in the RW pedigree. *Diabetes* 1994;43:40–46

54. Byrne MM, Sturis J, Menzel S, et al. Altered insulin secretory responses to glucose in diabetic and nondiabetic subjects with mutations in the diabetes susceptibility gene MODY3 on chromosome 12. *Diabetes* 1996;45:1503–1510

55. Steele AM, Shields BM, Shepherd M, Ellard S, Hattersley AT, Pearson ER. Increased all-cause and cardiovascular mortality in monogenic diabetes as a result of mutations in the HNF1A gene. *Diabet Med* 2010;27:157–161

56. Pearson ER, Liddell WG, Shepherd M, Corrall RJ, Hattersley AT. Sensitivity to sulphonylureas in patients with hepatocyte nuclear factor-1alpha gene mutations: evidence for pharmacogenetics in diabetes. *Diabet Med* 2000;17: 543–545

57. Shepherd M, Shields B, Ellard S, Rubio-Cabezas O, Hattersley AT. A genetic diagnosis of HNF1A diabetes alters treatment and improves glycaemic control in the majority of insulin-treated patients. *Diabet Med* 2009;26:437–441

58. Shepherd M, Pearson ER, Houghton J, Salt G, Ellard S, Hattersley AT. No deterioration in glycemic control in HNF-1alpha maturity-onset diabetes of the young following transfer from long-term insulin to sulphonylureas. *Diabetes Care* 2003;26:3191–3192

59. Fajans SS, Brown MB. Administration of sulfonylureas can increase glucose-induced insulin secretion for decades in patients with maturity-onset diabetes of the young. *Diabetes Care* 1993;16:1254–1261

60. Østoft SH, Bagger JI, Hansen T, et al. Glucose-lowering effects and low risk of hypoglycemia in patients with maturity-onset diabetes of the young when treated with a GLP-1 receptor agonist: a double-blind, randomized, crossover trial. *Diabetes Care* 2014;37:1797–1805

61. Ellard S, Colclough K. Mutations in the genes encoding the transcription factors hepatocyte nuclear factor 1 alpha (HNF1A) and 4 alpha (HNF4A) in maturity-onset diabetes of the young. *Hum Mutat* 2006;27:854–869

62. Isomaa BB, Henricsson MM, Lehto MM, et al. Chronic diabetic complications in patients with MODY3 diabetes. *Diabetologia* 1998;41:467–473

63. Brackenridge A, Pearson ER, Shojaee-Moradie F, Hattersley AT, Russell-Jones D, Umpleby AM. Contrasting insulin sensitivity of endogenous glucose production rate in subjects with hepatocyte nuclear factor-1β and -1α mutations. *Diabetes* 2006;55:405–411

64. Pearson ER, Badman MK, Lockwood CR, et al. Contrasting diabetes phenotypes associated with hepatocyte nuclear factor-1α and -1β mutations. *Diabetes Care* 2004;27:1102–1107

65. Wildin RS, Ramsdell F, Peake J, et al. X-linked neonatal diabetes mellitus, enteropathy and endocrinopathy syndrome is the human equivalent of mouse scurfy. *Nat Genet* 2001;27:18–20

66. Temple IK, Gardner RJ, Mackay DJ, Barber JC, Robinson DO, Shield JP. Transient neonatal diabetes: widening the understanding of the etiopathogenesis of diabetes. *Diabetes* 2000;49:1359–1366

67. Gloyn AL, Pearson ER, Antcliff JF, et al. Activating mutations in the gene encoding the ATP-sensitive potassium-channel subunit Kir6.2 and permanent neonatal diabetes. *N Engl J Med* 2004;350:1838–1849

68. Babenko AP, Polak M, Cavé H, et al. Activating mutations in the *ABCC8* gene in neonatal diabetes mellitus. *N Engl J Med* 2006;355:456–466

69. Støy J, Edghill EL, Flanagan SE, et al. Insulin gene mutations as a cause of permanent neonatal diabetes. *Proc Natl Acad Sci U S A* 2007;104:15040–15044

70. Garin I, Edghill EL, Akerman I, et al. Recessive mutations in the INS gene result in neonatal diabetes through reduced insulin biosynthesis. *Proc Natl Acad Sci U S A* 2010;107:3105–3110

71. Greeley SAW, Naylor RN, Philipson LH, Bell GI. Neonatal diabetes: an expanding list of genes allows for improved diagnosis and treatment. *Curr Diab Rep* 2011;11:519–532

72. Allen HL, Flanagan SE, Shaw-Smith C, et al. *GATA6* haploinsufficiency causes pancreatic agenesis in humans. *Nat Genet* 2011;44:20–22

73. Njølstad PRP, Søvik OO, Cuesta-Muñoz AA, et al. Neonatal diabetes mellitus due to complete glucokinase deficiency. *N Engl J Med* 2001;344:1588–1592

74. Gloyn AL, Cummings EA, Edghill EL, et al. Permanent neonatal diabetes due to paternal germline mosaicism for an activating mutation of the *KCNJ11* Gene encoding the Kir6.2 subunit of the beta-cell potassium adenosine triphosphate channel. *J Clin Endocrinol Metab* 2004;89:3932–3935

75. Temple IK, James RS, Crolla JA, et al. An imprinted gene(s) for diabetes? *Nat Genet* 1995;9:110–112

76. Carmody D, Beca FA, Bell CD, et al. Role of noninsulin therapies alone or in combination in chromosome 6q24-related transient neonatal diabetes: sulfonyl-urea improves but does not always normalize insulin secretion. *Diabetes Care* 2015;38:e86–e87

77. Gloyn AL, Diatloff-Zito C, Edghill EL, et al. *KCNJ11* activating mutations are associated with developmental delay, epilepsy and neonatal diabetes syndrome and other neurological features. *Eur J Hum Genet* 2006;14:824–830

78. Klupa T, Skupien J, Mirkiewicz-Sieradzka B, et al. Efficacy and safety of sulfonyl-urea use in permanent neonatal diabetes due to KCNJ11gene mutations: 34-month median follow-up. *Diabetes Technol Ther* 2010;12:387–391

79. Iafusco D, Bizzarri C, Cadario F, et al. No β-cell desensitisation after a median of 68 months on glibenclamide therapy in patients with KCNJ11-associated perma-nent neonatal diabetes. *Diabetologia* 2011;54:2736–2738

80. Begum-Hasan J, Polychronakos C, Brill H. Familial permanent neonatal diabetes with *KCNJ11* mutation and the response to glyburide therapy—a three-year fol-low-up. *J Pediatr Endocrinol Metab* 2008;21:895–903

81. Slingerland AS, Nuboer R, Hadders-Algra M, Hattersley AT, Bruining GJ. Improved motor development and good long-term glycaemic control with sulfo-nylurea treatment in a patient with the syndrome of intermediate developmental delay, early-onset generalised epilepsy and neonatal diabetes associated with the V59M mutation in the *KCNJ11* gene. *Diabetologia* 2006;49:2559–2563

82. Shah RP, Spruyt K, Kragie BC, Greeley SAW, Msall ME. Visuomotor perfor-mance in KCNJ11-related neonatal diabetes is impaired in children with DEND-associated mutations and may be improved by early treatment with sulfonylureas. *Diabetes Care* 2012;35:2086–2088

83. Wambach JA, Marshall BA, Koster JC, White NH, Nichols CG. Successful sulfo-nylurea treatment of an insulin-naïve neonate with diabetes mellitus due to a *KCNJ11* mutation. *Pediatr Diabetes* 2010;11:286–288

84. Loomba-Albrecht LA, Glaser NS, Styne DM, Bremer AA. An oral sulfonylurea in the treatment of transient neonatal diabetes mellitus. *Clin Ther* 2009;31:816–820

85. Pearson ER, Flechtner I, Njølstad PR, et al. Switching from insulin to oral sulfonylureas in patients with diabetes due to Kir6.2 mutations. *N Engl J Med* 2006;355:467–477

86. Edghill EL, Flanagan SE, Patch A-M, et al. Insulin mutation screening in 1,044 patients with diabetes mutations in the INS gene are a common cause of neonatal diabetes but a rare cause of diabetes diagnosed in childhood or adulthood. *Diabetes* 2008;57:1034–1042

87. Polak M, Dechaume A, Cavé H, et al. Heterozygous missense mutations in the insulin gene are linked to permanent diabetes appearing in the neonatal period or in early infancy: a report from the French ND (Neonatal Diabetes) Study Group. *Diabetes* 2008;57:1115–1119

88. Colombo C, Porzio O, Liu M, et al. Seven mutations in the human insulin gene linked to permanent neonatal/infancy-onset diabetes mellitus. *J Clin Invest* 2008;118:2148–2156

89. Russo L, Iafusco D, Brescianini S, et al. Permanent diabetes during the first year of life: multiple gene screening in 54 patients. *Diabetologia* 2011;54:1693–1701

90. Rajan S, Kanakatti Shankar R, Eames SC, et al. In vitro processing and secretion of mutant insulin proteins that cause permanent neonatal diabetes. *Am J Physiol Endocrinol Metab* 2010;298:E403–E410

91. Hodish I, Liu M, Rajpal G, et al. Misfolded proinsulin affects bystander proinsulin in neonatal diabetes. *J Biol Chem* 2010;285:685–694

92. Meur G, Simon A, Harun N, et al. Insulin gene mutations resulting in early-onset diabetes: marked differences in clinical presentation, metabolic status, and pathogenic effect through endoplasmic reticulum retention. *Diabetes* 2010;59:653–661

93. Park SY, Ye H, Steiner DF, Bell GI. Mutant proinsulin proteins associated with neonatal diabetes are retained in the endoplasmic reticulum and not efficiently secreted. *Biochem Biophys Res Commun* 2010;391:1449–1454

94. Liu M, Haataja L, Wright J, et al. Mutant INS-gene induced diabetes of youth: proinsulin cysteine residues impose dominant-negative inhibition on wild-type proinsulin transport. *PLoS One* 2010;5:e13333

95. Bonfanti R, Colombo C, Nocerino V, et al. Insulin gene mutations as cause of diabetes in children negative for five type 1 diabetes autoantibodies. *Diabetes Care* 2009;32:123–125

96. Rubio-Cabezas O, Edghill EL, Argente J, Hattersley AT. Testing for monogenic diabetes among children and adolescents with antibody-negative clinically defined type 1 diabetes. *Diabet Med* 2009;26:1070–1074

97. Pörksen S, Laborie LB, Nielsen L, et al. Disease progression and search for monogenic diabetes among children with new onset type 1 diabetes negative for ICA, GAD- and IA-2 antibodies. *BMC Endocr Disord* 2010;10:16

98. Molven A, Ringdal M, Nordbø AM, et al. Mutations in the insulin gene can cause MODY and autoantibody-negative type 1 diabetes. *Diabetes* 2008;57:1131–1135

99. Boesgaard TW, Pruhova S, Andersson EA, et al. Further evidence that mutations in INS can be a rare cause of maturity-onset diabetes of the young (MODY). *BMC Med Genet* 2010;11:42

100. Garin I, Molven A, Perez de Nanclares G, et al. Permanent neonatal diabetes caused by creation of an ectopic splice site within the INS gene. *PLoS One* 2012;7:e29205

101. Raile K, O'Connell M, Galler A, et al. Diabetes caused by insulin gene (INS) deletion: clinical characteristics of homozygous and heterozygous individuals. *Eur J Endocrinol* 2011;165:255–260

102. Carmody D, Park S-Y, Ye H, et al. Continued lessons from the INS gene: an intronic mutation causing diabetes through a novel mechanism. *J Med Genet* 2015;52:612–616

103. Delépine M, Nicolino M, Barrett T, Golamaully M, Lathrop GM, Julier C. *EIF2AK3*, encoding translation initiation factor 2-alpha kinase 3, is mutated in patients with Wolcott-Rallison syndrome. *Nat Genet* 2000;25:406–409

104. Rubio-Cabezas O, Patch AM, Minton JA, Flanagan SE, Edghill EL, Hussain K, et al. Wolcott-Rallison syndrome is the most common genetic cause of permanent neonatal diabetes in consanguineous families. *J Clin Endocrinol Metab* 2009;94:4162–4170

105. Julier C, Nicolino M. Wolcott-Rallison syndrome. *Orphanet J Rare Dis* 2010;5:29

106. Senée V, Vattem KM, Delépine M, Rainbow LA, Haton C, Lecoq A, Shaw NJ, Robert J-J, Rooman R, Diatloff-Zito C, et al. Wolcott-Rallison Syndrome: clinical, genetic, and functional study of *EIF2AK3* mutations and suggestion of genetic heterogeneity. *Diabetes* 2004;53:1876–1883

107. Suzuki E, Evans T, Lowry J, et al. The human GATA-6 gene: structure, chromosomal location, and regulation of expression by tissue-specific and mitogen-responsive signals. *Genomics* 1996;38:283–290

108. Strom T. Diabetes insipidus, diabetes mellitus, optic atrophy and deafness (DID-MOAD) caused by mutations in a novel gene (wolframin) coding for a predicted transmembrane protein. *Hum Mol Genet* 1998;7:2021–2028

109. Inoue H, Tanizawa Y, Wasson J, et al. A gene encoding a transmembrane protein is mutated in patients with diabetes mellitus and optic atrophy (Wolfram syndrome). *Nat Genet* 1998;20:143–148

110. Fonseca SG, Fukuma M, Lipson KL, et al. WFS1 is a novel component of the unfolded protein response and maintains homeostasis of the endoplasmic reticulum in pancreatic beta-cells. *J Biol Chem* 2005;280:39609–39615

111. Cagalinec M, Liiv M, Hodurova Z, et al. Role of mitochondrial dynamics in neuronal development: mechanism for Wolfram syndrome. *PLoS Biol* 2016;14:e1002511

112. Zalloua PA, Azar ST, Delépine M, et al. WFS1 mutations are frequent monogenic causes of juvenile-onset diabetes mellitus in Lebanon. *Hum Mol Genet* 2008;17:4012–4021

113. Murphy R, Turnbull DM, Walker M, Hattersley AT. Clinical features, diagnosis and management of maternally inherited diabetes and deafness (MIDD) associated with the 3243A>G mitochondrial point mutation. *Diabet Med.* 2008;25:383–399

114. Katulanda P, Groves CJ, Barrett A, et al. Prevalence and clinical characteristics of maternally inherited diabetes and deafness caused by the mt3243A > G mutation in young adult diabetic subjects in Sri Lanka. *Diabet Med* 2008;25:370–374

115. Reinauer C, Meissner T, Roden M, et al. Low prevalence of patients with mitochondrial disease in the German/Austrian DPV diabetes registry. *Eur J Pediatr* 2016;175:613–622

116. Goto Y-I, Nonaka I, Horai S. A mutation in the tRNALeu(UUR) gene associated with the MELAS subgroup of mitochondrial encephalomyopathies. *Nature* 1990;348:651–653

117. Chae JH, Hwang H, Lim BC, Cheong HI, Hwang YS, Kim KJ. Clinical features of A3243G mitochondrial tRNA mutation. *Brain Dev* 2004;26:459–462

118. van den Ouweland JM, Lemkes HH, Ruitenbeek W, et al. Mutation in mitochondrial tRNA(Leu)(UUR) gene in a large pedigree with maternally transmitted type II diabetes mellitus and deafness. *Nat Genet* 1992;1:368–371

119. Guéry B, Choukroun G, Noël LH, et al. The spectrum of systemic involvement in adults presenting with renal lesion and mitochondrial tRNA(Leu) gene mutation. *J Am Soc Nephrol* 2003;14:2099–2108

120. Narbonne H, Perucca-Lostanlen D, Desnuelle C, Vialettes B, Saunières A, Paquis-Flucklinger V. Searching for A3243G mitochondrial DNA mutation in buccal mucosa in order to improve the screening of patients with mitochondrial diabetes. *Eur J Endocrinol* 2001;145:541–542

121. Frederiksen AL, Jeppesen TD, Vissing J, et al. High prevalence of impaired glucose homeostasis and myopathy in asymptomatic and oligosymptomatic 3243A>G mitochondrial DNA mutation-positive subjects. *J Clin Endocrinol Metab* 2009;94:2872–2879

122. Greeley SAW, John PM, Winn AN, et al. The cost-effectiveness of personalized genetic medicine: the case of genetic testing in neonatal diabetes. *Diabetes Care* 2011;34:622–627

123. Naylor RN, John PM, Winn AN, et al. Cost-effectiveness of MODY genetic testing: translating genomic advances into practical health applications. *Diabetes Care* 2014;37:202–209

124. Rubio-Cabezas O, Hattersley AT, Njølstad PR, et al. The diagnosis and management of monogenic diabetes in children and adolescents. *Pediatr Diabetes* 2014;15(Suppl. 20):47–64

125. American Diabetes Association. Standards of medical care in diabetes—2015: summary of revisions. *Diabetes Care* 2015;38 (Suppl. 1):S4

126. American Diabetes Association. Standards of medical care in diabetes—2017. *Diabetes Care* 2017;40(Suppl. 1):S11–S24.

127. Ellard S, Bellanné-Chantelot C, Hattersley AT; European Molecular Genetics Quality Network (EMQN). Best practice guidelines for the molecular genetic diagnosis of maturity-onset diabetes of the young. *Diabetologia* 2008;51:546–553

128. Ellard S, Allen HL, De Franco E, et al. Improved genetic testing for monogenic diabetes using targeted next-generation sequencing. *Diabetologia* 2013;56:1958–1963

129. Alkorta-Aranburu G, Carmody D, Cheng YW, et al. Phenotypic heterogeneity in monogenic diabetes: the clinical and diagnostic utility of a gene panel-based next-generation sequencing approach. *Mol Genet Metab* 2014;113:315–320

130. Bonnefond A, Philippe J, Durand E, et al. Highly sensitive diagnosis of 43 monogenic forms of diabetes or obesity through one-step PCR-based enrichment in combination with next-generation sequencing. *Diabetes Care* 2014;37: 460–467

Part I
Case Studies

Introduction

These 22 cases illustrate both the most important examples of monogenic diabetes and the difficulties in making a diagnosis as well as in obtaining genetic analysis. The most important aspect to recognize is when there is an actionable outcome to making a specific diagnosis. This includes both a change in therapy and the recognition that many of these conditions are dominantly inherited, so there likely will be more individuals, sometimes many more, to consider in the impact of making a genetic diagnosis. In some cases, the impact can be immediate and profound, such as in the use of sulfonylureas in neonatal diabetes caused by mutations in *KCNJ11* and *ABCC8* (Cases 1 and 2), or in young adult onset diabetes caused by HNF1A mutations (Case 12) that are also highly responsive to sulfonylureas. Where there might not be a change in treatment, there can be a change in how other organs are potentially impacted, such as the great vessels in *GATA6*, thyroid abnormalities with *GLIS3*, bone abnormalities with *EIF2AK3*, or variably presenting multi-organ involvement with mitochondrial diabetes (MELAS, MIDD, etc). In the case of Wolfram syndrome (WFS1), we simply do not yet know enough. In severe cases the outcome is often fatal, but milder cases are being uncovered where the outcome and progression is less certain. Making the diagnosis of this and many of the other cases changes the nature of the follow-up visits. In GCK-MODY2 (Case 11) limited follow-up may be useful just to remind the patient of their situation, except in the case of pregnancy or perhaps development of obesity. The growing recognition of these atypical cases makes it important that they can be considered and accurately and rapidly diagnosed, in a cost-effective manner. In addition to this volume, several websites are continuously updated to provide up-to-date information and consultation to the inquiring clinicians—and patients—www.diabetesgenes.org and www.monogenicdiabetes.org in particular. Please see Chapter 1 for specific references and discussion of most of the relevant gene mutations causing diabetes.

Case 1:
KCNJ11 – DEND: Neonatal Diabetes

Lisa R. Letourneau, MPH, RD;[1] May Sanyoura, PhD;[1] Laura Dickens, MD;[1] Siri Atma W. Greeley, MD, PhD;[1] Rochelle N. Naylor, MD;[1] Graeme I. Bell, PhD;[1] and Louis H. Philipson, MD, PhD[1]

Case

A now 11-year-old Caucasian female was born appropriate for gestational age at 38 weeks after an uncomplicated pregnancy and delivery. At four months of age, she presented to a community clinic with decreased activity and increased sleeping. No polyuria, polydipsia, or weight loss was reported by her caregivers. She was found to have elevated blood glucose of 635 mg/dL (35.3 mmol/L) and carbon dioxide 13 nmol/L, was diagnosed with insulin-dependent type 1 diabetes, and was admitted for diabetes education and stabilization of blood glucose. She was discharged on glargine 1 unit daily and aspart insulin corrections, 1 unit every 4–6 hours as needed for blood glucose above 400 mg/dL.

The patient had a past medical history significant for developmental delay and scoliosis. Caregivers reported concern for lack of communication/smiling, difficulty latching to feed, poor muscle tone, inability to hold head up, and inability to grab for objects at age 4 months. She was born with a turned foot and was later found to have scoliosis. Family and social history was unremarkable.

[1]Departments of Medicine and Pediatrics, The University of Chicago, Chicago, IL

At 3 years old, research-based genetic testing for neonatal diabetes was performed and revealed a heterozygous p.Val59Ala (V59A) *KCNJ11* mutation. Following genetic testing, she was transitioned off insulin and onto glyburide.

Since diagnosis, the patient has had multiple seizures, usually after unusual physical exertion such as in physical therapy. Her development has continued to be delayed. At age 5 years, she was not walking or talking. She was able to hop and scoot with some assistance.

At her last visit, she was taking glimepiride 1 mg (0.02 mg/kg) daily and glyburide 10 mg eight times daily (1.38 mg/kg) and had excellent glycemic control with an HbA_{1c} of 5.5%. Other medications included carbamazepine 10 mg TID and topiramate 25 mg twice daily. The topiramate appeared to be controlling her seizures well. She had made significant developmental progress with intensive physical therapy and caregiver support. At the time of the visit, she was walking unassisted, nearly completely toilet trained, interactive, and smiling. Follow-up is ongoing.

Discussion

Mutations in *KCNJ11* are the most common cause of permanent neonatal diabetes and are typically treatable with oral sulfonylurea medication, although the dose required may vary depending on the exact mutation (0.5–2.5 mg/kg/day).[1,2] *KCNJ11* V59A mutations are known to be associated with DEND syndrome (developmental delay, epilepsy, and neonatal diabetes).[3,4] DEND syndrome can be severe, as noted in this case, or more moderate (iDEND/intermediate DEND). The initiation of intensive therapy, including physical, occupational, and speech therapy, at an early age is critical to patient progress. Sulfonylurea therapy not only tightly manages blood glucose level, but may play a critical role in K_{ATP} channel activity in the brain.[5] Therefore, ensuring adequate total daily doses of sulfonylurea in patients with DEND syndrome is essential.

References

1.   Gloyn AL, Pearson ER, Antcliff JF, et al. Activating mutations in the gene encoding the ATP-sensitive potassium-channel subunit Kir6.2 and permanent neonatal diabetes. *N Engl J Med* 2004;350:1838–1849

2.   Pearson ER, Flechtner I, Njølstad PR, et al. Switching from insulin to oral sulfonylureas in patients with diabetes due to Kir6.2 mutations. *N Engl J Med* 2006;355:467–477

3.   Carmody D, Pastore AN, Landmeier KA, Letourneau LR, Martin R, Hwang JL, Naylor RN, Hunter SJ, Msall ME, Philipson LH, Scott MN, Greeley SA. Patients with KCNJ11-related diabetes frequently have neuropsychological impairments compared with sibling controls. *Diabet Med* 2016;33:1380–1386

4.   Landmeier KA, Lanning M, Carmody D, Greeley SA, Msall ME. ADHD, learning difficulties and sleep disturbances associated with KCNJ11-related neonatal diabetes. *Pediatr Diabetes* 24 August 2016 [Epub ahead of print]

5.   Shah RP, Spruyt K, Kragie BC, Greeley SAW, Msall ME. Visuomotor performance in KCNJ11-related neonatal diabetes is impaired in children with DEND-associated mutations and may be improved by early treatment with sulfonylureas. *Diabetes Care* 2012;35:2086–2088

Case 2:
ABCC8 Neonatal Diabetes

Lisa R. Letourneau, MPH, RD;[1] May Sanyoura, PhD;[1] Laura Dickens, MD;[1] Siri Atma W. Greeley, MD, PhD;[1] Rochelle N. Naylor, MD;[1] Graeme I. Bell, PhD;[1] and Louis H. Philipson, MD, PhD[1]

Case

A now 3-year-old Caucasian male was born small for gestational age at about 40 weeks, weight z-score -2.09, after a pregnancy remarkable for small intrauterine ultrasound measurements and an uncomplicated delivery. At 4 months of age, he presented to a community emergency room with two days of stuffy nose, noisy breathing, vomiting, and darkened, cold hands and lips. He was found to have elevated blood glucose of 758 mg/dL, HbA_{1c} 13.6% (potentially impacted by fetal hemoglobin), ketoacidosis (carbon dioxide 3 mmol/L), negative pancreatic islet autoantibodies (GAD65 0.00 nmol/L and insulin AB 0.0 nmol/L), and was diagnosed with diabetes. Intravenous insulin infusion was initiated at 0.1 unit/kg/h. He was discharged on multiple daily doses of insulin (MDI), including lantus 1.5 units at 8 A.M. and regular insulin corrections every 6 hours (0.5 unit for every 100 mg/dL >200 mg/dL).

The patient had no additional medical or surgical history, although the parents did retrospectively note that he was always considered a "thin" infant and often wet through his diapers. From birth to diabetes diagnosis, growth tracked along the third percentile weight-for-age on

---

[1]Departments of Medicine and Pediatrics, The University of Chicago, Chicago, IL

World Health Organization growth charts for males.[1] Development had been appropriate for age. Family and social history was unremarkable (Figure C2.1).

Commercial genetic testing for the most common neonatal diabetes genes was ordered and revealed a heterozygous c.631C>A (p.Gln211Lys) *ABCC8* mutation. At 7 months of age, he was transitioned off of insulin and onto glyburide. His initial glyburide regimen (2.5 mg tablet suspended at 1 mL solution) was as follows:

- 1.2 mL (3 mg) at 5 A.M.
- 1.2 mL (3 mg) at 11 A.M.
- 1.2 mL (3 mg) at 5 P.M.
- 1.0 mL (2.5 mg) at 10P.M.
- 0.2 mL (0.5 mg) at 2 or 3 A.M. (if he wakes up overnight)

His initial total daily dose was 1.47–1.53 mg/kg/day. Slight motor developmental delay was noted, so intensive physical and occupational therapy was initiated.

At age 1 year old, he was noted to have an abnormal brain MRI suggestive of metachromatic leukodystrophy, but further workup including blood tests and genetic testing for this were negative. Thus, he is said to have leukodystrophy NOS.

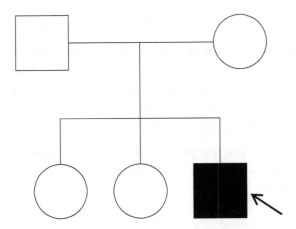

Figure C2.1 — Pedigree of a patient with *ABCC8*-related neonatal diabetes.

At his last visit, this patient had excellent glycemic control on glyburide with an HbA$_{1c}$ of 5.4%. His motor development had improved, including walking and running, but his speech was delayed. Follow-up is ongoing.

Discussion

Mutations in *ABCC8* can cause either permanent or transient neonatal diabetes. Patients with *ABCC8*-related neonatal diabetes, similar to *KCNJ11*, typically respond well to sulfonylureas such as glyburide.[2-5] However, less is known about the neurodevelopmental impact of this class of conditions. As shown in this case report, some patients with *ABCC8* mutations do have various developmental delays, including speech, motor, and cognitive delays.

References

1. WHO Multicentre Growth Reference Study Group. WHO Child Growth Standards based on length/height, weight and age. *Acta Paediatr Suppl* 2006;450:76–85

2. Proks P, Arnold AL, Bruining J, Girard C, Flanagan SE, Larkin B, Colclough K, Hattersley AT, Ashcroft FM, Ellard S. A heterozygous activating mutation in the sulphonylurea receptor SUR1 (*ABCC8*) causes neonatal diabetes. *Hum Mol Genet* 2006;15:1793–1800

3. Babenko AP, Polak M, Cavé H, et al. Activating mutations in the *ABCC8* gene in neonatal diabetes mellitus. *N Engl J Med* 2006;355:456–466

4. Ellard S, Flanagan SE, Girard CA, Patch AM, Harries LW, Parrish A, Edghill EL, Mackay DJ, Proks P, Shimomura K, Haberland H, Carson DJ, Shield JP, Hattersley AT, Ashcroft FM. Permanent neonatal diabetes caused by dominant, recessive, or compound heterozygous SUR1 mutations with opposite functional effects. *Am J Hum Genet* 2007;81:375–382

5. Greeley SA, Naylor RN, Philipson LH, Bell GI. Neonatal diabetes: an expanding list of genes allows for improved diagnosis and treatment. *Curr Diab Rep* 2011;11:519–532

Case 3:
INS – Insulin Gene Mutation in Neonatal Diabetes

Lisa R. Letourneau, MPH, RD;[1] May Sanyoura, PhD;[1] Laura Dickens, MD;[1] Siri Atma W. Greeley, MD, PhD;[1] Rochelle N. Naylor, MD; [1] Graeme I. Bell, PhD;[1] and Louis H. Philipson, MD, PhD[1]

Case

Here we describe the case of a family with a strong, linear history of diabetes diagnosed at less than 12 months of age. Linkage analysis, accompanied by Sanger sequencing, revealed a heterozygous mutation in the insulin gene in several family members (p.Gly32Ser). A case summary of the granddaughter (designated in pedigree with arrow, Figure C3.1) is discussed.

A now 9-year-old Caucasian-Hispanic female was born appropriate for gestational age at 37 weeks after an uncomplicated pregnancy and delivery. Blood glucose values on the day of birth were normal. Due to the strong family history of known INS gene mutations, caregivers checked the patient's blood glucose levels on a home glucometer from age 1 month to 4 months. The patient presented to a children's emergency room at age 4 months after home hyperglycemia and was found to have elevated blood glucose of 404 mg/dL (22.4 mmol/L) and HbA$_{1c}$ 9.8% (potentially impacted by fetal hemoglobin) without ketoacidosis (pH 7.433, HCO3 25.0 mm/L, carbon dioxide 24 mEq/L, beta-hydroxybutyrate 0.19 mmol/L). Multiple daily doses of insulin (MDI) were initiated, with total daily doses of about 0.31 unit/kg/day in the first six months of life. A detectable C-peptide of

---

[1]Departments of Medicine and Pediatrics, The University of Chicago, Chicago, IL

0.5 pmol/mL (reference range: 0.3–2.35) and detected insulin level of 5.1 (reference range: 3–20) were found. Genetic testing was performed and confirmed the presence of the *INS* p.Gly32Ser mutation.

The patient had no additional medical or surgical history. Growth and development has been normal. Family history was remarkable for a strong, linear history of diabetes diagnosed under age 12 months, suggestive of an autosomal dominant inheritance pattern (Figure C3.1). Her paternal great-grandmother was diagnosed at 11 months old. Her paternal grandmother was diagnosed at age 2 months, while her father was diagnosed at 12 months. Four years after the birth of this patient, a sister was born who also carries this mutation. Social history was remarkable for barriers to medication adherence.

Other relevant labs include: negative pancreatic islet autoantibodies at diagnosis (GAD65 0.00 nmol/L, insulin AB <3 % bound, IA-2 negative),

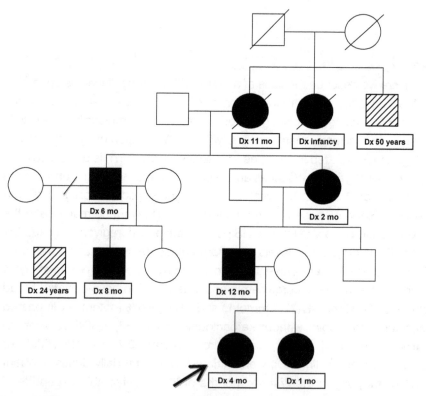

Figure C3.1 — Pedigree of a family with INS-related neonatal diabetes.

continually present but low C-peptide levels (0.11 pmol/mL at age 3 years and 0.13 pmol/mL at age 3.5 years), and continually present but low insulin levels (1.3 at age 3 years and 1.0 at age 3.5 years).

Glycemic control was consistently suboptimal from initiation of insulin to age 3.5 years. Therefore, she transitioned to continuous subcutaneous insulin infusion therapy at 42 months old. The patient is currently managed on an insulin pump with average total daily dose of 0.82 unit/kg/day. Follow-up is ongoing.

Discussion

INS mutations are the second most common cause of permanent neonatal diabetes, yet are variable in their presentation and age at diagnosis.[1-4] Insulin therapy remains the best treatment for this form of neonatal diabetes. Advancing diabetes technology, including continuous subcutaneous insulin infusion pumps and continuous glucose monitors, can be critically important to optimizing glycemic control safely in infants and young children.[5] This patient began insulin therapy fairly early on, which may have helped contribute to her low but present C-peptide and insulin levels. This family is an excellent example of the benefit of early, targeted, family-based genetic testing.

References

1. Støy J, Edghill EL, Flanagan SE, Ye H, Paz VP, Pluzhnikov A, Below JE, Hayes MG, Cox NJ, Lipkind GM, Lipton RB, Greeley SA, Patch AM, Ellard S, Steiner DF, Hattersley AT, Philipson LH, Bell GI; Neonatal Diabetes International Collaborative Group. Insulin gene mutations as a cause of permanent neonatal diabetes. *Proc Natl Acad Sci U S A* 2007;104:15040–15044

2. Edghill EL, Flanagan SE, Patch AM, Boustred C, Parrish A, Shields B, Shepherd MH, Hussain K, Kapoor RR, Malecki M, MacDonald MJ, Støy J, Steiner DF, Philipson LH, Bell GI, Hattersley AT, Ellard S; Neonatal Diabetes International Collaborative Group. Insulin mutation screening in 1,044 patients with diabetes: mutations in the INS gene are a common cause of neonatal diabetes but a rare cause of diabetes diagnosed in childhood or adulthood. *Diabetes* 2008;57:1034–1042

3. Støy J, Greeley SA, Paz VP, Ye H, Pastore AN, Skowron KB, Lipton RB, Cogen FR, Bell GI, Philipson LH; United States Neonatal Diabetes Working Group. Diagnosis and treatment of neonatal diabetes: a United States experience. *Pediatr Diabetes* 2008;9:450–459

4. Støy J, Steiner DF, Park SY, Ye H, Philipson LH, Bell GI. Clinical and molecular genetics of neonatal diabetes due to mutations in the insulin gene. *Rev Endocr Metab Disord* 2010;11:205–215

5. Marin MT, Coffey ML, Beck JK, Dasari PS, Allen R, Krishnan S. A novel approach to the management of neonatal diabetes using sensor-augmented insulin pump therapy with threshold suspend technology at diagnosis. *Diabetes Spectr* 2016;29:176–179

Case 4:
STAT3 and Neonatal Diabetes

David W. Hansen, MD, MPH;[1] Juan C. Sanchez, MD;[1] and Tamara S. Hannon, MD[1]

Case

The patient is a 9-month-old Hispanic female who was noted in the days and weeks after birth to have fluctuating circulating plasma glucose concentrations.

Gestation and Birth History

She was born at 37 weeks estimated gestational age via vaginal delivery with APGAR scores of 6 and 5 at 1 and 5 minutes, respectively. The pregnancy was complicated by pregnancy-induced hypertension and severe intrauterine growth restriction resulting in her birth weight of 1.25 kg (−4.19 SD), birth length of 39.0 cm (−3.98 SD), and head circumference of 28.5 cm (−2.90 SD). She was started on respiratory support with oxygen via high flow nasal cannula. A sepsis workup with antibiotic initiation was commenced along with intravenous fluids containing dextrose (6 mg/kg/min). She also received a packed red blood cell transfusion for a hematocrit of 29%. Her physical exam included overriding sutures, normal anterior fontanelle, low-set ears, and a prominent forehead. The remainder of the exam was unremarkable except for pronounced jaundice.

---

[1]Indiana University School of Medicine and Riley Hospital for Children, Indianapolis, IN

Hospital Course – The First Month

On day 2 of life, circulating plasma glucose concentrations continued to rise to >400 mg/dL and dextrose in the IV fluids was discontinued. C-peptide was <0.1 mg/mL, insulin 0.50 mcU/mL, and cortisol 20.2 mcg/dL. A central glucose was not taken at the time of these labs, but the point of care glucometer readings before and after these results were 352 and 331 mg/dL. Her glucose concentration returned to normal and dextrose was subsequently added back into the fluids and continued to be titrated based on her plasma glucose concentration. IV fluids were replaced with expressed breast milk on day 5 of life. At that point, her plasma glucose concentration was 242 mg/dL. The C-peptide was <0.1 mg/mL, and insulin was 2.15 mcU/mL. The patient was noted to be hypoglycemic within a few hours to 34 mg/dL and fluids with dextrose were restarted. The amount of dextrose continued to be titrated for acceptable circulating glucose concentrations until day 10 of life when an insulin drip was initiated due to continued high blood glucose concentrations. Genetic testing for monogenic diabetes was sent at this time.

Maintaining appropriate blood glucose levels was challenging and the patient was on and off an insulin drip for the next few months. She continued to have feeding intolerance and poor weight gain, which necessitated parenteral nutrition. In addition to her hyperglycemia, she was noted to have increased bilirubin levels on day 4 of life to total bilirubin 6.9 and direct of 3.5. Her oxygen was weaned to room air by this point.

Hospital Course – The Remaining Months

At 6 weeks of age, results of the monogenic test showed a mutation in *ABCC8* gene, c.2858A>C, which resulted in a Gln for Pro exchange. The area of the mutation was in a part of the gene considered to be nonfunctioning and consequently was not thought to be significant. However, other patients with an *ABCC8* mutation had responded to sulfonylureas, so a trial of glyburide therapy was initiated per protocol at 0.2 mg/kg/day.[1]

Over the next few weeks she required parenteral nutrition as she suffered from continued feeding intolerance, abdominal distention, and concern for sepsis. The glyburide trial was discontinued at 8 weeks of age at a dose of 0.92 mg/kg/day with her blood glucose concentrations continuing to run consistently >200 mg/dL with concurrent insulin therapy.

Insulin pump therapy was started at 4 months of age (weight 2.5 kg) with U100 insulin. She did well in terms of the pump site and insulin delivery, but there was difficulty keeping her blood glucose within range. Large variations in her blood glucose resulted from small changes with her basal rates and boluses. In discussion with the pharmacy, diluted insulin was pursued. The pharmacy obtained a diluent from the insulin manufacturer and U10 diluted insulin was started around 5 months of age (weight 2.6 kg). Her weight gain during the month prior to this change was suboptimal. A continuous blood glucose monitor was placed and gave reliable readings consistent with fingerstick blood glucose. Around this time, whole exome sequencing was sent, including samples from mother and father for further analysis.

She had a G-tube placed at 6 months of age (weight 3.0 kg). The volume of oral therapy for hypoglycemia was too much to be practical in a hypoglycemic situation, so mini-glucagon rescue was utilized for hypoglycemic incidents.

Whole Exome Sequencing Results and Other Testing

Whole exome sequencing showed a heterozygous *STAT3* mutation. Specifically, *STAT3* p.E616Q: p.Glu616Gln (GAA>CAA): c.1846 G>C in exon 20 in the *STAT3* gene. Neither mother nor father harbored this mutation. The E616Q variant had not been previously reported, based on the NHLBI Exome Sequencing Project. It is thought that this is likely a pathological variant, responsible for the constellation of findings in this patient.

Discussion and Follow-up

Both *STAT3* activating and inactivating mutations have been seen. Inactivating mutations produce hyper-IgE syndrome,[2] musculoskeletal and coronary vascular anomalies, whereas activating mutations are known to cause early-onset autoimmune disease. This can include autoimmune enteropathy, neonatal diabetes, interstitial lung disease, juvenile-onset arthritis, thyroid dysfunction, short stature, and eczema.[3]

Diabetes-related autoantibodies were sent at 7 months of life and GAD65 and islet cell antigen 2 antibodies were negative, while insulin antibodies were positive. Immunodeficiency screening was performed, and she was found to have a mild polyclonal gammopathy. She tested positive for anti-enterocyte antibody and was subsequently started on inhaled budesonide. After this, she tolerated increasing enteral feeds. She was discharged from the hospital at 8 months of age (weight 4.0 kg). Since that time, she has been screened for adrenal insufficiency. 21-hydroxylase antibodies were negative, and cortisol after a hypoglycemic event was 26.5 mcg/dL, an appropriate response. The most recent HbA_{1c} was 6.9%. She has continued use of inhaled steroid therapy, but more recently started having issues with loose stools. Endoscopy was performed and the biopsy showed continued mild villi blunting and increased patchy intraepithelial lymphocytes. Future treatment possibilities include increasing steroid administration, rituximab, monoclonal antibodies, or even allogeneic transplantation.

Special thanks to Dr. Charles Vanderpool, Dr. Siri Greeley, and Dr. Robert Nelson for their excellent care and input on this patient.

References

1. Pearson ER, Flechtner I, Njolstad PR, et al. Switching from insulin to oral sulfonylureas in patients with diabetes due to Kir6.2 mutations. *N Engl J Med* 2006;355:467–477

2. Haapaniemi E, Kaustio M, Rajala HLM, et al. Autoimmunity, hypogammaglobulinemia, lymphoproliferation, and mycobacterial disease in patients with activating mutations in *STAT3*. *Blood* 2015;125:639–648

3. Milner JD, Vogel TP, Forbes L, et al. Early-onset lymphoproliferation and autoimmunity caused by germline STAT3 gain-of-function mutations. *Blood* 2015;125:591–599

Case 5:
GATA6 — Heart and Pancreas

Taylor Triolo, MD;[1] and Kimber Simmons, MD[1]

Case

TF is an ex full term, 72-day-old female, who initially presented to pediatric gastroenterology (GI) clinic for evaluation of failure to thrive. Her history was significant for intrauterine growth restriction, and she was born at 39 weeks via induced vaginal delivery. Placental evaluation was concerning for placental infarction. At birth, she had mild hypoglycemia that resolved without intervention, and she was discharged home with her mother. Feeding at home was initially difficult due to poor maternal breast milk supply requiring supplementation with formula, but she was able to fully breastfeed by 2 weeks of age. Her primary care provider (PCP) followed her for frequent weight checks. Her weight gain was slow after birth, and her weight dropped to <1st percentile despite feeding every 1.5–2 hours with a reported post-feed weight increase of 2 oz (Figure C5.1). Her PCP evaluated her poor weight gain with an ultrasound and upper GI for pyloric stenosis, which were normal. TF was then referred to the pediatric GI clinic for failure to thrive. Her mother reported that TF frequently had noisy breathing and worked hard to breathe when feeding, but there were no color changes or apparent fatigue. On evaluation in GI clinic, a chest x-ray was ordered due to noticeable tachypnea. Her initial chest x-ray

[1]Barbara Davis Center for Childhood Diabetes, University of Colorado, Denver, CO

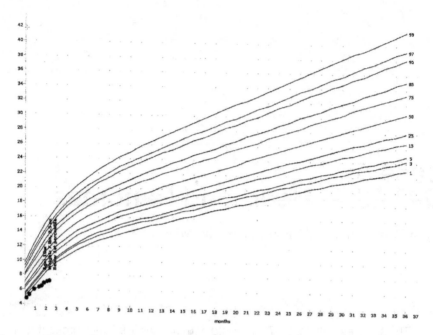

Figure C5.1—Growth chart showing significant failure to thrive (weight for age).

(Figure C5.2) showed cardiomegaly with prominent pulmonary vasculature and pulmonary edema bilaterally. She was urgently referred to cardiology, and an echocardiogram that day showed truncus arteriosus type 1 with a main pulmonary artery present that arose from the truncal root, a large atrial septal defect, and an interrupted aortic arch. A patent ductus arteriosus was present that perfused the left subclavian and descending aorta. She was admitted to the cardiac intensive care unit. Initial lab evaluation included a complete metabolic panel with blood glucose of 113 mg/dL (6.3 mmol/L). She was started on total parenteral nutrition (TPN) D12.5% with a glucose infusion rate (GIR) of 6 mg/kg/min and was noted to have significantly elevated blood glucoses up to 536 mg/dL (29.8 mmol/L).

Initial Management

To achieve normal blood glucoses (60s–80s), her medical team decreased the dextrose in her TPN to 2% with a GIR of 0.7 mg/kg/min. With adequate nutrition and euglycemia being important pre-surgical targets, dextrose was increased, and she required an insulin drip of between 0.03 and 0.5 unit/kg/h

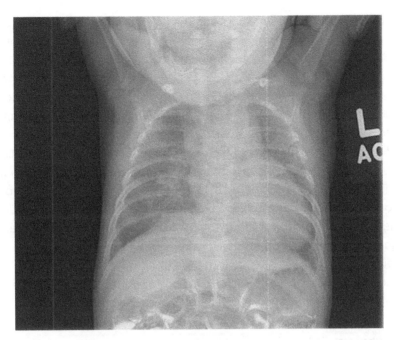

Figure C5.2—Initial chest radiograph for patient TF. Interpreted as, "The cardiac silhouette is moderately enlarged and pulmonary vasculature appears prominent bilaterally."

in order to maintain euglycemia on an adequate GIR. Once her truncus and interrupted aortic arch were repaired, she continued to have hyperglycemia although not as dramatic as on presentation. For 5 days she required titration of an insulin drip for times when her blood glucose was above 200 mg/dL (11.1 mmol/L). Plans were being made to initiate pump therapy, but by day 6 postoperatively she had fasting blood glucose ranging from 54–166 mg/dl (3–9 mmol/L). Although she was not requiring insulin, her persistent mild hyperglycemia prompted us to send genetic testing for both the patient and her parents. The family was asked to check blood glucose weekly upon discharge and call if >200 mg/dL (11.1 mmol/L).

Diagnostic Workup

The differential diagnosis of TF's persistent hyperglycemia included stress-related hyperglycemia due to her procedure and critical illness; poor gut perfusion with related pancreatic insufficiency due to her congenital heart disease; and neonatal diabetes due to a monogenic mutation. Specifically, we were concerned for a genetic mutation in *GATA6*, a transcription factor involved in organogenesis, which has been reported in children with congenital heart defects and neonatal diabetes. Initial workup included imaging of the pancreas to look for agenesis and testing for exocrine insufficiency. An abdominal ultrasound showed a partially visualized pancreas with no obvious abnormalities and nonvisualization of the gallbladder with a normal biliary duct. A stool elastase was less than 50 ug E/g stool, indicating pancreatic insufficiency. C-peptide was 2.0 ng/mL, indicating she had some endogenous insulin production. Genetic testing for monogenic forms of neonatal diabetes was sent for both the patient and her parents. Sequence analysis, through the University of Exeter, identified a heterozygous p.Arg456His missense mutation in her *GATA6* gene, which has previously been reported to be pathogenic.[1] Neither parent carried this mutation and her mutation was thought to have arisen *de novo*.

Discussion

Neonatal diabetes is defined as onset of diabetes in a child less than 6 months of age and is a monogenic disease that results in either agenesis or dysgenesis of the pancreas or lack of insulin production or secretion. Pancreatic agenesis is a very rare cause of neonatal diabetes that can occur with mutations in *PDX1* and PTF1A. *GATA6* is a gene only recently implicated in pancreatic agenesis and is now the most common known cause of pancreatic agenesis.[1]

GATA6 functions as a DNA-binding domain and is involved in organogenesis. It is a transcription factor with two GATA zinc fingers. Mutations in *GATA6* affect the DNA binding surface. Heterozygous missense mutations, frameshift insertions or deletions, and splicing mutations in *GATA6* have all been implicated in previously unknown causes of pancreatic agenesis.[1] Given its role in organogenesis, extrapancreatic features including congenital heart disease, hypothyroidism, hepatobiliary malformations, gut abnormalities, pituitary dysfunction, and neurocognitive defects have also been reported.

In Lango Allen's initial study of 27 patients with pancreatic agenesis, 15 had a mutation in *GATA6*.[1] In a follow-up study of 171 subjects with unknown genetic causes of neonatal diabetes, an additional 9 patients were found to have *GATA6* mutations.[2] In the total cohort of 795 subjects with neonatal diabetes, 29 subjects (3%; 24 probands and 5 parents) had a *GATA6* mutation.[2] There was a large spectrum in phenotypes between the subjects, with some presenting with neonatal diabetes due to complete pancreatic agenesis and some with adult-onset diabetes without exocrine insufficiency. In addition to pancreatic dysfunction, cardiac malformations were seen in 83% of subjects with a *GATA6* mutation. Case reports have shown novel *GATA6* mutations associated with permanent neonatal diabetes due to pancreatic agenesis associated with a wide range of congenital heart defects, including atrial septal defects with mitral valve stenosis or pulmonary valve stenosis, ventricular septal defects, and severe truncus arteriosus.[3–5]

While our patient TF is doing well and currently off of insulin, she will likely develop a need for insulin during childhood given her history of hyperglycemia, marked exocrine insufficiency, and history of poor perfusion. Table C5.1 shows the range of clinical characteristics that can be present in *GATA6* mutations and their manifestations, if any. TF's parents are currently monitoring blood glucose levels weekly two hours after a meal. Her family will monitor her blood glucoses daily during illnesses or more frequently if additional surgeries are required.

Table C5.1—Clinical Characteristics That Can Be Present in *GATA6* Mutations and Their Manifestations

Clinical Characteristics of GATA6 Mutations	TF's Results	Treatment Plan
Pancreatic agenesis or dysgenesis causing neonatal diabetes and/or exocrine insufficiency	Hyperglycemia to 536 mg/dL requiring insulin drip with continued subtle abnormalities in blood glucose levels post cardiac surgery Fecal elastase <50 ug E/g stool	• Pancreatic enzyme replacement • Blood glucose monitoring • Not yet requiring insulin
Heart malformation	Truncus arteriosus Type I with a main pulmonary artery, ASD, and interrupted aortic arch. Now repaired.	Follow-up per cardiology recommendations
Hepatobiliary malformations	Abdominal US: Nonvisualization of the gallbladder with normal caliber common bile duct CMP: LFTs, bilirubin in range	No intervention needed per consultation with GI

(Continued)

Table C5.1 — (Continued)

Clinical Characteristics of GATA6 Mutations	TF's Results	Treatment Plan
Gut abnormalities (hernias, malrotation, perforation, etc.)	Not present	Education for symptoms that should prompt evaluation
Pituitary dysgenesis	Cortisol (fasting) 10.1 mcg/dL; thyroid function normal on newborn screen; normal sodium and urine output	Will continue to monitor growth and pubertal development
Thyroid abnormalities	Newborn screen normal	Thyroid labs every 6 months (until 3–5 years of age)
Developmental delay and/or seizures	Not present at this time	Refer for early intervention with close monitoring of development

References

1. Lango Allen H, Flanagan SE, Shaw-Smith C, De Franco E, Akerman I, Caswell R, et al. GATA6 haploinsufficiency causes pancreatic agenesis in humans. *Nat Genet* 2012;44:20–22

2. De Franco E, Shaw-Smith C, Flanagan SE, Shepherd MH, International NDMC, Hattersley AT, et al. GATA6 mutations cause a broad phenotypic spectrum of diabetes from pancreatic agenesis to adult-onset diabetes without exocrine insufficiency. *Diabetes* 2013;62:993–997

3. Stanescu DE, Hughes N, Patel P, De Leon DD. A novel mutation in GATA6 causes pancreatic agenesis. *Pediatr Diabetes* 2015;16:67–70

4. Bonnefond A, Sand O, Guerin B, Durand E, De Graeve F, Huyvaert M, et al. GATA6 inactivating mutations are associated with heart defects and, inconsistently, with pancreatic agenesis and diabetes. *Diabetologia* 2012;55:2845–2847

5. Chao CS, McKnight KD, Cox KL, Chang AL, Kim SK, Feldman BJ. Novel GATA6 mutations in patients with pancreatic agenesis and congenital heart malformations. *PloS One* 2015;10:e0118449

Case 6:
KCNJ11 R201C – Neonatal Diabetes

Laura Marie Nally, MD;[1] and Darrell M. Wilson, MD[1]

Case

Our patient presented to the emergency department (ED) at 4 months of age after one episode of nonbloody, nonbilious vomiting and abnormal breathing that had become more labored over the past 24 hours. No other symptoms were identified initially, but in retrospect, these first-time parents felt that she may have been consuming more breastmilk and urinating more frequently for about 3–4 weeks prior to arrival. She was born full term weighing 2.75 kg at birth. There was a remote history of type 2 diabetes in older family members. In the ED, the infant had dry mucous membranes and lips, increased work of breathing, and intermittent grunting. Blood gas revealed a pH of 6.83 with base excess of -30 and lactate level of 6.8 mmol/L. Electrolytes were normal with glucose of 553 mg/dL (30.7 mmol/L); there was an anion gap of 26 and beta-hydroxybutyrate level of 12.2 mmol/L. Insulin autoantibodies (GAD-65, ICA-512, insulin autoantibody) were negative. Urine was positive for glucose and ketones. HbA$_{1c}$ at presentation was 14.6%. An abdominal ultrasound showed a normal-appearing pancreas.

She was initially treated with an insulin drip in the pediatric intensive care unit and then transitioned briefly to insulin injections and then to an Animas insulin pump. She required a total daily dose of 0.5 unit/kg/day.

---

[1]Division of Endocrinology and Diabetes, Department of Pediatrics, Stanford University School of Medicine, Palo Alto, CA

Three months after starting the pump, her HbA$_{1c}$ decreased to 6.3%. She continued to develop normally without any neurological symptoms. The neonatal diabetes sequencing panel was sent and returned positive for a heterozygous *KCNJ11* mutation with a nucleotide change at the c.601C->T leading to an amino acid change of p.Arg201Cys (Figure C6.1). After genetic testing returned, the family was trained on the use of continuous glucose monitoring (CGM) and began to use it as a part of her diabetes management. Once familiar with CGM, she was started on 0.2 mg/kg/day of glyburide and gradually increased to 0.5 mg/kg/day prior to being completely transitioned off insulin over a four-week period using guidelines

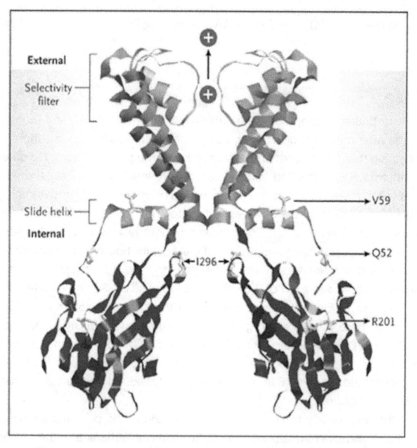

Figure C6.1—Location of the mutation in the patient along the internal portion of the Kir6.2 subunit at R201.

Modified from Gloyn et al.[6]

published by Hattersley and Pearson.[1] During the outpatient transition, the family had access to physicians at all times and were in frequent contact about glycemic levels and medication changes, frequently referring to CGM data in order to make safe, appropriate changes to the insulin regimen. HbA$_{1c}$, fasting C-peptide, CBC, and liver function tests were monitored as well as her growth and development.

Discussion and Follow-Up

Neonatal diabetes occurs in 1:89,000 to 300,000 live births.[2–4] Infants can be misdiagnosed as having diabetes leading to unnecessary insulin use. Heterozygous activating mutations in *KCNJ11* gene that encode the Kir6.2 subunit of the ATP-sensitive potassium channel cause 30–58% of diabetes presenting before 6 months of age (Table C6.1).[5] We present a case of neonatal diabetes presenting at 4 months of age involving a mutation in the *KCNJ11* gene that was responsive to treatment with oral sulfonylurea. A CGM system was used to safely transition the infant from insulin to oral sulfonylurea therapy in the outpatient setting.

The most optimal dosing of insulin for this particular patient involved 4 daily doses before meals and at bedtime with well-managed glucose levels approaching euglycemia (see Figure C6.2 and Figure C6.3). After the first

Table C6.1 — Glucose Trends and Treatment from Time of Diagnosis

Months from Diagnosis	HbA$_{1c}$ (%)	Glucose Average +/– Standard Dev (mg/dL)	Fasting C-peptide (ng/ml)	Dose of Insulin or Sulfonylurea
0	14.6		<0.1	Insulin injections 0.5 units/kg/day
1	8.8	215 +/– 94		CSII 0.5 units/kg/day
3	6.5	190 +/– 80		CSII 0.5 units/kg/day
4	6.3	183 (CGM 52% in range, 1% low)		Glyburide 0.4 mg/kg/day
7	5.1	129 (CGM 81% in range, 4% low)	1.8	Glyburide 0.5 mg/kg/day
11	5	114 +/– 25	1.5	Glyburide 0.5 mg/kg/day

This table shows the hemoglobin A1C, glucose average, C-peptide levels, and change in insulin and sulfonylurea dosing during the transition from insulin to sulfonylurea. "In range" was defined as 70–180 mg/dL; low was defined as >70 mg/dL.

month of therapy, her CGM data showed that she had an estimated HbA$_{1c}$ of 6.2% with 81% of the time spent in a target range of 70–180 mg/dL, 3% of the time spent hypoglycemic (<70 mg/dL), and 16% hyperglycemic (>180 mg/dL). After 4 months of glyburide therapy, her HbA$_{1c}$ decreased to 5.1%. Now 17 months old, she is growing and developing normally. On a dose of 0.5 mg/kg/day of glyburide, her most recent HbA$_{1c}$ was 5% without any significant hypoglycemia. She continues to be monitored by a CGM at all times because the family has found this helpful in preventing hypoglycemia and treating unforeseen hyperglycemia by dosing earlier or increasing her glyburide dose.

To date, the patient has continued to have excellent glycemic control. She had one episode of fever and a complete blood cell count (CBC) was performed due to reports of transient leukopenia; however, her results were normal. Liver function tests have been monitored and remained normal. No adverse reactions to glyburide have been suspected to date. Neurological exams remain normal. The family has opted to continue using a CGM for her diabetes management.

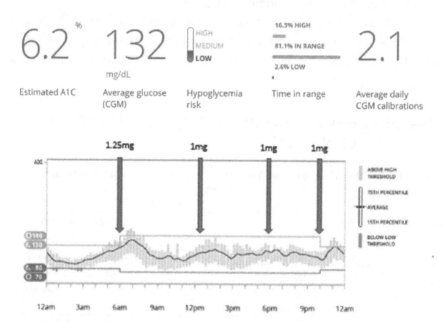

Figure C6.2—CGM tracing of glucose values over the first month of glyburide therapy.

Arrows denote the estimated times that the glyburide was given and the doses that the infant received.

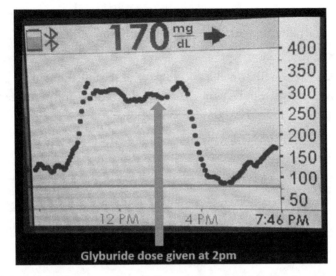

Figure C6.3—CGM tracing of the patient's blood glucose levels prior to and after her glyburide dose was given at 2 P.M.

The family reported that glyburide typically started to lower her blood sugars 1–2 hours after the dose was given and tended to last about 5–6 hours before her blood glucose started increasing again.

References

1. Hattersley A, Pearson E. Transferring patients with diabetes due to a Kir6.2 or SUR1 mutation from insulin to sulphonylureas [article online], 2012. Available from: http://www.diabetesgenes.org/content/transferring-patients-diabetes-due-kir62-mutation-insulin-sulphonylureas. Accessed May 2017

2. Slingerland A, Shields BM, Flanagan SE, et al. Referral rates for diagnostic testing support an incidence of permanent neonatal diabetes in three European countries of at least 1 in 260,000 live births. *Diabetologia* 2009;52:1683–1685

3. Stanik J, Gasperikova D, Paskova M, et al. Prevalence of permanent neonatal diabetes in Slovakia and successful replacement of insulin with sulfonylurea therapy in *KCNJ11* and *ABCC8* mutation carriers. *J Clin Endocrinol Metab* 2007;92:1276–1282

4. Grulich-Henn J, Wagner V, Thon A, et al. Entities and frequency of neonatal diabetes: data from the Diabetes Documentation and Quality Management System (DPV). *Diabet Med* 2010;27:709–712

5. Pearson ER, Flechtner I, Njolstad PR, et al. Switching from insulin to oral sulfo-nylureas in patients with diabetes due to Kir6.2 mutations. *N Engl J Med* 2006;355:467–477

6. Gloyn AL, Pearson ER, Antcliff JK, et al. Activating mutations in the gene encoding the ATP-sensitive potassium-channel subunit Kir6.2 and permanent neonatal diabetes. *N Engl J Med* 2004;350:1838–1849

Case 7:
PDX1 – Pancreatic Agenesis

May Sanyoura, PhD;[1] Lisa R. Letourneau, MPH, RD;[1] Laura Dickens, MD;[1] Siri Atma W. Greeley, MD, PhD;[1] Rochelle N. Naylor, MD;[1] Graeme I. Bell, PhD;[1] and Louis H. Philipson, MD, PhD[1]

Summary of: "Neonatal diabetes mellitus with pancreatic agenesis in an infant with homozygous IPF-1 Pro63fsX60 mutation" by Thomas IH, Saini NK, Adhikari A, Lee JM, Kasa-Vubu JZ, Vazquez DM, Menon RK, Chen M, Fajans SS*

Case

A male infant was born at 37-weeks gestation with a birth weight of 1.56 kg. Pregnancy was complicated as the mother was diagnosed with gestational diabetes. He was delivered by Caesarean section because of oligohydramnios and intrauterine growth retardation. Initial blood glucose levels were 110 mg/dL that quickly rose to 378 mg/dL after 24 hours. He was started on an intravenous insulin drip and received between 1/2 to 1 unit of regular insulin a day. Urine ketones were negative. At 8 days of life, the following measures were recorded: blood glucose was 346 mg/dL, C-peptide <0.5 ng/mL, insulin <2 µU/mL, GAD-65, and insulin autoantibodies were negative. Physical examination was unremarkable and did not reveal dysmorphic features or physical abnormalities. He was continued on the insulin drip and fed continuously with Neosure 22 kcal/oz 3

---

[1]Departments of Medicine and Pediatrics, The University of Chicago, Chicago, IL
*This case was previously published.[1]

weeks later and despite significant intake of formula, he had persistent weight loss and foul-smelling stools. Reducing substances were present in the stool. Stool elastase levels were <50 μg elastase/g stool, indicating severe exocrine pancreatic insufficiency, and treatment was initiated with pancreatic enzymes. Ultrasound examination only revealed the head of the pancreas. His growth and weight gain improved on insulin and pancreatic enzyme replacement. Family history is significant for diabetes. The mother had gestational diabetes with both of her pregnancies and was treated with insulin. The father was diagnosed with hyperglycemia at the age of 15 and is on oral agents. Both maternal and paternal grandparents are treated for type 2 diabetes. Genetic testing of genes associated with neonatal diabetes identified a homozygous 1-base deletion in *PDX1* (c.188delC, p.Pro63fsX60). Both parents were found to be carriers.[1]

Discussion

Pancreas duodenum homeobox-1 (*PDX1*) is a pancreas-specific transcription factor that regulates embryonic pancreas development, expression of genes essential for glucose metabolism, and the differentiation, survival, and function of β-cells in the pancreas.[2] Mutations in the *PDX1* gene are associated with multiple metabolic phenotypes in humans. Homozygous mutations in *PDX1* are associated with neonatal diabetes, pancreas agenesis, intrauterine growth retardation, and exocrine pancreas deficiency.[3] Heterozygous mutations in *PDX1* are associated with type 2 diabetes (MODY 4) indicating that partial deficiency leads to severe β-cell dysfunction and increased β-cell death.[4,5]

References

1. Thomas IH, Saini NK, Adhikari A, Lee JM, Kasa-Vubu JZ, Vazquez DM, Menon RK, Chen M, Fajans SS. Neonatal diabetes mellitus with pancreatic agenesis in an infant with homozygous IPF-1 Pro63fsX60 mutation. *Pediatr Diabetes* 2009;10:492–496

2. Babu DA, Deering TG, Mirmira RG. A feat of metabolic proportions: PDX1 orchestrates islet development and function in the maintenance of glucose homeostasis. *Mol Genet Metab* 2007;92:43–55

3. Stoffers DA, Zinkin NT, Stanojevic V, Clarke WL, Habener JF. Pancreatic agenesis attributable to a single nucleotide deletion in the human IPF1 gene coding sequence. *Nat Genet* 1997;15:106–110

4. Stoffers DA, Ferrer J, Clarke WL, Habener JF. Early-onset type-II diabetes mellitus (MODY4) linked to IPF1. *Nat Genet* 1997;17:138–139

5. Brissova M, Blaha M, Spear C, Nicholson W, Radhika A, Shiota M, Charron MJ, Wright CV, Powers AC. Reduced PDX-1 expression impairs islet response to insulin resistance and worsens glucose homeostasis. *Am J Physiol Endocrinol Metab* 2005;288:E707–E714

Case 8:
Neonatal Diabetes and Congenital Hypothyroidism: *GLIS3*

May Sanyoura, PhD;[1] Lisa R. Letourneau, MPH, RD;[1] Laura Dickens, MD;[1] Siri Atma W. Greeley, MD, PhD;[1] Rochelle N. Naylor, MD;[1] Graeme I. Bell, PhD;[1] and Louis H. Philipson, MD, PhD[1]

Case

A Libyan female was born at full term with a weight of 2.4 kg and head circumference of 34 cm to first-degree consanguineous parents. Intrauterine growth retardation was noted during pregnancy. Six weeks after birth, she was admitted to the hospital with hypovolemic shock and found to have blood glucose levels of 1,020 mg/dL without significant acidosis or ketosis. The patient was started on IV insulin and subsequently switched to subcutaneous insulin therapy. Target blood glucose levels have been easy to achieve with intermittent doses of long-acting insulin.

At five months of age, TSH was found to be elevated on two different occasions, 10.7 and 10.4 µIU/ml, respectively (normal range: 0.45–5.6 µIU/ml) with normal free thyroxine (T4) 15.9 (normal range: 9.0–20.0 pmol/L). The patient was started on levothyroxine replacement (12.5 mcg daily) with adequate TSH suppression. No overt clinical signs of hypothyroidism were observed on physical examination. Thyroid gland anatomy and echotexture appearance were normal on ultrasound scan. Abdominal ultrasound scan performed at age of 6 months showed normal morphology of the liver, pancreas, and both kidneys. Other laboratory tests revealed normal liver

---

[1]Departments of Medicine and Pediatrics, The University of Chicago, Chicago, IL

and kidney function. Dilated ophthalmic examination was negative for any abnormalities. The patient is now 13 months old with normal developmental milestones. Liver and kidney function tests remain normal. Her most recent HbA$_{1c}$ was 6.5%. Next generation sequencing of all known genes associated with permanent neonatal diabetes identified a homozygous change in GLIS3 (c.1924A>T) leading to a substitution of serine to cysteine at position 642 (Ser642Cys). Both parents were tested and confirmed to be carriers.

Discussion

GLIS3, a zinc finger transcription factor, is expressed in early embryogenesis and plays a critical role as both a repressor and activator of transcription by interacting with specific nucleotide sequences in the promoter region of target genes.[1] Mutations in GLIS3 are associated with a rare syndrome characterized by congenital hypothyroidism and neonatal diabetes (NDH).[2] Patients with NDH exhibit diminished levels of triiodothyronine (T3) and T4, along with elevated levels of thyroid stimulation hormone (TSH) and thyroglobulin (TG).

Mutations in GLIS3 have been identified in more than ten families and include frame shifts resulting in premature termination, large deletions encompassing the 5' UTR, exons 1–2, 1–4, 5–9, or 9–11, and missense mutations.[3] Aside from the presentation of neonatal diabetes and hypothyroidism, additional features may include glaucoma, liver fibrosis, cystic kidneys, mental retardation, osteopenia, deafness, and pancreatic exocrine insufficiency.[2–4] The variability in phenotype among affected patients may be attributed to the tissue expression of variable-length GLIS3 transcripts. Larger transcripts (7.5 kb) are predominately expressed in the pancreas, thyroid, and kidney, with smaller transcripts (0.8–2 kb) expressed in the heart, kidney, liver, and skeletal muscle.[2] Therefore, severe truncating mutations have the potential to cause widespread damage. This case describes a novel missense mutation that resulted in neonatal diabetes and congenital hypothyroidism. This mutation falls outside of the zinc finger and known functional domains of the protein, which may explain the less severe phenotype.

In conclusion, thyroid function should be tested and GLIS3 sequenced in newborn infants with intrauterine growth retardation and who develop hyperglycemia in the first week of life.

References

1. Beak JY, Kang HS, Kim YS, Jetten AM. Functional analysis of the zinc finger and activation domains of GLIS3 and mutant GLIS3(NDH1). *Nucleic Acids Res* 2008;36:1690–1702

2. Senee V, Chelala C, Duchatelet S, Feng D, Blanc H, Cossec JC, Charon C, Nicolino M, Boileau P, Cavener DR, Bougneres P, Taha D, Julier C. Mutations in GLIS3 are responsible for a rare syndrome with neonatal diabetes mellitus and congenital hypothyroidism. *Nat Genet* 2006;38:682–687

3. Dimitri P, Habeb AM, Gurbuz F, Millward A, Wallis S, Moussa K, Akcay T, Taha D, Hogue J, Slavotinek A, Wales JK, Shetty A, Hawkes D, Hattersley AT, Ellard S, De Franco E. Expanding the clinical spectrum associated with GLIS3 mutations. *J Clin Endocrinol Metab* 2015;100:E1362–1369

4. Dimitri P, Warner JT, Minton JA, Patch AM, Ellard S, Hattersley AT, Barr S, Hawkes D, Wales JK, Gregory JW. Novel GLIS3 mutations demonstrate an extended multisystem phenotype. *Eur J Endocrinol* 2011;164:437–443

Case 9:
EIF2AK3: Wolcott-Rallison Syndrome

May Sanyoura, PhD;[1] Lisa R. Letourneau, MPH, RD;[1] Laura Dickens, MD;[1] Sally S. Ladsaria, BS;[1] Siri Atma W. Greeley, MD, PhD;[1] Rochelle N. Naylor, MD;[1] Graeme I. Bell, PhD;[1] and Louis H. Philipson, MD, PhD[1]

Case

A Pakistani female was born at full term with a weight of 3,260 kg to first-degree consanguineous parents. At 9 weeks of age, she developed a high fever, was taken to the emergency room, and was found to be in severe DKA with extreme dehydration (blood glucose 796 mg/dL). Neurologically, she appeared normal. An abdominal ultrasound was completed; the pancreas appeared normal. She had low C-peptide levels at diagnosis and was negative for type 1 diabetes–associated autoantibodies. This patient was reported to have frequent cough and fever and underwent evaluation by Immunology. She was not found to have any immunodeficiencies, but was found to have normocytic, normochromic anemia.

Family history was significant for consanguinity (parents are first cousins) and adult-onset diabetes in the maternal and paternal grandfathers. A previous sibling died at 40 days old.

Genetic testing was ordered at 5 months of age, and it identified a homozygous 2 base pair deletion in *EIF2AK3* (c.1564_1565del, p.Trp522Glufs*34). Insulin pump therapy was initiated, and glycemic control improved (Figure C9.1). At 7 months of age, bone X-rays for epiphyseal dysplasia were negative. At 9 months of age, she began using a continuous glucose monitor (CGM).

[1]Departments of Medicine and Pediatrics, The University of Chicago, Chicago, IL

At a follow-up visit at 13 months old, she continued on her insulin pump and CGM, using an average of 4 units per day (~0.45 unit/kg/day, 70% basal/30% bolus). She was meeting developmental milestones, including cruising well. Her weight was 37th percentile-for-age and her length was 49th percentile-for-age based on World Health Organization (WHO) growth charts.[2] At a follow-up visit at 23 months old, she continued on her insulin pump and CGM, using an average of 6.3 units per day (~0.65 unit/kg/day, 52% basal/48% bolus). Her weight had decreased to the 11th percentile-for-age and her length had decreased to the 3rd percentile-for-age based on WHO growth charts, likely related to a decrease in caloric intake.[2] The family met with a registered dietitian to make a more structured meal plan. Further follow-up is ongoing.

Discussion

Wolcott-Rallison syndrome (WRS) is a rare autosomal recessive disorder characterized by early-onset diabetes, skeletal dysplasia (specifically multiple epiphyseal dysplasia), osteoporosis, and growth retardation.[3] Other clinical findings and manifestations may include central hypothyroidism, hepatic dysfunction, renal insufficiency, central nervous system abnormalities, cardiorespiratory defects, hypothalamic-pituitary dysfunction, neutropenia,

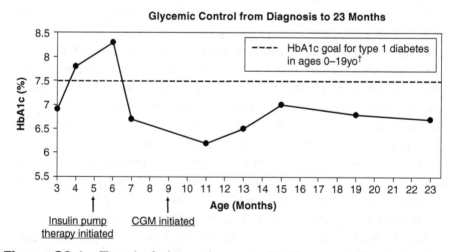

Figure C9.1—Trend of glycemic control before and after introduction of insulin pump therapy and CGM.

[†]HbA$_{1c}$ <6 months are underestimated due to fetal hemoglobin.
Source: Suzuki S et al.[1]

and exocrine pancreatic insufficiency.[4,5] WRS is caused by mutations in the gene encoding eukaryotic translation initiation factor 2α kinase 3 (*EIF2AK3*), also known as PKR-like endoplasmic reticulum kinase (PERK).[6] PERK is an endoplasmic reticulum transmembrane protein, which plays a key role in translation control during the unfolded protein response. Studies in animal models showed that loss of PERK activity leads to cell death in multiple tissues and is associated with skeletal, pancreatic, and growth defects that are similar to those seen in WRS.[7]

WRS is considered the most common cause of permanent neonatal diabetes in consanguineous pedigrees. *EIF2AK3* should be tested in all patients with isolated neonatal diabetes diagnosed before 6 months of age who are from known consanguineous families or countries with high consanguinity rates.

References

1. Suzuki S, Koga M, Amamiya S, Nakao A, Wada K, Okuhara K, et al. Glycated albumin but not HbA$_{1c}$ reflects glycaemic control in patients with neonatal diabetes mellitus. *Diabetologia* 2011;54:2247–2253

2. WHO Multicentre Growth Reference Study Group. WHO Child Growth Standards based on length/height, weight and age. *Acta Paediatr Suppl* 2006;450:76–85

3. Wolcott CD, Rallison ML. Infancy-onset diabetes mellitus and multiple epiphyseal dysplasia. *J Pediatr* 1972;80:292–297

4. Habeb AM. Frequency and spectrum of Wolcott-Rallison syndrome in Saudi Arabia: a systematic review. *Libyan J Med* 2013;8:21137

5. Julier C, Nicolino M. Wolcott-Rallison syndrome. *Orphanet J Rare Dis* 2010;5:29

6. Delepine M, Nicolino M, Barrett T, Golamaully M, Lathrop GM, Julier C. EIF2AK3, encoding translation initiation factor 2-alpha kinase 3, is mutated in patients with Wolcott-Rallison syndrome. *Nat Genet* 2000;25:406–409

7. Harding HP, Zeng H, Zhang Y, Jungries R, Chung P, Plesken H, Sabatini DD, Ron D. Diabetes mellitus and exocrine pancreatic dysfunction in perk-/- mice reveals a role for translational control in secretory cell survival. *Mol Cell* 2001;7:1153–1163

Case 10:
Transient Neonatal Diabetes

Elizabeth O. Buschur, MD;[1] and Kathleen Dungan, MD, MPH[1]

Case

"Sarah" is a 24-year-old woman who was diagnosed with transient neo-natal diabetes (TND) at birth. She was born to a 30-year-old gravida 1 (G1) mother who had diet-controlled gestational diabetes. She was born at 41–42 weeks gestation and weighed 5 lb 3 oz. She was immediately found to have hyperglycemia and was started on insulin. She was hospitalized for her first two weeks of life and remained on insulin until about 3 months of age, at which time hyperglycemia resolved and insulin was discontinued.

She then developed polydipsia and polyphagia and was diagnosed with diabetes again at age 17 with a blood glucose of greater than 400 mg/dL and HbA$_{1c}$ 16%. Initial physical exam noted tacky mucous membranes but was otherwise unremarkable. Urinalysis showed 2+ glucosuria. Urine ketones were negative, serum acetone was negative, serum bicarbonate was 27 mmol/L, venous pH was 7.34, insulin antibody level <53, and glu-tamic acid decarboxylase antibody-65 (GAD-65) was negative. Thyroid testing was normal (TSH 4.5 mIU/mL, free T4 1.1 ng/dL). She immediately started insulin and eventually transitioned to an insulin infusion pump. In retrospect, she and her family noted that she had polyuria for about 3 years prior to rediagnosis of diabetes. She also always complained of a raven-ous appetite. She developed mild nonproliferative retinopathy (two small

[1]The Ohio State University Division of Endocrinology, Diabetes, & Metabolism, Columbus, OH

microaneurysms) in the right eye after having diabetes for only 18 months. She also reports transient paresthesias in her toes bilaterally, though her peripheral neurologic exam was normal.

Her family history includes gestational diabetes in her mother, without subsequent development of diabetes thus far, and coronary artery disease in her maternal grandmother. There is no other family history of diabetes or autoimmune disease. Sarah graduated college and works full time.

Sarah had MODY evaluation that was negative. She also had genetic testing at the age of 20 years showing partial hypomethylation at the Transient Neonatal Diabetes locus. Sarah's parents did not have the same hypomethylation, indicating *de novo* duplication of paternal 6q24. She tested negative for other causes of TND including *KCNJ11* and *ABCC8* gene mutations. Her family members also tested negative for these genetic mutations.

Sarah uses an insulin pump with continuous glucose monitoring to manage her diabetes. She had no apparent honeymoon period following diagnosis of diabetes. HbA$_{1c}$ values are typically close to goal with minimal hypoglycemia (Figure C10.1). She has had no severe hypoglycemia. She has never had diabetic ketoacidosis. Glucoses range from 60–200 mg/dL at times postprandially without extreme fluctuations despite missing boluses (Figure C10.2). She has had repeat laboratory studies showing normal lipids, urine protein values, thyroid testing, and basic metabolic panel. When glucose was 100 mg/dL, C-peptide was 1.4 ng/dL (reference

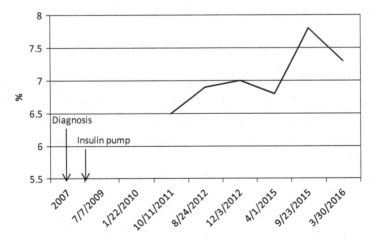

Figure C10.1—Timeline and HbA$_{1c}$ trends.

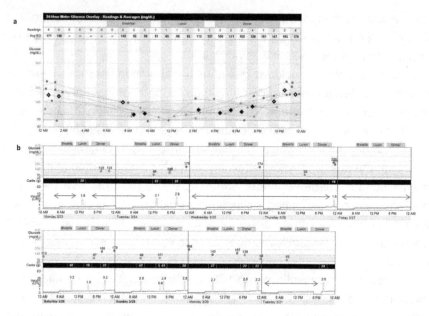

Figure C10.2—14-day self-monitored glucose profile.

range 0.2–2.7). Physical exam is unremarkable including normal weight (57 kg, body mass index 21 kg/m²), thyroid exam, and intact monofilament and vibratory sensation in the feet. She has no apparent abnormal features.

Discussion

Neonatal diabetes (ND) is defined as diabetes diagnosed within the first 6 months of life that requires treatment.[1] ND can be transient (TND) or permanent (PND). ND is a rare cause of monogenic diabetes; the estimated prevalence of ND is 1 in 89,000–500,000 live births.[2,3] TND typically resolves within a few months and may recur during adolescence or as an adult. TND typically affects males and females equally.[4] Patients with TND commonly have intrauterine growth retardation, are less likely to have diabetic ketoacidosis, and have lower insulin requirements than those with PND.[3]

ND results from a single gene mutation in over 80% of patients with more than 20 genes identified.[1] These mutations more often lead to impaired insulin secretion rather than altered insulin sensitivity.[5] One fourth of patients with TND have mutations of KCNJ11, *ABCC8*, INS, or HNF1B, whereas about 70% have abnormalities of the TND locus on chromosome 6q24. The majority of cases of TND are associated with three distinct aberrations leading to overexpression of the imprinted genes PLAGL1 and HYMAI, including paternal uniparental disomy of chromosome 6 (UPD6pat), paternally inherited duplication of 6q24, and maternal hypomethylation of the differentially methylated region (DMR) of 6q24.[1,4] Hypomethylation may be epigenetic and exclusively affecting the DMR in TND, while hypomethylation in other cases affects multiple imprinted loci.[4]

Neonates with 6q24 abnormalities are typically born with moderate intrauterine growth retardation and develop severe hyperglycemia without ketosis during the first week of life. About one-third of affected neonates are born prior to 37 weeks gestation.[4] For the majority of patients with TND, hyperglycemia resolves by a median age of 12 weeks.[1] During remission, transient hyperglycemia may recur during illnesses and diabetes may recur around puberty, although cases of earlier relapse around age 4 years have been seen.[1,6] Clinically, hyperglycemia in these patients is similar to early type 2 diabetes and may respond to noninsulin therapies, including sulfonylureas. If insulin is needed, doses are typically lower than in patients with type 1 diabetes, as with Sarah (0.25 unit/kg/day).[1]

Patients with ND may have a number of extrapancreatic manifestations. In a case series of 163 patients with TND, the most common congenital malformations were macroglossia and umbilical hernia, with less frequent reported abnormalities including dysmorphic facial features, renal abnormalities, cardiac malformations, clinodactyly, polydactyly, short finger abnormalities, and hypothyroidism. Congenital anomalies occurred less frequently among patients with 6q24 duplication compared to hypomethylation subgroups.[4]

In conclusion, TND is a rare cause of monogenic diabetes. Although hyperglycemia is often transient and resolves within the first few months of life, diabetes may recur. Therefore, long-term follow-up of patients with a history of TND and education for patients and families is imperative, since microvascular complications may occur, as demonstrated in this case. Since TND is a rare cause of diabetes, further research is needed to understand the pathophysiology and develop effective management strategies. Patient registries have been created in the United Kingdom and the United States.

References

1. Rubio-Cabezas O, Ellard S. Diabetes mellitus in neonates and infants: genetic heterogeneity, clinical approach to diagnosis, and therapeutic options. *Horm Res Paediatr* 2013;80:137–146

2. Grulich-Henn J, Wagner V, Thona A, et al. Entities and frequency of neonatal diabetes: data from the Diabetes Documentation and Quality Management System (DPV). *Diabet Med* 2010;27:709–712

3. Polak M, Cave H. Neonatal diabetes mellitus: a disease linked to multiple mechanisms. *Orphanet J Rare Dis* 2007;2:12

4. Docherty LE, Kabwama S, Lehmann A, et al. Clinical presentation of 6q24 transient neonatal diabetes mellitus (6q24 TNDM) and genotype-phenotype correlation in an international cohort of patients. *Diabetologia* 2013;56:758–762

5. Murphy R, Ellard S, Hattersley AT. Clinical implications of a molecular genetic classification of monogenic beta-cell diabetes. *Nat Clin Pract Endocrinol Metab* 2008;4:200–213

6. Shield, JP, Temple IK, Sabin M, et al. An assessment of pancreatic endocrine function and insulin sensitivity in patients with transient neonatal diabetes in remission. *Arch Dis Child Fetal Neonatal Ed* 2004;89:F341–343

Case 11:
GCK-MODY

May Sanyoura, PhD;[1] Lisa R. Letourneau, MPH, RD;[1] Laura Dickens, MD;[1] Siri Atma W. Greeley, MD, PhD;[1] Rochelle N. Naylor, MD;[1] Graeme I. Bell, PhD;[1] and Louis H. Philipson, MD, PhD[1]

Case

A 13-year-old white male presented to a university hospital for a second opinion about diabetes management. He was diagnosed with diabetes at age 8 years after presenting with urinary frequency. Fasting blood glucose was found to be mildly elevated ranging from 120–140 mg/dL and oral glucose tolerance testing showed fasting blood glucose of 130 mg/dL and 2-hour blood glucose of 206 mg/dL. The patient was started on metformin 500 mg once daily, which was gradually increased to 500 mg b.i.d. He was monitored by HbA$_{1c}$, which remained stable around 6.5% with no change to metformin dose.

Additional past medical history was notable for obesity with BMI consistently above the 90th percentile for age. Pubertal development had occurred normally. The patient had no surgical history. Family history was remarkable for multiple maternal relatives with diabetes. His mother had a BMI of 29 and a longstanding history of mildly elevated HbA$_{1c}$ in the mid 6% range with a peak of 7.5%. She was on treatment with glimepiride with most recent HbA$_{1c}$ of 6.6%. The patient's maternal grandfather had a similar history of mild hyperglycemia and was on treatment

[1]Departments of Medicine and Pediatrics, The University of Chicago, Chicago, IL

with pioglitazone. The patient's maternal great-grandmother was 93 years old with a history of mild diabetes, off medication due to side effects of hypoglycemia, with no known diabetes-related complications. The patient's social history was unremarkable. Medications included metformin 500 mg b.i.d. He had no allergies to medications.

On examination, vital signs were BP 109/67, pulse 75. BMI was 28.37 kg/m^2, corresponding to the 97.57 percentile based on CDC 2-20 Years BMI-for-Age data.[1] Physical exam showed generalized obesity, tanner 4–5 pubic hair, and pubertal testes. Labs showed HbA$_{1c}$ of 6.5%. The patient was referred for genetic testing, and research-based Sanger sequencing revealed c.667G>A (p.Gly223Ser) heterozygous mutation in the GCK gene. His mother also underwent genetic testing and was found to have the same mutation.

Based on these results, the patient was advised that it would be reasonable to attempt discontinuation of metformin as it was not clear that his glycemia was being improved by this treatment. His obesity did raise concern for the future potential for developing type 2 diabetes. He was counseled on dietary changes and increased physical activity and will be followed regularly for clinical monitoring.

Discussion

GCK-MODY is characterized by mildly elevated fasting blood glucose and glycated hemoglobin levels. This condition affects approximately 1 in every 1,000 people and is the most common cause of MODY in the U.S. National Monogenic Diabetes Registry.[2,3] Pharmacologic therapy in GCK-MODY is generally not recommended, except in some pregnancy cases, as it does not significantly alter glycemic control.[4,5] These slightly elevated blood glucose levels are not associated with typical diabetes-related complications.[6] This patient's clinical history was suspicious for GCK-MODY due to his strong family history of mild fasting hyperglycemia without significant long-term diabetes-related complications. His elevated BMI at diagnosis was not typical for monogenic diabetes, but this fact alone should not deter genetic testing in the appropriate clinical scenario.

References

1. Centers for Disease Control and Prevention. Clinical Growth Charts [Internet], 2000. Available from https://www.cdc.gov/growthcharts/clinical_charts.htm

2. Carmody D, Naylor RN, Bell CD, Berry S, Montgomery JT, Tadie EC, Hwang JL, Greeley SA, Philipson LH. GCK-MODY in the US National Monogenic Diabetes

Registry: frequently misdiagnosed and unnecessarily treated. *Acta Diabetol* 2016;53:703–738

3. Osbak KK, Colclough K, Saint-Martin C, et al. Update on mutations in glucoki-nase (GCK), which cause maturity-onset diabetes of the young, permanent neona-tal diabetes, and hyperinsulinemic hypoglycemia. *Hum Mutat* 2009;30:1512–1526

4. Stride A, Shields B, Gill-Carey O, et al. Cross-sectional and longitudinal studies suggest pharmacological treatment used in patients with glucokinase mutations does not alter glycaemia. *Diabetologia* 2014;57:54–56

5. Chakera AJ, Spyer G, Vincent N, Ellard S, Hattersley AT, Dunne FP. The 0.1% of the population with glucokinase monogenic diabetes can be recognized by clini-cal characteristics in pregnancy: the Atlantic Diabetes in Pregnancy cohort. *Dia-betes Care* 2014.;37:1230–1236

6. Steele AM, Shields BM, Wensley KJ, Colclough K, Ellard S, Hattersley AT. Preva-lence of vascular complications among patients with glucokinase mutations and prolonged, mild hyperglycemia. *JAMA* 2014;311:279–286

Case 12:
HNF1A – MODY

May Sanyoura, PhD;[1] Lisa R. Letourneau, MPH, RD;[1] Laura Dickens, MD;[1] Siri Atma W. Greeley, MD, PhD;[1] Rochelle N. Naylor, MD;[1] Graeme I. Bell, PhD;[1] and Louis H. Philipson, MD, PhD[1]

Case

A 14-year-old Hispanic male presented to a university hospital for a second opinion about diabetes management. He was diagnosed with diabetes at age 12 years after presenting with fatigue and polydipsia and found to have elevated blood glucose of 270 mg/dL and 3+ urinary ketones. He was admitted to a children's hospital and hydrated with intravenous fluids, then started on subcutaneous insulin with NPH 4 units in the morning and aspart 1.5 units before breakfast and before dinner. Labs were significant for HbA$_{1c}$ of 6.4%, negative diabetes antibodies, and negative thyroid and adrenal autoantibodies. In the first two years after diagnosis, he remained on the same dose of NPH and aspart was reduced to 1 unit before breakfast. He had no episodes of diabetic ketoacidosis (DKA). The patient reported fasting blood glucose ranging from 90–115 mg/dL, preprandial blood glucose of 100–120 mg/dL, and bedtime blood glucose 100–200 mg/dL.

The patient had no additional medical or surgical history. Growth, weight gain, and pubertal development all occurred normally. Family history was remarkable for diabetes in multiple family members. His mother was diagnosed with type 1 diabetes at 12 years of age and had history

---

[1]Departments of Medicine and Pediatrics, The University of Chicago, Chicago, IL

of two episodes of DKA while off insulin for several months. His maternal grandfather had a diagnosis of type 2 diabetes with complications including retinopathy and bilateral below the knee amputations. A maternal aunt also had a history of gestational diabetes. Social history was unremarkable. He had no allergies to medications.

On examination, vital signs were blood pressure 132/66 mmHg, pulse 76. BMI was 18.34 kg/m^2, corresponding to 36.71 percentile based on CDC 2–20 years BMI-for-age data.[1] Physical exam showed Tanner 4–5 pubic hair, pubertal testes, and mild lipohypertrophy on the abdomen. Labs showed HbA$_{1c}$ of 6.2%, C-peptide of 0.34 pmol/mL, and negative GAD65, Znt8, and islet antigen 2 antibodies. Genetic testing was arranged and research-based Sanger sequencing revealed c.476G>A (p.Arg159Gln) heterozygous mutation in the HNF1A gene, consistent with a diagnosis of HNF1A-MODY. His mother was also tested and found to have the same mutation.

Over the next 18 months, he required slight increases to his insulin regimen to NPH 5 units in the morning and aspart 1 unit before breakfast and before dinner. Nevertheless, his HbA$_{1c}$ increased from 6.9% up to peak of 7.7%. At that time, he was started on glyburide at half of a 1.25 mg tablet twice daily and insulin doses were decreased and ultimately discontinued.

Discussion

HNF1A mutations are a common cause of MODY and patients are often very sensitive to sulfonylurea therapy.[2-4] Several features of this patient's presentation were suspicious for monogenic diabetes, including family history of atypical diabetes, small insulin requirements for a pubertal male, detectable C-peptide, and negative diabetes antibodies. In this case, a genetic diagnosis allowed for targeted therapy for HNF1A-MODY with sulfonylureas.

References

1. Centers for Disease Control and Prevention. Clinical Growth Charts [Internet], 2000. Available from https://www.cdc.gov/growthcharts/clinical_charts.htm

2. Yamagata K, Oda N, Kaisaki PJ, et al. Mutations in the hepatocyte nuclear factor-1alpha gene in maturity-onset diabetes of the young (MODY3). *Nature* 1996;384:455–458

3. Bellanné-Chantelot C, Levy DJ, Carette C, et al. Clinical characteristics and diagnostic criteria of maturity-onset diabetes of the young (MODY) due to molecular anomalies of the HNF1A gene. *J Clin Endocrinol Metab* 2011;96:E1346–E1351

4. Shepherd M, Shields B, Ellard S, Rubio-Cabezas O, Hattersley AT. A genetic diagnosis of HNF1A diabetes alters treatment and improves glycaemic control in the majority of insulin-treated patients. *Diabet Med* 2009;26:437–441

Case 13:
HNF4A – MODY

May Sanyoura, PhD;[1] Lisa R. Letourneau, MPH, RD;[1] Laura Dickens, MD;[1] Siri Atma W. Greeley, MD, PhD;[1] Rochelle N. Naylor, MD;[1] Graeme I. Bell, PhD;[1] and Louis H. Philipson, MD, PhD[1]

Case

A 41-year-old white woman with a past medical history of gestational diabetes, hypertriglyceridemia, and obesity presented to a university hospital for a second opinion about diabetes management. She was initially diagnosed with gestational diabetes at age 26, approximately 12 weeks into pregnancy with her first child. Prepregnancy BMI was 22.1, and she gained 25 lb during pregnancy. She was treated with metformin, glyburide, and insulin over the ensuing years with HbA$_{1c}$ ranging from 8–10%. She reportedly had good response to glyburide, but it was stopped for unclear reasons and treatment continued with insulin alone.

Additional past medical history included elevated triglycerides as high as 15,247 mg/dL and recurrent pancreatitis. Hypertriglyceridemia responded well to treatment with statins, fenofibrate, and pioglitazone and recent triglyceride level was significantly improved at 147 mg/dL. Surgical history was significant for two caesarean sections. Family history was remarkable for multiple family members with diabetes spanning five generations, including the patient's mother, daughter, and maternal grandmother. Social history was noncontributory;

[1]Departments of Medicine and Pediatrics, The University of Chicago, Chicago, IL

she reported occasional alcohol intake. Medications included insulin glargine 50 units daily, simvastatin 80 mg daily, and fenofibrate 145 mg daily. She had no known allergies to medications.

On examination, vital signs were BP 129/83, pulse 101. BMI was 31. Physical exam was normal. Laboratory results included HbA_{1c} of 8.4%. Research-based Sanger sequencing revealed a heterozygous splice mutation c.493-1G>A in the *HNF4A* gene. Based on these results, she was restarted on glyburide at 2.5 mg b.i.d.

At follow-up one month later, her HbA_{1c} remained elevated at 8.7%, but she was tolerating glyburide well and had reduced her insulin from 50 units to 30 units daily. Her glyburide was increased to 5 mg b.i.d. and at next follow-up 18 months later, her HbA_{1c} had improved to 7.0% and insulin requirements decreased to 15 units daily. At the most recent clinic follow-up, her HbA_{1c} had increased to a peak of 9.6% in the setting of poor medication compliance and 15 lb weight gain. Treatment with GLP-1 agonist is now being considered.

A brief history of the patient's daughter was obtained. She was diagnosed with diabetes at age 14 after a screening HbA_{1c} was checked during a routine physical because of her strong family history of diabetes. HbA_{1c} was 9.1% and urine/serum ketone testing was negative. She was started on insulin and continued for 1 year, then glyburide was added. She was ultimately able to be treated with low-dose glyburide alone and has maintained HbA_{1c} in the low 7% range. Genetic testing of the patient's daughter also revealed c.493-1G>A (splice mutation).

Discussion

Mutations in *HNF4A* are a less common cause of MODY that may respond to sulfonylurea therapy.[1-3] This case illustrates several classic presenting features of HNF4A-MODY: young age at onset, normal BMI at diagnosis, multigenerational family history, and good glycemic response to sulfonylurea treatment. Appropriate diagnosis of the proband in this case allowed for early diagnosis and targeted treatment of her daughter.

References

1.   Yamagata K, Furuta H, Oda N, et al. Mutations in the hepatocyte nuclear factor-4 alpha gene in maturity-onset diabetes of the young (MODY1). *Nature* 1996;384:458–460

2. Ellard S, Colclough K. Mutations in the genes encoding the transcription factors hepatocyte nuclear factor 1 alpha (HNF1A) and 4 alpha (HNF4A) in maturity-onset diabetes of the young. *Hum Mutat* 2006;27:854–869

3. Pihoker C, Gilliam LK, Ellard S, et al. Prevalence, characteristics and clinical diagnosis of maturity onset diabetes of the young due to mutations in HNF1A, HNF4A, and glucokinase: results from the SEARCH for Diabetes in Youth. *J Clin Endocrinol Metab* 2013;98:4055–4062

Case 14:
MODY as a Possible Diagnosis

Ifrah Jamil, MD;[1] and Janice L. Gilden, MS, MD[1]

Case

A 41-year-old African-American female with history of bipolar disorder and hyperlipidemia was evaluated for diabetes and diagnosed at age 23.

Diabetes continues to be increasingly diagnosed among the youth, particularly among certain ethnic groups. The rate of new cases of type 1 and type 2 diabetes among people younger than 20 years of age is estimated to be almost 35 per 100,000 per year among all ethnicities, whereas this number is closer to 40 and 45 among Hispanics and non-Hispanic blacks, respectively.[1]

Our patient was initially treated for diabetes with oral therapy including metformin, but her blood glucose levels were not well controlled. She was therefore started on insulin approximately 2 years after diagnosis of diabetes. Her regimen consisted of regular insulin and NPH insulin. In her mid-30s, the patient had an uncomplicated pregnancy. Soon after she was evaluated by an endocrinologist and placed on insulin pump therapy for uncontrolled type 1 diabetes. She was seen by a primary care physician for the next 2 years. Of note, the patient's bipolar disease, diagnosed prior to that of type 1, was treated with various regimens, including divalproex and bupropion. She provided differing facts at times, regarding the treatment and control of her diabetes.

[1]Rosalind Franklin University of Medicine and Science/Chicago Medical School and Captain James A. Lovell Federal Health Care Center, North Chicago, IL

Many antipsychotic medications are associated with weight gain and increased risk of diabetes. Although originally thought that the increased risk of diabetes was secondary to weight gain, reports of acute hyperglycemia after initiation of certain antipsychotic medications suggest otherwise.[2] The specific effects of mental health medications on glucose metabolism are still unknown, but are believed to be related to insulin resistance.[3]

The patient was evaluated at our institution at age 41, while continuing with insulin pump therapy. Since the diagnosis of diabetes, she had lost approximately 30 pounds, unintentionally. She reported a recurrent history of hypoglycemia and hypoglycemia unawareness requiring progressive decreases in her insulin requirements. During initial evaluation, she was found to have the following insulin pump settings: single basal rate of 0.3 units/h, blood glucose target 70–140 mg/dL (3.9–7.8 mmol/L), insulin to carbohydrate ratio of 10, and correction factor of 40 mg/dL (2.2 mmol/L).

Her family history is significant for diabetes: father, two paternal uncles, paternal grandfather, paternal grandmother, paternal great-grandmother and maternal grandfather. Ages of onset are unknown. The patient's BMI at time of encounter was 26 kg/m^2 (18.5–24.9). Examination was significant for vitiligo of the extremities.

After discovering a strong family history of diabetes, the clinician should consider the diagnosis of maturity-onset diabetes of the young (MODY). MODY is an autosomal dominant disorder, distinguished by an early age of onset without autoantibodies and typically treated without insulin. Diagnosing MODY can be difficult, as these patients have various underlying genetic mutations and present with a wide spectrum of clinical characteristics.[4] However, many of these patients are misdiagnosed as having type 1 or type 2 diabetes.

After initial evaluation, we considered discontinuing the patient's insulin pump. However, she was hesitant to make this change. Therefore, her insulin pump basal rate was decreased to 0.2 unit/h, and she was again counseled by an interdisciplinary team on medical nutrition therapy, hypoglycemia prevention, and hypoglycemia treatment. Despite these interventions, the patient continued to experience frequent hypoglycemic episodes, mostly attributed to an unpredictable schedule and erratic eating patterns. Routine laboratory testing revealed normal renal and liver function with a glycosylated hemoglobin (HbA$_{1c}$) of 7.8% (4.0–6.0%) without evidence of anemia, microalbuminuria, or thyroid dysfunction. Over the course of four months, the HbA$_{1c}$ decreased to 7.1%.

A continuous blood glucose monitoring system was used to further evaluate for nocturnal hypoglycemia and hypoglycemia unawareness (Figure C14.1). Over 4 days, 14 glucose meter values ranged from 57–184 mg/dL (3.2–10.2 mmol/L), and 814 sensor values ranged from 64–304 mg/dL (3.5–16.9 mmol/L). Her insulin requirements remained low and due to hypoglycemic patterns, her insulin pump basal rate was decreased to 0.1 unit/hr.

A 2-hour postprandial C-peptide level was 1.14 ng/mL (0.80–3.85) with a corresponding glucose level of 150 mg/dL (70–99 mg/dL or 3.9–5.5 mmol/L). Repeated 2-hour postprandial C-peptide and glucose levels

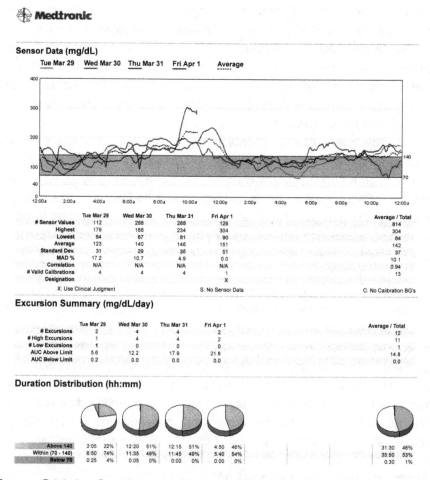

Figure C14.1—Continuous Glucose Monitoring Profiles.

were 2.36 ng/mL and 318 mg/dL (17.6 mmol/L), respectively. Glutamic acid decarboxylase antibody level was 1.0 unit/mL (≤1.0 unit/mL).

Based on our evaluation, we concluded that this patient, who initially was diagnosed and treated as having type 1 diabetes, has type 2 diabetes with insulin resistance. She was transitioned to metformin extended release, and her insulin pump was discontinued. She continues to do well on metformin. However, we are considering a trial of additional antihyperglycemic agents, such as DPP-IV inhibitors, to control postprandial hyperglycemia. The hypoglycemia resolved after discontinuing insulin.

Discussion

Distinguishing type 1 from type 2 diabetes can be difficult, especially when the history is unclear, as highlighted in this case. This patient was treated 20 years for diabetes by different providers. History of mental illness and recurrent hypoglycemia complicated the condition further. Given the young age of onset of diabetes in our patient, weight-neutral status, and evidence of vitiligo, one should also entertain the possibility of type 1 diabetes. However, further investigation should include evaluation for autoimmunity, as well as response to noninsulin therapy. As our investigation moved forward, it became apparent that this patient did have some endogenous insulin production. A minority of antibody-positive patients with type 1 diabetes are able to produce small amounts of C-peptide, even after disease duration of 30 to 40 years.[5] However, this patient had moderate C-peptide levels and significant postprandial hyperglycemia, typical of type 2 diabetes. More importantly, a trial of antihyperglycemic agents continued to control her diabetes.

It is important for the clinician to be aware and question historical diagnoses, particularly when the history is unclear. Clinical evidence can direct one into an alternate diagnostic pathway. Consideration of personal, social, and biological factors is necessary in order to obtain a correct diagnosis and more importantly to determine treatment.

This research was supported in part by the Captain James A. Lovell Federal Health Care Center.

References

1.   Centers for Disease Control and Prevention. *National Diabetes Statistics Report: Estimates of Diabetes and Its Burden in the United States, 2014.* Atlanta, GA: US Department of Health and Human Services, 2014

2. Lipscombe L., Lévesque L, Gruneir A, et al. Antipsychotic drugs and hyperglyce-
    mia in older patients with diabetes. *Arch Intern Med* 2009;169:1282–1289

3. American Diabetes Association, American Psychiatric Association, American
    Association of Clinical Endocrinologists, and North American Association for
    the Study of Obesity. Consensus development conference on antipsychotic drugs
    and obesity and diabetes. *Diabetes Care* 2004;27:596–601

4. Fajans S, Bell G, Polonsky K. Molecular mechanisms and clinical pathophysiol-
    ogy of maturity-onset diabetes of the young. *N Engl J Med* 2001;345:971–980

5. Wang L, Lovejoy N, Faustman D. Persistence of prolonged C-peptide production
    in type 1 diabetes as measured with an ultrasensitive C-peptide assay. *Diabetes
    Care* 2012;35:465–470

Case 15:
Could This Be MODY vs. Type 2?

Bushra Z. Osmani, MD;[1] Janice L. Gilden, MS, MD;[1] Alvia Moid, DO;[1] and Charles Harris, BS[1]

Case

A 23-year-old Caucasian man was referred to the Diabetes/Endocrine Clinic for evaluation and management of newly diagnosed diabetes. He was recently admitted to general medicine with a random blood glucose value of 275 mg/dL (15.28 mmol/L) that was discovered incidentally on laboratory testing. The patient complained of an eight-month history of polyuria, polydipsia, and fatigue. During hospitalization, his fingerstick blood glucose ranged from 179–291 mg/dL (9.94–16.17 mmol/L). Table C15.1 shows laboratory tests performed during inpatient hospitalization.

The patient was discharged home with the diagnosis of type 2 diabetes, taking insulin therapy and metformin 500 mg twice a day. Past medical history was unremarkable. He drinks alcohol socially. He noted weight loss of 80 pounds over the past 2–4 years, which he attributed to more intense physical exercise and a healthier diet. The increased thirst and urination over the past 1–2 years had improved after initiation of insulin.

His mother (diagnosed during pregnancy and currently using insulin), maternal grandfather, and maternal great-grandmother had been diagnosed with diabetes (ages of onset and type of diabetes unknown).

---

[1]Rosalind Franklin University of Medicine and Science/Chicago Medical School and Captain James A. Lovell Federal Health Care Center, North Chicago, IL

Table C15.1 — Laboratory Results

Laboratory Test	Result
Glycosylated Hemoglobin (HbA$_{1c}$)	12.4% (normal: 4.0–6.0%)
Glutamic Acid Decarboxylase (GAD) Antibodies	Negative
Fasting C-Peptide Level	0.91 (normal: 0.81–3.85)
High Density Lipoprotein - Cholesterol (HDL-C)	31 (normal: >40)
Arterial Blood pH on Admission	7.424 (normal: 7.38–7.46)
Urine Ketones	80 mg/dL (normal: negative)

Physical examination was significant for BMI of 25 kg/m^2, with no evidence of acanthosis nigricans, skin tags, xanthoma, muscle wasting, or peripheral neuropathy.

The patient received intensive diabetes self-management education by the Diabetes team. Based on his current blood glucose levels, his insulin dose was adjusted to 10 units of detemir insulin nightly, 2 units of aspart insulin with meals, and metformin 500 mg twice a day. Genetic testing for MODY was advised but the patient refused.

Discussion

According to the American Diabetes Association criteria, a diagnosis of diabetes can be made if either the fasting plasma glucose (FPG) is ≥126 mg/dL (7.0 mmol/L), or 2-hour plasma glucose (2-h PG) is ≥200 mg/dL (11.1 mmol/L) during a 75 g oral glucose tolerance test, or glycosylated hemoglobin (HbA$_{1c}$) is ≥6.5%, or a random plasma glucose level is ≥200 mg/dL (11.1 mmol/L) in individuals with symptoms of hyperglycemia. For FPG, 2-h PG, and HbA$_{1c}$, results should be confirmed by repeat testing unless there is unequivocal hyperglycemia.[1]

According to the above, our patient meets the criteria for diagnosis of diabetes since he had a random blood glucose level of greater than 200 mg/dL (11.1 mmol/L) with symptoms of polyuria, polydipsia, and weight loss, and an HbA$_{1c}$ >6.5%.

The diagnosis of MODY should be considered in this patient due to the onset of nonobese diabetes occurring in young age (age is 23 years) with no signs of insulin resistance, and with diabetes in at least four generations of his family.

MODY is characteristically seen in younger patients (<25 years), with lack of autoantibodies, and has an autosomal dominant transmission. One to two percent of all diabetes cases diagnosed in Europe are MODY.[2]

One study observed that more than 80% of patients are incorrectly diagnosed with type 1 diabetes (T1D) and type 2 diabetes (T2D) at presentation, and there is a delay of 12 years from the time of diagnosis with diabetes to the time that they are actually identified as MODY.[3]

Optimal treatments for T1D, T2D, and MODY differ. Therefore, it is important to distinguish among these entities. Furthermore, there is a 50% probability of first-degree relatives inheriting the same mutation, which confers a greater than 95% risk of developing MODY.[4]

MODY can result from mutations in at least 13 different genes that cause pancreatic β-cell dysfunction, pancreatic endocrine and exocrine dysfunction, insulin gene mutation, insulin secretion defect, and ATP-sensitive potassium channel dysfunction. Mutations in glycolytic enzyme glucokinase (GCK) and hepatocyte nuclear factor (HNF1A, HNF4A, and HNF1B) genes are the most common causes of MODY, and respectively account for 32%, 52%, 10%, and 6% of the cases of MODY in the U.K. (Table C15.2).[5]

Patients with MODY 3 have mutations in the HNF1A gene, which is the most common cause in Europe, North America, and Asia. Mutations in the HNF1A gene can result in progressive β-cell dysfunction leading to diabetes in early adult life.[5] Patients usually have normal blood glucose levels in childhood, but progressively develop defects of insulin secretion, eventually leading to a diagnosis of diabetes in the second to fifth decades of life.[4] Since these patients may have severe hyperglycemia that worsens over time, the risks of microvascular and macrovascular complications are similar to T1D and T2D. These patients are sensitive to sulfonylurea therapy, which is recommended as first-line treatment.[5]

Patients with MODY 2 have mutations in the GCK enzyme. These patients present with mild fasting hyperglycemia with an HbA_{1c} in the range of 5.8–7.6%. They usually have no symptoms and may be discovered during routine screening such as during pregnancy. These patients may not require treatment after pregnancy because there are no long-term complications.[5]

Patients with MODY 1 have HNF4A gene mutations and present similarly to those with HNF1A mutations. An estimated 10–29% of patients who test negative for HNF1A mutations, are found to have HNF4A mutations. These patients do not have glycosuria, and a clue to diagnosing this condition can be low levels of apolipoproteins. These patients respond to sulfonylurea therapy.[5]

In our patient, we can consider a mutation in either the HNF1A gene or the HNF4A gene. He presented in early adult life (age 23 years) with

Table C15.2—MODY Gene Mutations

MODY Gene	Age of Onset	Features	Management
HNF1A	Adolescence or early adulthood	• Progressive β-cell failure • Increasing hyperglycemia • Glycosuria • Increased risk for micro and macrovascular complications of diabetes • High HDL-C	• Sulfonylureas • May eventually require insulin
GCK	Commonly discovered during routine screening during pregnancy or during insurance physicals	• Mild, stable fasting hyperglycemia • Generally asymptomatic • Usually maintain HbA$_{1c}$ <8% • Not at risk to develop diabetes-related complications	• Lifestyle modifications— dietary control and increased physical activity • Insulin may be required during pregnancy
HNF4A	Adolescence or early adulthood	• Progressive β-cell failure • Family history of diabetes • Absence of insulin resistance or obesity • Presents similarly to HNF1A mutation • Low HDL-C • Higher birth weight • Transient neonatal hypoglycemia	• Sulfonylureas
HNF1B	Adolescence or early adulthood	• Renal disease • Pancreatic atrophy • Genital tract abnormalities in females • Abnormal liver function tests • Low birth weight	• Insulin

signs and symptoms of hyperglycemia, as well as HbA$_{1c}$ of 12.4%. He has a strong family history of diabetes, which favors both of these conditions, and no signs of insulin resistance. Although the patient reports that this weight loss was intentional, we cannot rule out the possibility that this was secondary to diabetes or to a combination of intentional efforts and diabetes. The diagnosis of HNF1A mutation is further supported by the fact that he had glycosuria. However, low levels of HDL-C support the diagnosis of HNF1A mutation.

In order to confirm this diagnosis, genetic testing is required. However, our patient had moved and previously refused genetic testing. Ideally, he should have been treated with sulfonylurea therapy. We recommended that he continue the current treatment (insulin and metformin) until continuity of care with an endocrinologist was obtained. He was counseled on the importance of genetic testing and genetic counseling, as this could have an impact on the management of his diabetes and the management of diabetes for the rest of his family.

This case illustrates the challenge that is faced by many physicians in diagnosing and identifying patients with MODY or its genetic variants. There is a lack of awareness by providers, as well as difficulty obtaining genetic testing and the high costs involved. However, it is important to identify an accurate diagnosis due to important clinical implications for proper treatment, as well as monitoring for chronic complications, and the need for genetic counseling.

This research was supported in part by the Captain James A. Lovell Federal Health Care Center.

References

1. American Diabetes Association. Standards of medical care in diabetes—2017. *Diabetes Care* 2017;40(Suppl. 1):S11–S24

2. Ledermann HM. Maturity-onset diabetes of the young (MODY) at least ten times more common in Europe than previously assumed? *Diabetologia* 1995;38:1482

3. Shields BM, Hicks S, Shepherd MH, Colclough K, Hattersley AT, Ellard S. Maturity-onset diabetes of the young (MODY): how many cases are we missing? *Diabetologia* 2010;53:2504–2508

4. Thanabalasingham G, Owen KR. Diagnosis and management of maturity onset diabetes of the young (MODY). *BMJ* 2011;343:d6044

5. Kim SH. Maturity-onset diabetes of the young: what do clinicians need to know? *Diabetes Metab J* 2015;39:468–477

Case 16:
Misclassification of MODY 3 as Type 1

Li Song, MD;[1] Jacqueline Nicole McNulty, PharmD;[2] and Ildiko Lingvay, MD[1,3]

Case

A 31-year-old Hispanic man presented to clinic for management of uncontrolled type 1 diabetes (T1D). He was diagnosed at age 10 when he was hospitalized for a ruptured appendix. He was started on insulin and told that he would be insulin dependent for his lifetime. He has been off insulin intermittently for as long as one year due to financial difficulty; however, he never developed diabetic ketoacidosis (DKA). Patient subsequently developed left foot osteomyelitis due to a nonhealing wound necessitating left transmetatarsal amputation at age 27, diabetic peripheral neuropathy, severe proliferative retinopathy in both eyes at age 29, and progressive chronic kidney disease to stage 5 with nephrotic-range proteinuria at age 31. He developed hypertension and hyperlipidemia with the onset of nephrotic syndrome. Family history was significant for diabetes in his sister, parents, and maternal grandfather, all with thin to normal body habitus (Figure C16.1). He was initially on a basal-bolus insulin regimen;

[1]Department of Internal Medicine, Division of Endocrinology, University of Texas Southwestern Medical Center, Dallas, TX

[2]Department of Pharmacy, Global Diabetes Program, Parkland Health & Hospital System, Dallas, TX

[3]Department of Clinical Sciences, University of Texas Southwestern Medical Center, Dallas, TX

however, he frequently missed insulin because of the burden of needing multiple daily injections. He was switched to twice-daily premixed insulin 70/30, but he still often forgot his injections. His other medications included lisinopril, amlodipine, carvedilol, furosemide, sodium bicarbonate, calcium acetate, and atorvastatin. His vital signs showed blood pressure 141/95, weight 66 kg, and BMI 21 kg/m². Physical examination revealed a thin man with diminished sensation to vibration and monofilament on both feet and no evidence of acanthosis nigricans. Laboratory studies showed hemoglobin (Hgb) A1C ranged over the past 10 years 9.5–14.4%, and on the most recent testing: HbA_{1c} 11.0%, glucose 197 mg/dL, Hgb 8.5 g/dL, creatinine 7.26 mg/dL, urine protein to creatinine ratio 9.8, LDL cholesterol 119 mg/dL, and triglyceride 118 mg/dL. His autoantibodies against glutamic acid decarboxylase, islet cell, and insulinoma-associated protein 2 were negative. C-peptide was 2.6 ng/mL (1.1–4.4) concomitant with a glucose level of 197 mg/dL.

MODY was suspected, thus a MODY NextGen Sequencing was obtained.[1] The result showed two heterozygous mutations in the hepatocyte nuclear factor 1α (HNF1A) gene. One is a missense variant c.716C>T (p.Ala239Val) with uncertain clinical significance. The other is a novel mutation c.527_528del that is predicted to result in a premature protein termi-

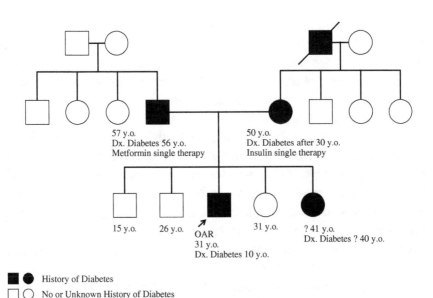

Figure C16.1 — Pedigree of the patient's (OAR) family. Crossed symbol indicates deceased individual.

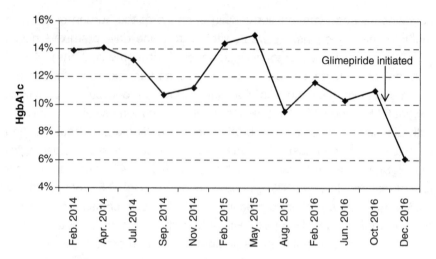

Figure C16.2—HgbA1c trend of the patient.

nation. A trial of glimepiride 1 mg daily was started with discontinuation of insulin. At his 6-week follow-up, his HbA$_{1c}$ improved from 11% to 6.1% and he reported no hypoglycemia (Figure C16.2).

Discussion

Maturity-onset diabetes of the young (MODY) is a monogenic diabetes that accounts for 1–2% of all diabetes.[2] It is suspected in nonobese patients who are diagnosed with diabetes before age 25 and have an extensive family history of diabetes in at least 3 successive generations suggesting an autosomal dominant inheritance pattern.[2] It is often misdiagnosed as T1D due to patients' young age and thin body habitus. The distinction between MODY and T1D is important because the therapy and surveillance of hyperglycemia-related complications may be different. We present a young man with MODY 3, which for 20 years was misdiagnosed as T1D. During this time, he was treated with multiple daily insulin injections with limited compliance due to financial difficulty and being overwhelmed by the number of injections, thus he was exposed to the deleterious effects of hyperglycemia for two decades, leading to multiple hyperglycemia-related microvascular complications.

Our patient was diagnosed with T1D at age 10; however, he had multiple features suggestive of a different form of diabetes. He never had diabetic ketoacidosis despite long periods of not taking insulin. Multiple family members were thin and had diabetes. He had negative T1D-associated autoantibodies and a detectable C-peptide after 20 years of presumed T1D. These features presented an opportunity to the health-care workers to reconsider his initial diagnosis; however, it was missed. Unfortunately, about 10% of MODY are initially diagnosed as T1D.[3] A correct diagnosis can have significant implication regarding therapy and surveillance for hyperglycemia-related complications. MODY 1, 2, and 3 are due to mutations in HNF4α (HNF4A), glucokinase, and HNF1A, respectively. They account for 90% of all MODY cases. Patients with MODY 2 have stable and mild hyperglycemia that does not require treatment. They are not at risk for hyperglycemia-related complications.[2] Patients with MODY 1 and 3 have a delayed and decreased insulin secretion in response to glucose, and a lower renal threshold for reabsorption of glucose (MODY 3). They have glycosuria before hyperglycemia, fasting normoglycemia, and postprandial hyperglycemia. They have progressive disease and are at risk for hyperglycemia-related complications. They are very sensitive to sulfonylurea therapy.[2]

The age of MODY 3 onset is early in our patient. This could be due to acute stress from perforated appendix at the time of diagnosis on the background of genetic predisposition. His HNF1A mutation c.527_528del is predicted to result in a premature protein termination and likely pathologic. The missense variant c.716C>T (p.Ala239Val) was shown to result in decreased transactivation activities compared to wild type; however, it does not exert a dominant negative effect when coexpressed with a wild type HNF1A.[4,5] Both of these mutations are heterozygous in our patient; however, if they are located on two separate alleles, he may be predisposed to an early onset of disease. Screening his family would help discern the inheritance pattern, but it is not feasible due to socioeconomic constraints.

It is uncertain whether an earlier diagnosis of MODY 3 would have prevented all his microvascular complications. However, it would have led to an earlier implementation of sulfonylurea therapy, which is more affordable and convenient than insulin injections, thus conducive to better compliance and quality of life.

For the health-care workers, multiple factors likely contributed to this missed opportunity to improve the care for the patient, including the lack of familiarity with MODY, anchoring on the established diagnosis without questioning its validity, failure in obtaining a thorough history, and the cost of genetic testing. In conclusion, we emphasize the importance of a thorough history in every patient with diabetes and a high index of suspicion for other types of diabetes when clinical features are atypical for T1D or type 2 diabetes.

References

1. Prevention Genetics. Maturity onset diabetes of the young (MODY) sequencing panel [Internet]. Available at https://www.preventiongenetics.com/testInfo.php?sel=test&val=Maturity+Onset+Diabetes+of+the+Young+%28MODY%29+Sequencing+Panel

2. Fajans SS, Bell GI. MODY: history, genetics, pathophysiology, and clinical decision making. *Diabetes Care* 2011;34:1878–1884

3. Siddiqui K, Musambil M, Nazir N. Maturity onset diabetes of the young (MODY)–history, first case reports and recent advances. *Gene* 2015;555:66–71

4. Gu N, Suzuki N, Takeda J, et al. Effect of mutations in HNF-1alpha and HNF-1beta on the transcriptional regulation of human sucrase-isomaltase in Caco-2 cells. *Biochem Biophys Res Commun* 2004;325:308–313

5. Tonooka N, Tomura H, Takahashi Y, et al. High frequency of mutations in the HNF-1alpha gene in non-obese patients with diabetes of youth in Japanese and identification of a case of digenic inheritance. *Diabetologia* 2002;45:1709–1712

Case 17:
Wolfram Syndrome WFS1

Jennifer Sarhis-Avigdor, MD;[1] and Eda Cengiz, MD, MHS[1]

Case

A 5-year-old Caucasian male born from a nonconsanguineous marriage, by normal delivery, and with no history of chronic disease or concern for developmental delay, presented with glucosuria during a routine health-care visit. The patient was diagnosed with type 1 diabetes (T1D) after having a confirmatory blood glucose of 400 mg/dL with negative urine ketones and was started on daily insulin injection therapy. Renal function, hepatic function, and thyroid function were normal. He was transitioned to insulin pump therapy at age 7 and was requiring 0.9 unit/kg/day insulin (40% basal/60% bolus).

Four years after diabetes onset, he was diagnosed with sensorineural hearing loss picked up on routine health screening. At that time, he also complained of difficulty seeing the blackboard in school and was diagnosed with bilateral optic atrophy upon dilated fundoscopic exam. Subject's diagnosis with optic nerve atrophy concomitant with sensorineural deafness and diabetes called the diagnosis of T1D into question and led to re-evaluation of his case to explore a likely diagnosis of Wolfram syndrome (WS).

In the patient, genetic analysis of the coding region of the WFS1 gene revealed two mutations: c.387G>A, p.Trp129stop mutation and c.1620G>A, p.Trp540stop mutation, consistent with a diagnosis of WS

[1]Division of Pediatric Endocrinology, Yale School of Medicine, New Haven, CT

Type 1. Father was a confirmed carrier of the c.387G>A, p.Trp129 stop mutation, and mother was a confirmed carrier of the c.1620G>A, p.Trp540 stop mutation. His sibling had two normal alleles. The family was referred for genetic counseling.

Additional testing was ordered to detect organ system abnormalities associated with WS. Gonadotrophin, testosterone, and insulin-like growth factor levels were within normal range for his age. Magnetic resonance imaging of the brain was significant for small optic nerves and an otherwise normal brain structure. Retroperitoneal ultrasound to evaluate for bladder and renal structure and function showed a parenchymal band dividing the renal sinus on the left, suggestive of partial versus complete duplication of the collecting system without hydronephrosis, ureteric dilation, renal calculi, or thickened bladder wall.

Our subject struggled with enuresis and urinary frequency that would wax and wane with time. He had normal water deprivation test results and vasopressin levels at baseline, therefore he was not started on desmopressin acetate (DDAVP) until a few years after the diagnosis of WS. Daily tamsulosin treatment was initiated by urology to facilitate bladder emptying based on urodynamic study findings.

He is currently 20 years of age and had normal growth and pubertal progression. He is on insulin pump therapy and has been keeping his HbA$_{1c}$ levels in the 6.0–6.9% range.

Discussion

Wolfram Syndrome is a rare, progressive neurodegenerative genetic disorder inherited in an autosomal recessive pattern with an estimated prevalence of 1 in 500,000 people worldwide.[1] It is commonly referred to as DIDMOAD syndrome, which captures the key features of the disease: diabetes insipidus, diabetes (juvenile onset), optic atrophy, and deafness.[2]

Two types of WS exist. Type 1 is caused by homozygous or compound heterozygous mutation in the gene encoding wolframin (WFS1; 606201) on chromosome 4p. Type 2 is caused by a mutation in the CISD2 gene (WFS2; 604928) on chromosome 4q22-q24. Such individuals do not have diabetes insipidus but can develop gastrointestinal ulcers.[2]

WS Type 1 is due to a defective production of the protein wolframin secondary to mutations in the WFS1 gene. Wolframin is located in the endoplasmic reticulum of the pancreas, brain, heart, bones, muscles, lung, liver, and kidneys and regulates calcium homeostasis within cells. The disrupted calcium balance at the cellular level due to Wolframin dysfunction ultimately leads to cellular apoptosis.[3] The β-cells of the pancreas are usually affected first, leading to diabetes as the initial manifestation before 10 years of age as seen in our patient. Patients may present with ketoacidosis; however, the course of diabetes is milder with lower prevalence of microvascular complications as compared to T1D.[2]

Our patient developed optic atrophy within the first decade of life consistent with the median age of presentation. While diabetic retinopathy is rare, ophthalmologic symptoms can progressively worsen. Yearly eye examination, including visual acuity, color vision testing, fundoscopy, visual field, and optical coherence tomography scan, is recommended. Retinal thinning has been shown to be a reliable marker for the disease progression.[4]

Sensorineural hearing loss is seen in 66% of patients with WS and is detected in the second decade of life, unlike our subject who was diagnosed at 9 years of age. Hearing impairment in WS is typically progressive and mainly affects the higher frequencies.[2]

Central diabetes insipidus affects approximately 72% of WS Type 1 patients with a median age at onset of 15.5 years and responds to oral or nasal DDAVP therapy.[2]

A spectrum of urological abnormalities has been described in WS, such as large atonic bladder, a low capacity, high-pressure bladder with sphincter dyssynergia, and hydroureteronephrosis. Yearly assessment of renal function, measurement of postvoid residual urine volume by renal ultrasound, and urodynamic testing are recommended.[4]

The onset of neurologic abnormalities occurs between the first and second decades as a result of general brain atrophy with involvement of brainstem and cranial nerves. Central hypogonadism and delayed pubertal progression have been attributed to hypothalamic dysfunction and are more common in males.[1] Other manifestations of WS that have been described but not observed in our subject are cerebellar ataxia, peripheral neuropathy, dementia, psychiatric illness, cardiovascular and gastrointestinal autonomic neuropathy, and central apnea.[2,4]

Conclusion

Patients with WS usually present with diabetes as their initial manifestation of the disease. It is therefore critical for the endocrinologist to recognize other presenting symptoms as components of the syndrome and not merely as separate entities. Patients with confirmed WS should be managed through a multidisciplinary approach by multiple specialists to screen for associated features of the disease and to address issues related to the affected organ system.

There is still no cure for WS, and early mortality, often by age 30, is due to diabetes, renal, neurological, or respiratory complications, or the combination.[4] Patient registries have been established to determine disease progress and explore potential treatments to prolong and improve the quality of life of patients with WS.[2]

References

1. Wolfram Syndrome [Internet], 2016. NIH U.S. National Library of Medicine. Available from https://ghr.nlm.nih.gov/condition/wolfram-syndrome. Accessed 26 September, 2016

2. Tranebjærg L, Barrett T, Rendtorff ND. WFS1-Related Disorders. In *GeneReviews* [Internet]. Pagon RA, Adam MP, Ardinger HH, et al., Eds. Seattle, WA: University of Washington, Seattle, 1993–2016

3. Kumar S. Wolfram syndrome: important implications for pediatricians and pediatric endocrinologists. *Pediatr Diabetes* 2010;11:28–37

4. Urano F. Wolfram syndrome: diagnosis, management, and treatment. *Curr Diab Rep* 2016;16:6

Case 18:
Mitochondrial Diabetes

Catherine Sullivan, MD;[1] and Sara Alexanian, MD[1]

Case

A 37-year-old African-American male was initially seen by our inpatient diabetes consult team for management when he was transferred from an outside hospital with new-onset headaches, altered mental status, and worsening seizures. He had a prior history of traumatic brain injury and seizures, although he had been seizure free for 6 years prior to this presentation. Initially, there was concern for herpes simplex encephalitis due to left temporal lobe hyperintensities on magnetic resonance imaging. Ultimately, an infectious and immunologic workup was inconclusive, and he was discharged from the hospital with encephalitis of unknown etiology. His medical history was additionally notable for a five-year history of type 2 diabetes, migraines, and progressive bilateral hearing loss.

He presented again to the neurology service two months later due to worsening symptoms as well as blurred vision and transient, bilateral, left greater than right, cranial VI nerve palsies. His lactate concentration was noted to be mildly elevated even when clinically stable. At the same time, his mother had been admitted for stroke-like symptoms. His constellation of headache, worsening seizures, ophthalmoplegia, hearing loss, and diabetes, as well as development of similar symptoms in his mother, raised the concern for mitochondrial encephalomyopathy, lactic acidosis, and

---

[1]Section of Endocrinology, Diabetes, Nutrition and Weight Loss, Boston University Medical Center, Boston, MA

stroke-like episodes (MELAS). Genetic testing was therefore performed, which revealed that he was heteroplasmic for the A3243G point mutation, confirming the diagnosis.

Regarding his diabetes history, he was diagnosed at age 32 and initially treated with insulin, plus metformin and glyburide. He had a normal BMI of 21 kg/m^2 and weight of 59 kg. His HbA$_{1c}$ in 2008 was 10.7% and a few months later improved to 6.6% on low-dose glipizide and metformin. Following the diagnosis of MELAS, however, metformin was discontinued due to the increased risk of lactic acidosis. His glycemic control varied from 7–10.8% over the next 7 years. This was in part due to a progressive decline in memory and functional status and an inability to take medications and eat consistently. Following his MELAS diagnosis, he was trialed on Humalog mix 75/25 with his largest meal plus glipizide; however, due to concerns over safety on full insulin replacement therapy and poor control with this regimen, his regimen was changed to glargine insulin plus glipizide and sitagliptin for a few years. Unfortunately, at the age of 43 he developed recurrent strokes and worsening cardiac function with progressive cognitive decline requiring 24-hour care in a rehabilitation facility where his diabetes was managed with basal-bolus insulin therapy at approximately 0.6 unit/kg total daily dose. He died at the age of 44 in the setting of progressive cardiac and renal failure.

Discussion

It is estimated that 1 in 5,000 individuals are affected by mitochondrial disorders.[1] The mitochondria support multiple important metabolic functions in the cell, including oxidative phosphorylation, the citric acid cycle, fatty acid oxidation, and apoptosis. Oxidative phosphorylation involves a multi-step process of electron donation along the respiratory chain of the mitochondrion to generate heat and adenosine triphosphate (ATP). Mutations in mitochondrial DNA (mtDNA) may affect the production of ATP but also involve deregulation of other cellular processes due to alterations in signaling molecules.[2] A mutation initially affects only one cell; however, during multiple divisions there will be a random division of the mitochondria to daughter cells that will have either predominantly wild-type or mutant mitochondria. Cells with a mixed population are considered to have heteroplasmy.[2] The degree of heteroplasmy in specific organs may contribute to the multiple clinical manifestations observed in individuals with MELAS and other mitochondrial disorders, and can explain why even among family members. Consequently, the disease presentation can be varied.

For example, a higher amount of heteroplasmy in the β-cells of the pancreas may contribute to development of diabetes in some cases of MELAS, whereas other individuals are not affected.[2] Mitochondrial DNA is inherited through the oocyte, with mutations passed down maternally, an important consideration when diagnosing these conditions.

MELAS is characterized by multi-organ dysfunction, including stroke-like episodes, dementia, seizures, lactic acidosis, hearing difficulties, myopathies, diabetes, thyroid dysfunction, and short stature. Because mitochondria are essential for production of ATP, mitochondrial diseases preferentially affect organs with high energy utilization, including the endocrine system.[1] Most cases of MELAS present in childhood or early adolescence with the majority of cases identified before the age of 40.[3] Initial presentation of the disease includes headaches, seizures, stroke-like episodes, vomiting, muscle weakness, and short stature.[3,4] The seizures are associated with alterations in consciousness, which may be partially reversible. However, over time, repeated episodes result in progressive decline in mental and physical capabilities contributing to the morbidity and mortality of this condition. Hearing impairments are reported in over 75% of cases. Less commonly, diabetes is one of the initial presenting manifestations, but can be present in up to 21–38% of cases.[1,3]

The diagnosis of MELAS is based on clinical features and can be confirmed with genetic testing. Approximately 80% of MELAS cases are due to mutations in the MT-TL1 gene, encoding tRNA leucine 1, with the most common variant being the mtDNA A3243G mutation.[4] Other common variants in the MT-TL1 gene reported in MELAS include T3271C and A3252G mutations. Variants in the MT-ND5 gene, which encodes the NADH-ubiquinone oxidoreductase subunit 5, have also been reported in isolated MELAS cases or those with "overlap syndromes."[4] It should be noted that in some cases of MELAS the mutation may not be identified in blood testing and urine or other tissue sampling may be required to confirm the diagnosis.[1] The A3243G mutation is also associated with maternally inherited diabetes with deafness, or MIDD.[1]

The pathogenesis of diabetes in MELAS includes impairment of insulin secretion from the β-cells, insulin resistance in peripheral tissues, as well as increased gluconeogenesis.[5,6] Diabetes severity, as well as the intensity and choice of treatment modality, varies widely along a continuum, with some individuals managed by diet and lifestyle modifications alone and others requiring full insulin replacement. However, most will progress to full insulin deficiency in a short period of time.[2,7] Early-onset diabetes, without evidence of β-cell autoimmunity and with lack of obesity or other signs of insulin resistance as well as maternal inheritance, are some clues to suggest mitochondrial diabetes. The typical clinical features associated with MELAS and the presence of sensorineural hearing impairment can additionally aid in making the diagnosis and distinguishing between other inherited forms of diabetes, such as MODY or other mitochondrial disorders associated with diabetes, some of which are listed in Table C18.1.

Table C18.1 — Mitochondrial Disorders Associated with Diabetes

Mitochondrial Disorder and Common Mutations[a]	Clinical Features	Associated Prevalence of Diabetes
MELAS -A3243G (80% of cases) -T3271C -A3252G	Encephalomyopathy Seizures (associated with transient hemiparesis or blindness) Vomiting Migraines Cognitive decline Myopathy: Lactic acidosis, ragged-red fibers on muscle biopsy Stroke-like episodes Exercise intolerance or proximal limb weakness Sensorineural hearing loss Cardiomyopathy, cardiac conduction abnormalities	21–38% [1,3]
MIDD -A3243G	Sensorineural hearing loss Macular pattern dystrophy Myopathy Cardiomyopathy Short stature	38%[1]
Kearns Sayre Syndrome (KSS) (Can also present as more mild form: isolated chronic progressive external ophthalmoplegia, CPEO) -Large deletions of mtDNA (typically sporadic)	Age of onset <20 years Chronic progressive external ophthalmoplegia Cardiac conduction abnormalities Hearing loss Short stature Dementia Extremity weakness Hypocalcemia with hypoparathyroidism Growth hormone deficiencies	11–14%

Table C18.1—(*Continued*)

Mitochondrial Disorder and Common Mutations[a]	Clinical Features	Associated Prevalence of Diabetes
Myoclonic epilepsy with ragged-red fibers (MERRF) -A8344G	Myoclonus Myopathy Spasticity Lipomas Muscle tissue: ragged-red fibers	10%[1,7]
-C12258A[b]	Constipation Dysarthria Fatigue	[1]
MELAS-like phenotype -mutations in nuclear gene *POLG*, which encodes mtDNA polymerase gamma	Various disorders, some common feature include Epilepsy Ophthalmoplegia Hepatic failure Ataxia	11-66%[1,7]

[a] Common mutations listed, other mutations have been reported.
[b] 2 reported cases, both with development of diabetes.
MELAS, mitochondrial encephalomyopathy with lactic acidosis and stroke-like episodes; MIDD, maternally inherited diabetes and deafness; mtDNA, mitochondrial DNA.

Treatment of diabetes in MELAS patients should focus on improving insulin sensitivity via physical exercise, avoiding risk factors for lactic acidosis (including the use of metformin), and recognizing that patients will often develop complete insulin dependence. Some studies have suggested that coenzyme Q10 and L-carnitine therapies may improve mitochondrial function in patients with MELAS. However, there are no approved therapies for mitochondrial conditions.[1] Complications impacting diabetes care include inability to self-manage the disease, especially when managing the cognitive or physical impairments related to the neurologic manifestations of this condition.

References

1. Karaa A, Goldstein A. The spectrum of clinical presentation, diagnosis, and management of mitochondrial forms of diabetes. *Pediatr Diabetes* 2015;16:1–9

2. Maassen JA, van Essen E, van den Ouweland JM, Lemkes HH. Molecular and clinical aspects of mitochondrial diabetes mellitus. *Exp Clin Endocrinol Diabetes* 2001;109:127–134

3. El-Hattab AW, Adesina AM, Jones J, Scaglia F. MELAS syndrome: clinical manifestations, pathogenesis, and treatment options. *Mol Genet Metab* 2015;116:4–12

4. DiMauro S, Hirano M. MELAS. In *GeneReviews* [Internet]. Pagon RA, Adam MP, Ardinger HH, et al., Eds. Seattle, WA: University of Washington, Seattle, p. 1993–2016

5. El-Hattab AW, et al. Glucose metabolism derangements in adults with the MELAS m.3243A>G mutation. *Mitochondrion* 2014;18:63–69

6. Velho G, Byrne MM, Chement K, et al. Clinical phenotypes, insulin secretion and insulin sensitivity in kindreds with maternally inherited diabetes and deafness due to mitochondrial tRNALeu(UUR) gene mutation. *Diabetes* 1996;45:478–487

7. Whittaker RG, Schaefer AM, McFarland R, et al. Prevalence and progression of diabetes in mitochondrial disease. *Diabetologia* 2007;50:2085–2089

Case 19:
Mitochondrial Diabetes:
m.3243A>G Mutation

Brandon P. Galm, MD;[1] Sandra Sirrs, MD;[2] and Roseanne O. Yeung, MD, MPH[1]

Case

A 41-year-old Caucasian woman had screening blood work that showed asymptomatic hyperglycemia. She had been identified with the m.3243A>G mutation for mitochondrial encephalomyopathy, lactic acidosis, and stroke-like episodes (MELAS) on family screening when her mother presented with stroke-like episodes. Our patient had sensorineural hearing loss requiring cochlear implantation, exertional myalgias, and elevated lactate (2.6 mmol/L).

She received diabetes education and started metformin prior to our evaluation. She developed severe lethargy and was switched to gliclazide, but stopped this due to foot pain. She was not taking any antihyperglycemic therapy when she was seen in our clinic. Home glucose monitor readings revealed fasting glucose levels between 156 and 189 mg/dL (8.7 to 10.5 mmol/L) and 2-hour postprandial levels between 156 and 250 mg/dL (8.7 to 13.9 mmol/L).

Past medical history was significant for hypertension. Her family history is shown in Figure C19.1.

[1]Division of Endocrinology and Metabolism, Department of Medicine, University of Alberta, Edmonton, Alberta, Canada

[2]Division of Endocrinology and Metabolism, Department of Medicine, University of British Columbia, Vancouver, British Columbia, Canada

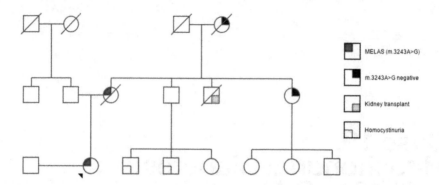

Figure C19.1—Pedigree. Arrowhead indicates the proband. Crossed symbols indicate deceased individuals.

Medications included hydrochlorothiazide, valsartan, vitamin K, levo-carnitine, coenzyme Q10, and a multivitamin.

On examination, her weight was 47.9 kg and height was 158.1 cm (BMI 19.2 kg/m^2). Blood pressure was 132/92 mmHg. She had mild proximal and distal muscle weakness of all four limbs, difficulties with tandem gait, and mild dysmetria. Examination was otherwise unremarkable. There was no acanthosis nigricans. Ophthalmologic evaluation showed no retinal dystrophy or diabetic retinopathy (Table C19.1).

She was started on repaglinide 0.5 mg with meals and has tolerated this without hypoglycemia. With treatment, fasting glucose levels were 108 to 115 mg/dL (6.0 to 6.4 mmol/L), 2-hour postprandial levels were 85 to 133 mg/dL (4.7 to 7.4 mmol/L), and HbA$_{1c}$ was 5.2%.

Discussion

Primary mitochondrial diseases affect about 1 in 10,000 individuals.[1,2] These disorders lead to impaired ATP production and reduced capacity to deal with reactive oxygen species. Organs with high energy requirements are most affected, including the nervous system, skeletal and cardiac muscle, retina, kidney, gastrointestinal tract, and pancreatic β-cell. Because only oocytes contribute mitochondria to the zygote, disorders of mitochondrial DNA (mtDNA) are maternally inherited. However, many mitochondrial proteins are also encoded by nuclear DNA, and thus inheritance of mitochondrial disorders may also be autosomal or X-linked.[2]

The most common primary mitochondrial disorder is caused by the m.3243A>G mutation in mtDNA.[2] In its severe form, this can lead to MELAS;

Table C19.1 — Investigations at the Time of Evaluation

Parameter	Measurement	Reference Range
Fasting glucose (mmol/L)	10.1	3.3–6.0
Hemoglobin A1C (%)	7.7	4.3–6.1
Lactate (mmol/L)	3.7	0.5–2.2
Creatine kinase (units/L)	117	<200
Creatinine (μmol/L)	36	50–105
Estimated GFR (ml/min/1.73m²)	128	>59
Total cholesterol (mmol/L)	4.54	<6.2
Triglycerides (mmol/L)	3.87	<1.70
HDL cholesterol (mmol/L)	1.01	>1.10
LDL cholesterol (mmol/L)	1.77	
Urine albumin to creatinine ratio (mg/mmol)	2.39	<2.8
Stimulated C-peptide* (nmol/L)	1.57	0.3–1.32

*30 minutes after a mixed meal

in its milder form, m.3243A>G can manifest as maternally inherited diabetes and deafness (MIDD). Phenotypic heterogeneity is common with mitochondrial disorders and the same mutation within the same family can present very differently. Other mitochondrial disorders result from various point mutations or copy-number variants and may also be associated with mitochondrial diabetes.[1,2]

Mitochondrial forms of diabetes (mD) are estimated to account for about 1% of all diabetes. Of these, about 85% are thought to be due to the m.3243A>G mutation, although this high proportion related to a single mutation may represent ascertainment bias. These monogenic forms of diabetes often present insidiously like type 2 diabetes, although some patients may present acutely in ketoacidosis. While the penetrance of diabetes with the m.3243A>G mutation is high, the age of onset is variable, with a mean of 37 years. The underlying pathophysiologic defect is thought to be insulin deficiency due to reduced ATP generation within pancreatic β-cells, although insulin resistance may contribute in some patients.[1]

Neurologic findings are common in patients with mitochondrial disorders and include seizures, dementia, developmental delay, ataxia, stroke-like episodes, movement disorders, and neuropathies. Sensorineural hearing loss develops in many patients. Ophthalmologic examination may show a distinctive macular-pattern retinal dystrophy as well as ptosis, external ophthalmoplegia, and optic atrophy. Other common manifestations include cardiomyopathy, pre-excitation syndromes, myopathy, chronic kidney disease, proteinuria, and gastrointestinal dysmotility. The most common nondiabetic endocrine manifestation is short stature due to hypothalamic growth hormone releasing hormone deficiency. Rarely, patients may have hypothalamic hypogonadism or secondary hypothyroidism.[1,2]

The diagnosis of mitochondrial disorders is challenging and may involve a combination of clinical characteristics, mode of inheritance, biochemical features (such as elevated lactate levels or abnormal urine organic acid analysis), pathological findings (such as alterations in staining for oxidative enzymes), and genetic testing. Some mtDNA mutations, including m.3243A>G, are readily detected using mitochondrial DNA isolated from peripheral blood leukocytes, while other mtDNA defects and those involving nuclear DNA may require DNA extraction from tissues such as muscle, heart, or brain.[1,2]

Lifestyle modification and education are important for managing patients with mitochondrial disorders. Metformin has not been recommended as first-line antihyperglycemic therapy due to the theoretical risk of lactic acidosis; however, limited data suggest that it may be used safely in patients with MELAS with monitoring of lactate levels.[1,3] Sulfonylureas are usually recommended as first-line pharmacotherapy.[2] Meglitinides would also be expected to be beneficial given a similar mechanism of action, as is demonstrated in our case. While insulin secretagogues may be useful, patients with mD often require insulin earlier (mean 2 to 4 years after diagnosis) as compared to patients with type 2 diabetes.[1] Thiazolidinediones are often avoided due to the theoretical risk of mitochondrial toxicity. Incretin agents have been used in some cases, but have not been thoroughly evaluated.[2]

Treatment of cardiovascular risk factors in mitochondrial disorders should be considered. Data suggest that young adults with MELAS syndrome may have higher rates of hypertension.[4] Theoretical concerns have been raised about statin therapy due to reduced levels of coenzyme Q10; however, several reports have shown no increase in adverse events or disease progression in those with mitochondrial disorders.[1,5] Some have recommended that statins may be used cautiously in those at high cardiovascular risk, although it is important to consider that cardiovascular outcome data are lacking in this population and that stroke-like episodes and cardiomyopathy may be due to the underlying metabolic disorder and not typical atherosclerosis.[1]

References

1. Murphy R, Turnbull DM, Walker M, Hattersley AT. Clinical features, diagnosis and management of maternally inherited diabetes and deafness (MIDD) associated with the 3243A>G mitochondrial point mutation. *Diabet Med* 2008;25:383–399

2. Schaefer AM, Walker M, Turnbull DM, Taylor RW. Endocrine disorders in mitochondrial disease. *Mol Cell Endocrinol* 2013;379:2–11

3. Hannah-Shmouni F, Sirrs S, Mattman A. Metformin therapy and lactate levels in adult patients with MELAS and diabetes mellitus. Abstract SAT-1040 presented at the 96th Annual Meeting and Expo of the Endocrine Society, 21–24 June 2014, Chicago, IL

4. Hannah-Shmouni F, Sirrs S, Mezei MM, Waters PJ, Mattman A. Increased prevalence of hypertension in young adults with high heteroplasmy levels of the MELAS m.3243A>G mutation. *JIMD Rep* 2014;12:17–23

5. Hannah-Shmouni F, Al-Sarraf A, Frohlich J, Mezei MM, Sirrs S, Mattman A. Safety of statin therapy in patients with mitochondrial diseases. *J Clin Lipidol* 2013;7:182

Case 20: mDNA3243A>G

Anja L. Frederiksen, MD;[1,2] and Henning Beck-Nielsen, MD[2,3]

Case 1

The female index patient (IV:1) developed diabetes aged 28 (Figure C20.1). At the time of diagnosis, the glutamic acid decarboxylase (GAD)-65 antibody titer was negative, plasma C-peptide was 735 nmol/L (reference range 130–760), and HbA$_{1c}$ was 8.9% (reference range 4.3–6.3); her BMI was 17.0 kg/m^2. She was initially treated with sulfonylurea with very good response. Twelve years later, she was diagnosed with bilateral sensorineural hearing impairment (HI), which prompted her consultant to reevaluate her family history. This included a healthy sister, while their mother was diagnosed with diabetes at age 27 and later with HI treated with cochlear implant at age 40. Two maternal uncles and an aunt had all been diagnosed with what initially clinically presented as a type 2 diabetes and HI, between ages 50 and 60. Subsequently, genetic screening identified the mDNA3243A>G mutation, thereby confirming the clinical diagnosis of maternally inherited diabetes and deafness (MIDD).

[1]Department of Clinical Genetics, Odense University Hospital (OUH), Odense, Denmark
[2]Department of Clinical Research, University of Southern Denmark, Odense, Denmark
[3]Department of Endocrinology, OUH, Denmark

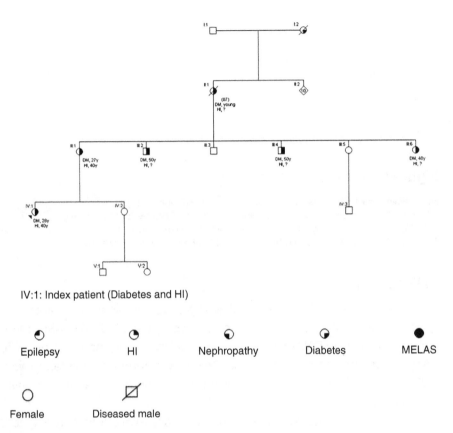

IV:1: Index patient (Diabetes and HI)

Epilepsy   HI   Nephropathy   Diabetes   MELAS

Female   Diseased male

Figure C20.1 — Family tree, case 1. Crossed symbols indicate deceased individuals.

Case 2

Two sisters (III:1 and III:2) were diagnosed with diabetes, at ages 19 and 26, and with bilateral sensorineural HI, at ages 26 and 36. Their BMIs were 20 and 22 kg/m^2 and both women were treated with low-dose insulin therapy. There was a strong family history of maternal diabetes and HI, and the genetic testing uncovered the mDNA3243A>G. Apart from retinitis pigmentosa and mild distal neuropathy, they had no late complications of diabetes. In the following years, the eldest sister developed ataxia, myopathy, and stroke-like episodes. She died at age 52. A third sister was diagnosed with HI. Several relatives were later diagnosed with mitochondrial-associated symptoms including myopathy, epilepsy, and ptosis (Figure C20.2).

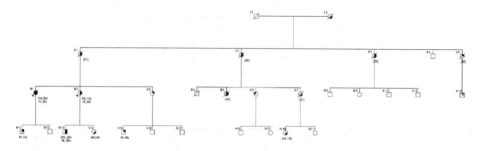

Figure C20.2—Family tree, case 2.

Index patients: III:1 (Diabetes, HI, and MELAS) and III:2 (Diabetes, HI).
II:1 (Diabetes, HI, encephalopathy), II:2 (Diabetes, HI), II:3 (Diabetes and HI), II:5 (HI)
III:3 (HI); III:5 (Diabetes, HI, gastrointestinal symptoms), III:6 (Epilepsy); III:7 (Diabetes); III:12 (Ptosis)
IV1: (HI and nephropathy), IV:3 (Diabetes, HI), IV:4 (Diabetes) and IV:10 (Diabetes)

Discussion

The two cases illustrate the clinical pictures observed in families with monogenetic mitochondrial diabetes caused by the mDNA3243A>G. Mitochondrial DNA (mDNA) defects are recognized to be diabetogenic. The most frequent mutation, mDNA3243A>G, was reported in a family with diabetes and HI by van den Ouweland et al., who proposed the acronym MIDD.[1]

Since mitochondrial diabetes may clinically mimic a type 1 or type 2 diabetes, it is challenging to properly recognize this rare subtype. However, if patients with diabetes have a family history of maternal diabetes or they present with comorbidities such as bilateral HI, cardiomyopathy, myopathy, migraine, ptosis, or strokes at an early age, the mitochondrial diabetes entity should be considered.

Patients may present with a "classic" MIDD phenotype more commonly; however, many individuals display a cluster of clinical features associated with the mutation. The considerable phenotypic variations can partially be explained by several important characteristics of the mitochondria, the essential intracellularly located organelle. Mitochondria hold their own circular 16 kilo-base genome mDNA, which is strictly inherited in the maternal lineage. Each organelle holds 2–10 copies of the mDNA and each cell has 100–1,000 mitochondria. Moreover, human cells can contain both mutated and wild-type mDNA in variable ratios, also called heteroplasmy. The mitochondrial genome encodes core proteins of the respiratory chain, holding the key function of aerobic adenosine triphosphate (ATP) production through an oxidative phosphorylation process. Tissues with high energy demands are more susceptible to impaired ATP supplies, and mutation in the mDNA may cause mitochondrial disease including diabetes.[2]

Diabetes may develop insidiously or in rare cases debut with ketoacidosis at any age; still, the majority of mDNA3243A>G-associated diabetes cases develop in midlife. The patients are mostly lean with a lower than average BMI and present with negative islet cell antibodies and normal or high levels of C-peptide.[3] The pathophysiological events prior to the development of diabetes are still only partly understood, and it is debated whether the impaired glucose homeostasis is due to diminished insulin secretion or insulin resistance.[4]

Generally, at the time of diagnosis, insulin treatment is not required and many patients can initially be treated with sulfonylurea in low dose while treatment with metformin should be used with caution as the mDNA3243A>G is associated with increased risk of lactic acidosis. The majority of patients will, however, progress to require additional treatment with insulin, dipeptidyl peptidase 4 (DPP4) inhibitors, or glucagon-like peptide (GLP)-1 receptor agonists.

Late complications of diabetes in MIDD appear to have a different profile compared with type 1 and type 2 diabetes. Nephropathy and neuropathy are independently associated with mitochondrial disease and mDNA3243A>G, but more commonly presented in patients with mitochondrial disease who develop diabetes. In contrast, diabetic retinopathy seems to occur less frequently while retinitis pigmentosa is a frequent finding.[3]

The mDNA3243A>G was initially identified in subjects presenting with mitochondrial encephalomyopathy, lactic acidosis, and stroke-like episodes (MELAS), hence termed the "MELAS mutation." Tissues with high metabolic rates are highly susceptible to the mDNA3243A>G, and morbidities accordingly include cardiomyopathy, which demands heart transplantation, epilepsy, migraine, ptosis, nephropathy, and gastrointestinal complaints. The patients may present with any of these symptoms prior to the development of diabetes and HI.

The phenotypic presentations vary considerably both among family members and between families. Some MIDD patients have a severe phenotype with multiple mDNA3243A>G-associated comorbidities while their siblings remain unaffected. This is partly explained by the level of heteroplasmy as high mutation loads are associated with earlier onset of symptoms and more severe phenotype. However, the level of heteroplasmy cannot be employed for predicting the exact phenotype. When suspecting MIDD, the genetic diagnostics can be done by blood sample screening, though levels of heteroplasmy may be nondetectable and thus, alternatively, buccal mucosa, urine sediment, or muscle biopsy may be required to establish the correct diagnosis.

Genetic counseling with information on the nature, inheritance, and implication of the genetic disorder should be offered to patients and family members when diagnosing mitochondrial diabetes. Surveillance programs, including echocardiography and screening for diabetes, may be beneficial as cardiomyopathy may be "silent" initially and, apparently, unaffected mutation positive subjects may have impaired glucose tolerance.[5]

The mitochondrial diabetes subtype should be considered when seeing an "atypical" diabetes patient with HI or comorbidity or when the patient presents with a maternal history of diabetes and HI. Furthermore, it should be emphasized that the family history must be reevaluated on a regular basis. The variable phenotypic presentations challenge the pattern recognition and, consequently, the correct diagnosis is often delayed.

References

1. van den Ouweland JM, Lemkes HH, Ruitenbeek W, Sandkuijl LA, de Vijlder MF, Struyvenberg PA, et al. Mutation in mitochondrial tRNA(Leu)(UUR) gene in a large pedigree with maternally transmitted type II diabetes mellitus and deafness. *Nat Genet* 1992;1:368–371

2. Friedman JR, Nunnari J. Mitochondrial form and function. *Nature* 2014;505:335–343

3. Massin P, Dubois-Laforgue D, Meas T, Laloi-Michelin M, Gin H, Bauduceau B, et al. Retinal and renal complications in patients with a mutation of mitochondrial DNA at position 3,243 (maternally inherited diabetes and deafness). A case-control study. *Diabetologia* 2008;51:1664–1670

4. Lindroos MM, Borra R, Mononen N, Lehtimäki T, Virtanen KA, Lepomäki V, et al. Mitochondrial diabetes is associated with insulin resistance in subcutaneous adipose tissue but not with increased liver fat content. *J Inherit Metab Dis* 2011;34:1205–1212

5. Frederiksen AL, Jeppesen TD, Vissing J, Schwartz M, Kyvik KO, Schmitz O, et al. High prevalence of impaired glucose homeostasis and myopathy in asymptomatic and oligosymptomatic 3243A>G mitochondrial DNA mutation-positive subjects. *J Clin Endocrinol Metab* 2009;94:2872–2879

Case 21:
Maternally Inherited Diabetes and Deafness: 23-Year Follow-Up

Iram Ahmad, MD;[1] and Irl B. Hirsch, MD[1]

Case

We present the case of LH, a 59-year-old female who has been followed by our clinic for 23 years. In 1993, at the age of 36 years, she presented to our emergency department in hyperglycemic crisis without ketonuria while 6 weeks postpartum. She had a past history of Hashimoto's thyroiditis with hypothyroidism and presumptive IgA nephropathy with proteinuria. During her pregnancy, she was diagnosed with gestational diabetes and was treated with insulin. Earliest BMI documented on accessible records was at 2 years postpartum and was 23 kg/m^2, but by her history, her BMI has always been in the normal range. Her family history was significant for renal disease of unknown etiology and deafness in her mother. There was no family history of diabetes. She was discharged with the presumptive diagnosis of type 1 diabetes and referred to our clinic to initiate insulin therapy. Antibodies to GAD were found to be negative on two occasions. There was a question of compliance with insulin therapy, yet her fasting glucose levels were consistently in the 120–130 mg/dL range. Due to this, fasting C-peptide was measured and found to be 2.8 ng/mL (reference 1.0–5.0 ng/mL). Due to her normal BMI, history of Hashimoto's thyroiditis, and lack of family history of diabetes she was presumed to have Latent Autoimmune Diabetes of Adults (LADA), although there was concern as she was GAD

[1]The University of Washington School of Medicine, Division of Metabolism, Endocrinology, and Nutrition, Seattle, WA

antibody negative and her insulin requirements were rising. Because of this, it was decided to give her a trial of metformin, but it resulted in abdominal cramping and documented lactate accumulation.

In 2001 at the age of 44, she developed class III to IV unstable angina. Myocardial infarction was ruled out and further evaluation requiring a percutaneous coronary intervention to the right coronary artery, which required another procedure a year later due to restenosis. She tolerated statins but developed two life-threatening upper gastrointestinal bleeds due to her antiplatelet therapy.

Over the course of her care, she became increasingly insulin resistant, later necessitating U-500 insulin, which was infused via an insulin pump. In 2008, during a routine phone call by a provider in our clinic to review results, she interrupted and asked the provider to stay on hold until she could find her hearing aids. At that time, the provider realized that this patient indeed fit the criteria for maternally inherited diabetes and deafness (MIDD). To date, she has had regular retinal eye exams, which have showed some uveitis but normal maculae without hyperpigmentation. Her BMI over the course of her care has ranged from 22–24 kg/m². Her son (with whom she was pregnant shortly before establishing care in our diabetes clinic) also has deafness and glucose intolerance, but does not yet have diabetes. She has a daughter who appears to exhibit no signs or symptoms of MIDD. When our patient was diagnosed with her diabetes, both children tested negative for islet cell antibodies, but GAD testing was not commercially available at that time.

Discussion

MIDD is a form of monogenic diabetes that was first described in 1992 and results most commonly from an A to G substitution at position 3242 of the mitochondrial DNA encoding the gene for tRNA^Leu denoted as m.3243A>G.[1] It is part of the spectrum of disorders associated with this point mutation, which includes mitochondrial encephalomyopathy, lactic acidosis, and stroke-like episodes (MELAS) and progressive external ophthalmoplegia (PEO).

The m.3243A>G point mutation promotes abnormal dimerization of the mitochondrial tRNA^Leu tertiary structure, which causes deficiencies in complex 1 and 4 of the respiratory chain within the mitochondria. This can cause dysfunction in many organ systems with high metabolic activity, including but not limited to macular pattern retinopathy, strokes, cerebral and cerebellar atrophy, congestive heart failure, focal segmental glomerulosclerosis, bilateral sensorineural deafness, and diabetes. Insulin resistance as seen in our patient can be severe. Premature coronary artery disease, which our patient has, is not a usual feature of MIDD as coronary angiograms are usually normal, but reduction in cardiac ATP synthesis causes myocyte hypertrophy and failure.[2]

There is high heteroplasmy of the m.3243A>G mutation in tissues with low mitogenic activity, such as muscle, which suggests that the main defect leading to diabetes is altered glucose uptake by the muscle. Hepatic gluconeogenesis may also be dysregulated due to high lactate influx into the liver.[3] As a result, metformin, which has a higher risk of lactic acidosis (which did develop in our patient), should be avoided. Statin therapy should also be avoided in patients with MIDD and myopathy, as HMG Co-A reductase inhibitors can also reduce levels of coenzyme Q10, which counteracts the enhanced release of free radicals and impairment of the mitochondrial respiratory chain by mutant mitochondria. It should be noted that the effect of statin in lowering coenzyme Q levels is reversible.[4]

Diagnosis specifically of MIDD is based on the presence of one or more of the following criteria: 1) maculopathy, 2) hearing impairment (which is decreased perception of frequencies of 5 kHz), 3) maternal heritability of diabetes/impaired fasting glucose, and 4) normal body mass index.[4] Given its rarity and variable presentation, it is often mistaken for type 1 or type 2 diabetes, which can lead to mismanagement of these patients, often lifelong. The phenotypic variability is not well understood, and only a small subset of the patients with this mutation has pure MIDD. It has been suggested that male gender confers a higher risk of strokes. This may partly be due to heteroplasmy with varying proportions of mutant and wild-type DNA, but an analysis of 126 carriers of this mutation in Italy showed that heteroplasmy alone could not predict the stroke-like episodes or other clinical features such as hearing loss, diabetes, or PEO.[5]

Diabetes in MIDD is usually insidious in onset and is secondary to abnormal β-cell function, loss of β-cell mass, and insulin deficiency.[6] In pancreatic β-cells, the m.3243A>G mutation alters the ATP/ADP ratio, which determines the opening probability of the potassium ATP channel involved in insulin secretion. Patients are usually negative for the HLA-polymorphisms associated with type 1 diabetes. A small subset have islet cell or GAD antibodies, but it is not agreed if this reflects coincidental type 1 diabetes or if the antibodies produced are a result of pancreatic β-cell destruction as a result of the m.3243A>G mutation. The degrees of insulin deficiency and insulin resistance are variable, and in some patients the insulin resistance can be severe.

The penetrance of diabetes has been estimated to be greater than 85% in carriers of the m.3243A>G mutation, but the age of onset is variable.[2] The mean age at diagnosis is 37 +/– 11 years, but as expected, the age of diagnosis falls in successive generations due to increased aware-ness. The patients described in the literature have been diagnosed at a wide range of ages, from 11 to 77 years.[2,4] The index of suspicion for MIDD should be raised in a strong familial history. Unlike MODY, which also dem-onstrates heritability, there should be a presence of maternal transmission and bilateral hearing impairment in both carriers. Patients with a type 2 diabetes–like phenotype can initially be treated by diet or sulfonylureas. The insulinopenia is progressive and most patients will eventually require insulin a few years after diagnosis, as our patient did.

The weakness of our case is that no renal biopsy was performed to confirm or rule out the initial presumptive diagnosis of IgA nephropathy, nor did the patient's insurance agree to cover the cost of mitochondrial DNA genetic testing to check for the m.3243A>G mutation (which costs $625.58 out of pocket at our institute at the time of this writing).

However, what this case does support is that MIDD is probably more common than appreciated. What this case illustrates first and foremost is that careful assessment of the patient and family history is key in differen-tiating MIDD from other forms of diabetes. There is a tendency for clini-cians to consider hearing impairment unrelated to the initial presentation of diabetes; however, deafness is indeed a clear feature in many syndromes, including MIDD. The patient's nephropathy was initially diagnosed as IgA nephropathy, but in retrospect, she never had a kidney biopsy to confirm this diagnosis and her proteinuria is almost certainly due to nephropathy from focal segmental glomerulosclerosis, which is a feature of MIDD. Since the phenotype can be variable between patients and individual features of the syndrome are not very specific, a family history is essential in order to appreciate the constellation of symptoms that make up this disorder, and ideally the gene defect should be tested for.

In summary, MIDD is likely more commonly seen than appreciated. It has a variable phenotype, but maternal transmission is required. Definitive diagnosis requires genetic testing, which unfortunately is not available to many patients. Nevertheless, a presumptive diagnosis can be made when maternal transmission of diabetes and deafness is clear, along with numer-ous other characteristics that have variable expression.

References

1.   van den Ouweland JM, Lemkes HH, Ruitenbeek W, Sandkuijl LA, de Vijlder MF, Struyvenberg PA, van de Kamp JJ, Maassen JA. Mutation in mitochondrial

tRNA(Leu)(UUR) gene in a large pedigree with maternally transmitted type II diabetes mellitus and deafness. *Nat Genet* 1992;1:368–371

2. Murphy R, Turnbull DM, Walker M, Hattersley AT. Clinical features, diagnosis and management of maternally inherited diabetes and deafness (MIDD) associated with the 3243A>G mitochondrial point mutation. *Diabet Med* 2008;25: 383–399

3. Maassen JA, 'T Hart LM, Van Essen E, Heine RJ, Nijpels G, Jahangir Tafrechi RS, Raap AK, Janssen GM, Lemkes HH. Mitochondrial diabetes: molecular mechanisms and clinical presentation. *Diabetes* 2004;53(Suppl. 1):S103–109

4. Naing A, Kenchaiah M, Krishnan B, Mir F, Charnley A, Egan C, Bano G. Maternally inherited diabetes and deafness (MIDD): diagnosis and management. *J Diabetes Complications* 2014;28:542–546

5. Mancuso M, Orsucci D, Angelini C, Bertini E, et al. The m.3243A>G mitochondrial DNA mutation and related phenotypes. A matter of gender? *J Neurol* 2014;261:504–510

6. Oka Y, Katagiri H, Yazaki Y, Murase T, Kobayashi T. Mitochondrial gene mutation in islet-cell-antibody-positive patients who were initially non-insulin-dependent diabetics. *Lancet* 1993;342:527–528

Case 22:
Glycogen Storage Type 1A Presenting with Type 2 Diabetes

Divya Sistla, MD;[1] Mary Korytkowski, MD;[2] and Sann Y. Mon, MD, MPH[2]

Case

A 28-year-old female Caucasian patient, born of a consanguineous marriage, was diagnosed at the age of 10 months with glycogen storage disease (GSD) 1A based on episodes of hypoglycemic seizures, lactic academia, hyperuricemia, and hepatomegaly. She has required significant dietary interventions to stabilize her blood glucose levels and avoid recurrent hypoglycemia. Her daily regimen includes a 45 g carbohydrate meal every 3 hours and gastric enteral nutrition (EN) overnight for 12 hours at a rate of 12 mL per hour. Her EN formulation consisted of Tolerex® (Nestle Health Care Nutrition, NJ, USA), 4 tablets of polycose, 6 ounces of water, and 7 tablespoons of cornstarch. She also takes allopurinol 300 mg once a day to control hyperuricemia.

GSD 1 or von Gierke disease is an autosomal recessive disorder caused by the deficiency of the glucose-6-phosphatase enzyme, the final step in gluconeogenesis. The estimated incidence of this disorder is 1 in 100,000 live births.[1] Clinical presentation typically appears at early infancy period, with hypoglycemia, lactic acidosis, hyperuricemia, hyperlipidemia, and hepatomegaly. Short stature and xanthomas can also be seen. Late

[1]Internal Medicine, UPMC McKeesport Hospital, McKeesport, PA
[2]Division of Endocrinology and Metabolism, University of Pittsburgh Medical Center, Pittsburgh, PA

manifestations may include delayed puberty, polycystic ovaries, gout, hepatic adenomas with risk for malignancy, renal failure, and osteoporosis.

At age 14, the patient was diagnosed with type 2 diabetes based on a laboratory A1C of 7% with negative GAD, insulin, and islet antibodies. Her physical exam was significant for a BMI of 34 kg/m² and acanthosis nigricans. An abdominal and pelvic ultrasound demonstrated hepatic steatosis with polycystic ovaries. She was able to lose 5% of her body weight after 6 months of lifestyle modifications, which included intensive dietary modification and moderate-intensity exercise. She achieved good glycemic control with 45 g of carbohydrate every 4 hours during the daytime and 70 g of glycoside at midnight (Figure C22.1).

Discussion

The coexistence of GSD type 1 and diabetes is rare. A case report from Israel suggested secondary diabetes as a late complication after recurrent pancreatitis in a patient with glycogen storage 1b.[2] One study postulated that insulin levels decline with age in patients with glycogen storage disease leading to correction of hypoglycemia and decreased glucose tolerance.[3] Altered activity of enzyme 11β-hydroxysteroid dehydrogenase is a possible mechanism of developing obesity and metabolic syndrome in GSD 1a.[3,4]

Nutrition plays a key role in maintaining normoglycemia without potential for medication-related side effects. A fructose, sucrose, and galactose-restricted diet has been used as treatment for GSD 1a. Intervals of fasting are strictly limited to prevent hypoglycemia.[5] A major challenge in patients

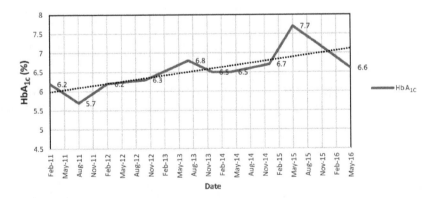

Figure C22.1—Showing the patient's glycemic trends over time.

with GSD 1 and diabetes is to optimize diet to maintain normoglycemia without increasing risk for hypoglycemia. A multidisciplinary care team, including endocrinologists and metabolic nutritionists, combined with counseling by medical genetists has been key to the success of this patient's management.

References

1.   Chou J, Jun HS, Mansfield BC. Type 1 glycogen storage diseases: disorders of the glucose-6-phosphatase/glucose-6-phosphate transporter complexes. *J Inherit Metab Dis* 2015;38:511–519

2.   Spiegel G, Rakover-Tenenbaum Y, Mandel H, Lumelski D, Admoni O, Horovitz Y. Secondary diabetes mellitus: late complication of glycogen storage disease type 1b. *J Ped Endocrin Metab* 2005;18:617–619

3.   Melis D, Rossi A, Pivonello R, et al. Glycogen storage disease type Ia (GSDIa) but not glycogen storage disease type Ib (GSDIb) is associated to an increased risk of metabolic syndrome: possible role of microsomal glucose 6-phosphate accumulation. *Orphanet J Rare Dis* 2015;10:1–8

4.   Wake DJ, Walker BR. 11 beta-hydroxysteroid dehydrogenase type 1 in obesity and the metabolic syndrome. *Mol Cell Endocrinol* 2004;215:45–54

5.   Shah KK, O'Dell SD. Effect of dietary interventions in the maintenance of normoglycaemia in glycogen storage disease type 1a: a systematic review and meta-analysis. *J Hum Nutr Diet* 2013;26:329–339

PART II:
Insulin Resistance, Genetic Defects in Insulin Action, and Diseases of Exocrine Pancreas

2
Insulin Resistance: Molecular Biology and Pathophysiology

Cecilia C. Low Wang, MD;[1] and Boris Draznin, MD, PhD[1]

Overview of Insulin Signaling

The biologic actions of insulin are mediated via its specific cell surface receptor, which initiates intracellular signaling cascades that ultimately lead to multiple physiologic effects of insulin.[1,2] The insulin receptor possesses an intrinsic tyrosine kinase activity, so interaction of the insulin molecule with the receptor results in autophosphorylation and a subsequent multitude of phosphorylation and dephosphorylation steps to bring about glucose uptake by key target tissues (adipose and skeletal muscle), suppression of lipolysis (in adipose tissue), glycogen synthesis, and inhibition of hepatic glucose production, among other actions.[1-3]

Insulin action can be divided into metabolic and mitogenic aspects, which generally result from distinct but interconnected signaling pathways.[3] Even though insulin resistance has emerged as an enormous health-care problem, trespassing the fields of obesity, diabetes, hypertension, and cardiovascular diseases, its molecular mechanism remains incompletely understood.[1,4] Clinically, the term "insulin resistance" implies that higher than normal concentrations of

[1]Division of Endocrinology, Diabetes and Metabolism, University of Colorado Anschutz Medical Campus School of Medicine, Denver, CO

DOI: 10.2337/9781580406666.02

insulin are required to maintain normoglycemia. In other words, insulin-resistant humans and animals develop compensatory hyperinsulinemia in order to ensure normal utilization of glucose by the insulin target tissues.[5] Physiologically, insulin is released from the pancreatic β-cells postprandially in order to maintain euglycemia. Insulin promotes glucose uptake in skeletal muscle and fat by stimulating translocation of glucose transporter 4 (GLUT 4) from the cytosol to the plasma membrane where it facilitates glucose transport.[6,7] Concomitantly, insulin stimulates intracellular utilization of glucose by many other tissues as well. Postabsorptively, the main physiological task of insulin is to suppress glucose production by the liver. Thus, if any one of these two main aspects of insulin action is impaired, one can encounter insulin resistance either at the level of skeletal muscle and fat or hepatic insulin resistance, both of which contribute to the total body insulin resistance.

The degree to which a given amount of insulin is able to result in metabolic actions of insulin is termed "insulin sensitivity." Thus, the terms "insulin sensitivity" or "insulin resistance" are applied exclusively to the metabolic action of insulin and tell us nothing about mitogenic potency or activity of this hormone. Different tissue types within the same individual or even different cell types within a single tissue may have differential sensitivities to insulin.[8-12] In the metabolic cascade of insulin signaling, the final effects of insulin action result in glucose uptake, utilization, and storage with a concomitant lowering of blood glucose levels, inhibition of glucose production in the liver, stimulation of lipogenesis, and inhibition of lipolysis.[13] The mitogenic cascade of insulin signaling promotes cell growth and differentiation, protein synthesis, and inhibition of protein degradation.[8]

On a cellular level, insulin plays an important role not only in the carbohydrate metabolism, but also in protein and lipid synthesis, ion fluxes, cell growth and differentiation, as well as in inhibition of lipolysis, protein degradation, and apoptosis. A possibility that not all aspects of insulin action are affected equally by insulin resistance gave rise to a concept of "selective insulin resistance." It also became apparent that many "metabolic" aspects of insulin action are mediated via stimulation of a distinct intracellular signaling pathway from the pathway involved in activation of the "mitogenic" aspects of insulin action.[9-12,14-19] Thus, on a cellular level, the term "insulin resistance" defines an inadequate strength of insulin signaling from the insulin receptor downstream to the final substrates of insulin action involved in multiple metabolic and mitogenic aspects of cellular function.[2,20]

If insulin binding to its receptor is the first step in the mechanism of insulin action, propagation of the signal generated by this binding event downstream to the signaling molecules represents the next steps in implementation of cellular response to insulin. Insulin signaling constitutes a complex system, and while signals are transmitted downstream via multiple phosphorylation and dephosphorylation steps, there are several feedback regulatory steps that guard against overstimulation.[21,22] Furthermore, enzymes and nonenzymatic proteins as well as other signaling molecules involved in propagation of insulin signaling can and frequently are affected by other intracellular mediators, including inflammatory molecules and lipids, which mainly result in inhibition of insulin action, with resulting insulin resistance.[23,24]

Even though there is redundancy in multiple sites of the insulin signaling system, defects in the insulin signaling cascade consisting of single inherited or multiple acquired mutations that block insulin action have been described in humans (see below), resulting in various phenotypic expressions of hyperglycemia and diabetes, which will be described later in this chapter. In some cases, impairment of insulin action can lead to the subtle clinical manifestations of mild insulin resistance and minimal hyperglycemia, while in other cases, patients may exhibit severe insulin resistance with or without overt diabetes.

Tyrosine Phosphorylation – Initial Steps in the Insulin Signaling Cascade

The cell surface insulin receptor (IR) is a heterotetrameric protein that consists of two extracellular α-subunits (135 kDa each) and two transmembrane β-subunits (95 kDa each) that possess intrinsic tyrosine kinase activity.[1,2,25-27] Insulin binding to the α-subunit of its receptor disinhibits the tyrosine kinase activity of the β-subunit, and promotes autophosphorylation of three regulatory tyrosine (Tyr) residues on the β-subunit (Tyr 1158, Tyr 1162, and Tyr 1163) along with phosphorylation of the insulin receptor substrate-1 (IRS1) and insulin receptor substrate-2 (IRS2) proteins and several other substrates, all of which provide docking sites for additional downstream signaling molecules.[28-31]

IRS proteins are large molecules comprising more than 1,200 amino acid residues that include an amino (NH2)-terminal pleckstrin homology domain (PH) that mediates cell membrane interactions, a phosphotyrosine binding (PTB) domain that binds to the specific phosphorylated motif NPXpY (Asn-Pro-X, with X being any amino acid, p indicating inorganic phosphate, and Y indicating Tyr) of the activated IR, and a carboxy (COOH)-terminal tail that contains multiple tyrosine and serine/threonine phosphorylation sites.[23,30–32] The COOH-terminal tail of IRS proteins contains approximately 20 tyrosine and 50 serine/threonine phosphorylation sites that function as on–off switches to propagate or inhibit insulin signaling to downstream molecules.[21–23]

Years of experimentation with disruption or deletions of IRS1 and IRS2 proteins have confirmed their major role in the metabolic pathways of insulin action, while phosphorylation of other proteins contributes minimally to the metabolic effects of insulin in comparison with the IRS-mediated signaling.[28–34] Tyrosine phosphorylation of IRS proteins by the tyrosine kinase activity of the IR generates binding sites for Src homology 2 (SH2) domain–containing proteins,[25,35] including the regulatory subunit of phosphatidylinositol 3-kinase (PI3K) p85, which attracts the catalytic subunit of PI3K p110 to the plasma membrane.[8,36–40] Recruitment of PI3K results in generation of phosphatidylinositol 3,4,5-triphosphate (PIP3), which activates 3-phosphoinositide-dependent protein kinase (PDK1)[18] and in turn promotes serine/threonine phosphorylation of Akt.[41] This step in the insulin signaling cascade initiates the transition from tyrosine phosphorylation signaling into the serine/threonine phosphorylation cascade.

Serine/Threonine Phosphorylation – The Second Line of Intracellular Insulin Signaling

First, it became apparent that serine phosphorylation of IRS proteins can reduce the ability of IRS proteins to attract PI 3-kinase, thereby minimizing its activation,[21–23,42–45] and can also lead to an accelerated degradation of IRS1 protein.[46] Thus, in contrast to a signal promoting tyrosine phosphorylation, excessive serine phosphorylation of IRS proteins could become detrimental for normal conductance of the metabolic insulin signaling downstream, causing insulin resistance. Serine phosphorylation of IRS proteins can occur in response to a number of intracellular serine kinases. Akt phosphorylation at the threonine 308 position (T308), which is undetectable in tissues lacking IRS proteins, appears to be among the first serine/threonine phosphorylation steps in the propagation of insulin signaling downstream.[21,47–51] This activation of Akt along with phosphorylation of PKCζ and PKCγ appears to be necessary for insulin-stimulated glucose uptake.[52,53] In addition to stimulatory phosphorylation of downstream molecules, Akt also promotes inhibitory phosphorylation of such proteins as AS 160, glycogen synthase kinase 3 (GSK3), and forkhead transcription factor O class member 1 (FOXO1).[54] The inhibitory phosphorylation of AS 160 releases the inhibition of glucose transporter (GLUT)-4–dependent glucose uptake, while inhibitory phosphorylation of GSK3 disinhibits glycogen synthase and promotes storage of glucose as glycogen.[55,56] In other words, dephosphorylated AS 160 inhibits translocation of GLUT4 to the plasma membrane. When insulin promotes its phosphorylation in the PI 3-K-dependent manner, this inhibition is removed and GLUT4 can be recruited to the plasma membrane, facilitating glucose uptake. Similarly, phosphorylation of GSK3 renders it inactive, allowing glycogen synthase to stimulate glycogen synthesis. Phosphorylation of FOXO1 by insulin is also PI 3-K-dependent. Phosphorylation of FOXO1 excludes it from the cell nucleus, so that it no longer promotes gene transcription. Thus, inhibitory phosphorylation of FOXO1 blocks gluconeogenic gene transcription, inhibiting gluconeogenesis, which is a major aspect of insulin action.[57]

In addition to promoting insulin signaling downstream, Akt activation of mTOR and S6 kinase 1 leads to serine phosphorylation of IRS proteins diminishing propagation of insulin signaling and exerting a negative feedback regulation of Akt activity. Thus, serine phosphorylation initiated by Akt functions as both a positive and a negative regulator of insulin signaling.[21–23, 42–44, 52–54, 58]

Insulin Resistance, Hyperglycemia, and Overt Diabetes

Lowering of blood glucose is the predominant effect of insulin observed in clinical practice. Physiologically, insulin stimulates glucose uptake by muscle and adipose tissue, protein and glycogen synthesis in liver and muscle, and lipid synthesis in liver and adipose tissue, while at the same time it inhibits fatty acid oxidation, glycogenolysis, gluconeogenesis, and apoptosis in insulin target tissues.

Defects in or loss of the insulin receptor protein or function result in severe insulin resistance accompanied by hyperglycemia that is frequently pronounced enough to meet criteria for diabetes. Loss of IRS1 and IRS2 also leads to inability to activate PI3K and Akt, and similarly results in severe insulin resistance with significant metabolic consequences.[59,60]

While certain serine/threonine phosphorylation steps promote insulin action as described above, a different set of serine/threonine phosphorylation steps result in feedback inhibition in the propagation of insulin signaling.[42–46,61,62]

For example, serine/threonine phosphorylation of specific residues of IRS proteins will convert them to an inactive state, inhibiting interaction with downstream signaling molecules. Activation of mTOR by nutrients, mitogen-activated protein kinases (MAPKs) by various growth factors, and c-Jun N-terminal kinase (JNK) by inflammatory mediators can all lead to serine/threonine phosphorylation of IRS proteins, causing varying degrees of insulin resistance.[43,61–79] Furthermore, hyperinsulinemia in and of itself has a significant effect to induce insulin resistance by stimulating serine/threonine phosphorylation of IRS proteins with subsequent inhibition of the PI3K and Akt steps of the insulin signaling cascade.[21–23,42,46] Thus, inactivation of PI3K/Akt signaling may represent a fundamental mechanism in the pathogenesis of insulin resistance associated with type 2 diabetes and obesity.

However, defects in insulin signaling leading to insulin resistance contribute differentially to the metabolic phenotype, depending upon the cell and tissue type in which this occurs, since some cells and tissue types may be more sensitive than the others to specific defects in insulin signaling. For example, patients with genetic defects in the IR that are generalized throughout the body have high adiponectin levels and manifest normal serum lipids.[79–81] These individuals do not tend to develop nonalcoholic fatty liver disease.[82,83] Conversely, patients with Akt mutations have marked dyslipidemia and fatty liver.[82]

On the other hand, prevailing hyperinsulinemia resulting from insulin resistance results in persistent activation of the Shc-Ras-MAPK signaling cascade, which maintains or even promotes the mitogenic effects of insulin and overgrowth of various tissues even while these same tissues exhibit insulin resistance as exhibited by diminished metabolic actions of insulin.[52, 84–86] This activation of mitogenic pathways of insulin signaling may lead to the increased risk for tissue overgrowth and malignancy, which is outside the scope of this discussion.[87–90]

Clinical Manifestations of Severe Insulin Resistance

Most patients with insulin resistance are obese, but a small number of patients exhibit a marked degree of severe insulin resistance (SIR) associated with a lean phenotype. These individuals develop hyperglycemia or overt diabetes due to genetic defects of the insulin receptor or other mediators of insulin action, absence of adipose tissue, or via acquired, immune-mediated mechanisms. The latter category includes autoantibodies against insulin or the insulin receptor, or autoimmune destruction of adipocytes leading to lipodystrophy.

The estimated prevalence of monogenic SIR is 0.1–0.5% of patients in hospital-based diabetes practices.[91] The following discussion will focus on those individuals with SIR due to genetic defects or immune-mediated mechanisms affecting the insulin signaling cascade.

Type B Insulin Resistance

Kahn et al.[92,93] proposed the categorization of lean patients with SIR as "type A" or "type B" in a series of publications from 1975. This was based on the absence (in type A) or presence (in type B) of insulin receptor antibodies. Patients with type A SIR have acanthosis nigricans and acne; females are hyperandrogenic, oligomenorrheic, and infertile, and are frequently found to have high serum testosterone levels. SIR type A usually manifests during adolescence.

SIR type B is distinguished by autoantibodies to the insulin receptor, with some patients manifesting immune activation as evidenced by elevated erythrocyte sedimentation rate, proteinuria, and elevated gamma globulin. Patients with type B insulin resistance have low levels of sex hormone–binding globulin, IGF binding protein 1, and adiponectin, with normal or low fasting triglyceride levels and absence of hepatic steatosis, features that are distinct from other SIR syndromes. Up to 20% of patients have identifiable insulin receptor mutations, usually heterozygous with autosomal dominant inheritance.

HAIR-AN

Around the time that these subtypes of SIR were described, a generic term for this constellation of clinical signs was coined: "HAIR-AN," which included hyperandrogenism, insulin resistance, and acanthosis nigricans.[94] These patients are usually obese and much less likely to have a single gene defect, in contrast to lean patients with type A or type B insulin resistance. Mutations in the insulin receptor are not commonly found in HAIR-AN patients, and the etiology of this condition remains unknown.

Donohue Syndrome

Both Donohue syndrome (formerly known as "leprechaunism") and Rabson-Mendenhall syndrome were originally described long before the identification of the insulin receptor.[91,95–97] They represent a spectrum of abnormalities caused by insulin receptor defects that are inherited in an autosomal recessive fashion. Overall prognosis in patients with both syndromes remains poor.

Donohue syndrome has congenital onset and is seen in infants who rarely survive beyond the first year of life because of infection but not diabetic keto-acidosis. Phenotypic features of this syndrome include severe intrauterine and postnatal retardation in linear growth, failure to thrive, lipoatrophy, impairment of muscle development, acanthosis nigricans, and dysmorphic features including large ears, globular eyes, and micrognathia. Patients display massive hyperinsulinemia that is associated with glucose intolerance or frank diabetes but also frequently manifest fasting hypoglycemia. Other features of Donohue syndrome include dysmorphic lungs, nephrocalcinosis, rectal prolapse, hirsutism, clitoromegaly in female infants, and penile enlargement in males. There is little to no residual insulin receptor function in affected individuals. It is unclear why individuals with Donohue syndrome do not develop diabetic ketoacidosis despite lacking a functional insulin receptor.

Rabson-Mendenhall Syndrome

Patients with Rabson-Mendenhall syndrome have less severe impairment of insulin receptor function.[59,60,91] The loss-of-function mutations in the insulin receptor are biallelic, with autosomal recessive inheritance. These individuals present in early childhood with SIR, acanthosis nigricans, diabetes, poor dentition and nail development, impaired linear growth, and soft tissue overgrowth. Fasting hypoglycemia and postprandial hyperglycemia resolve with time and persistent refractory hyperglycemia evolves. Many patients die from diabetic ketoacidosis or microvascular complications during the second decade of life.

Type A Insulin Resistance

The more common presentation of patients with insulin receptor defects includes oligomenorrhea, hyperandrogenism, and acanthosis nigricans in females around the time of puberty, with normoglycemia. Males may only exhibit acanthosis nigricans and occasionally also demonstrate hypoglycemia. Many remain undiagnosed, and diabetes may not be diagnosed until the fourth decade of life.

Overall, more than 100 allelic variants of the insulin receptor gene have been identified, causing the spectrum of SIR ranging from the most severe (Donohue syndrome) to the least severe (HAIR-AN).[60,91] Downstream defects in insulin signaling molecules have been described in only a handful of patients, including patients with heterozygous deletion or mutation of the

HMGA1 gene (a transcription factor that binds to sites in the insulin receptor promoter and allows transcription to occur), and a family with a heterozygous nonsense mutation in AS160. AS160 is a small GTPase-activating protein that plays a key role in activation of the GLUT4 transporter via the insulin signaling cascade.[60,98,99]

Diagnosis of Severe Insulin Resistance

Insulin resistance is accompanied by compensatory hyperinsulinemia, or high serum insulin concentrations. There is wide inter- and intra-individual variation in insulin concentrations, and the use of insulin concentration to quantify the degree of insulin resistance present in a particular individual does not take into account patients with decreasing β-cell function and resulting hyperglycemia. There is no clearly defined threshold for what is considered a "high" insulin concentration for the purposes of the diagnosis of SIR. For individuals with SIR who are completely insulin deficient, the dose of exogenous insulin required to achieve normoglycemia may be used as a surrogate to quantify degree of insulin resistance.

A diagnostic scheme for severe IR most likely due to a monogenic defect has been proposed by Semple et al.[60] In this scheme, the authors propose that patients with an exogenous insulin requirement of 3 units/kg/day or more who also exhibit absolute insulin deficiency and a lean phenotype (BMI of <30 kg/m^2) are more likely to have a monogenic defect causing the SIR. Although the authors do not state the threshold for absolute insulin deficiency, one might define this as a C-peptide level obtained after a period of good glycemic control to exclude the possible presence of glucotoxicity of <0.6 ng/mL, once patient adherence to insulin therapy has been confirmed. Another category of severe insulin resistance that is described in this scheme consists of patients who do not have diabetes, are lean (BMI <30 kg/m^2), and have a fasting insulin concentration of >250 pmol/L and/or peak insulin concentration on oral glucose tolerance testing of >1,500 pmol/L. The third category described by the authors consists of patients with partial β-cell compensation and/or obesity (BMI >30 kg/m^2), who are diagnosed by one or more of the following: a clinical history of ovarian hyperandrogenism, oligomenorrhea, a physical exam finding of acanthosis nigricans, and/or a physical exam finding of lipodystrophy.

Although there are no formal criteria for the diagnosis of SIR, most endocrinologists agree that very high levels of endogenous insulin (fasting over 150 pmol/L) in individuals with a BMI less than 30 kg/m^2 or exogenous insulin requirement of greater than 2–3 units per kg body weight per day justifies this term, particularly in the presence of such clinical features as acanthosis nigricans, oligomenorrhea, hyperandrogenism, or abnormal adipose distribution. The prevalence is believed to be around 0.1% among patients with diabetes.

Treatment Options for Severe Insulin Resistance

There are few data providing direct evidence to support the effectiveness of lifestyle changes in patients with SIR. This is mainly due to the rarity of patients with these syndromes and the lack of clinical trials in this area. However, extrapolating from data accumulated from management of common forms of insulin resistance, addressing obesity and diet with activity in patients with SIR is a key aspect of management, and helps ameliorate the underlying insulin resistance.

The use of insulin sensitizers such as thiazolidinediones or metformin to reduce hepatic glucose output may be considered and has been found to be effective to some degree in patients with SIR.[60]

U-500 insulin is often required because of the high doses of insulin needed to achieve glycemic control. There are small studies that support the use of U-500 therapy via continuous subcutaneous insulin infusion, or insulin pump therapy.[100,101]

For patients with severe defects caused by insulin receptor mutations, the use of recombinant human IGF-1 may improve glycemic control, but the mechanisms and ideal dosing are unclear.[102–105]

Management of diabetes in patients with Donohue syndrome usually consists of measures to prevent severe hypoglycemia and extreme hyperglycemia.[106]

Management of diabetes in patients with Rabson-Mendenhall syndrome can be challenging and requires exogenous insulin, frequently in very high doses.[100,101,107] U-500 insulin may be used in those requiring more than 200–300 units a day. Administration of leptin or IGF-1 (which acts by binding to either IGF-1 receptor or to a functioning insulin receptor) has been attempted in patients with Rabson-Mendelhall syndrome but without consistent substantial clinical benefit.[106]

References

1.   Olefsky JM. The insulin receptor: a multifunctional protein. *Diabetes* 1990;39: 1009–1016

2. Shulman GI. Cellular mechanism of insulin resistance. *J Clin Invest* 2000; 106:171–176

3. Wang CC, Goalstone ML, Draznin B. Molecular mechanisms of insulin resistance that impact on cardiovascular biology. *Diabetes* 2004;53:2735–2740

4. Reaven GM. Role of insulin resistance in human disease. *Diabetes* 1988;37:1595–1607

5. DeFronzo RA. The triumvirate: beta-cell, muscle, liver. A collusion responsible for NIDDM. *Diabetes* 1988;37:667–687

6. Bell GI, Burant CF, Takeda J, Gould GW. Structure and function of mammalian facilitative sugar transporters. *J Biol Chem* 1993;268:19161–19164

7. Shepherd PR, Kahn BB. Glucose transporters and insulin action—implications for insulin resistance and diabetes mellitus. *N Engl J Med* 1999;341:248–257

8. Draznin B. Molecular mechanisms of insulin resistance: serine phosphorylation of IRS-1 and increased expression of p85α – the two sides of a coin. *Diabetes* 2006;55:2392–2397

9. Jiang ZY, Lin YW, Clemont A, Feener EP, Hein KD, Igarashi M, Yamauchi T, White MF, King GL. Characterization of selective resistance to insulin signaling in the vasculature of obese Zucker (fa/fa) rats. *J Clin Invest* 1999;104:447–457

10. Cusi K, Maezono K, Osman A, Pendergrass M, Patti ME, Pratipanawatr T, DeFronzo RA, Kahn CR, Mandarino LJ. Insulin resistance differentially affects the PI 3-kinase- and MAP kinase-mediated signaling in human muscle. *J Clin Invest* 2000;105:311–320

11. Montagnani M, Golovchenko I, Kim I, Koh GY, Goalstone ML, Mundhekar AN, Johansen M, Kucik DF, Quon MJ, Draznin B. Inhibition of phosphatidylinositol 3-kinase enhances mitogenic action of insulin in endothelial cells. *J Biol Chem* 2002;277:1794–1799

12. Wang C, Gurevich I, Draznin B. Insulin affects vascular smooth muscle cell phenotype and migration via distinct signaling pathways. *Diabetes* 2003;52:2562–2569

13. Flakoff PJ, Jensen MD, Cherington AD. Physiologic action of insulin. In *Diabetes Mellitus: A Fundamental and Clinical Text*. 3rd ed. LeRoith D, Taylor SI, Olefsky JM, Eds. Philadelphia. Lippincott, Williams & Wilkins, 2004, p. 165–181

14. Cheatham B, Vlahos CJ, Cheatham L, et al. Phosphatidylinositol 3-kinase activation is required for insulin stimulation of pp70S6 kinase, DNA synthesis, and glucose transporter translocation. *Mol Cell Biol* 1994;14:4902–4911

15. Shepherd PR, Navé BT, Siddle K. Insulin stimulation of glycogen synthesis and glycogen synthase activity is blocked by wortmannin and rapamycin in 3T3-L1 adipocytes: evidence for the involvement of phosphoinositide 3-kinase and p70 ribosomal protein-S6 kinase. *Biochem J* 1995;305:25–28

16. Lazar DF, Wiese RJ, Brady MJ, et al. Mitogen-activated kinase kinase inhibition does not block the stimulation of glucose utilization by insulin. *J Biol Chem* 1995;270:20801–20807

17. Sutherland C, Waltner-Law M, Gnudi L, Kahn BB, Granner DK. Activation of the Ras mitogen-activated protein kinase-ribosomal protein kinase pathway is not required for the repression of phosphoenolpyruvate carboxykinase gene transcription by insulin. *J Biol Chem* 1998;273:3198–3204

18. Bandyopadhyay GK, Standaert ML, Zhao L, Yu B, Avignon A, Galloway L, Karnam P, Moscat J, Farese RV. Activation of protein kinase (α, β, and ξ) by insulin in 3T3-L1 cells: transfection studies suggest a role for PKC-zeta in glucose transport. *J Biol Chem* 1997;272:2551–2558

19. Sartipy P, Loskutoff DJ. Monocyte chemoattractant protein 1 in obesity and insulin resistance. *Proc Natl Acad Sci U S A* 2003;100:7265–7270

20. Ginsberg H. Insulin resistance and cardiovascular disease. *J Clin Invest* 2000;106:453–458

21. Birnbaum MJ. Turning down insulin signaling. *J Clin Invest* 2001;108:655–659

22. Aguirre V, Werner ED, Giraud J, Lee YH, Shoelson SE, White MF. Phosphorylation of Ser307 in insulin receptor substrate-1 blocks interactions with the insulin receptor and inhibits insulin action. *J Biol Chem* 2002;277:1531–1537

23. White MF. Insulin signaling in health and disease. *Science* 2003;302:1710–1711

24. Pessin JE, Saltiel AR. Signaling pathways in insulin action: molecular targets of insulin resistance. *J Clin Invest* 2000;106:165–169

25. Cheatham B, Kahn CR. Insulin action and the insulin signaling network. *Endocr Rev* 1995;16:117–141

26. Kasuga M, Karisson FA, Kahn CR. Insulin stimulates the phosphorylation of the 95,000-dalton subunit of its own receptor. *Science* 1982;215:185–187

27. Wilden PA, Siddle K, Haring E, Backer JM, White MF, Kahn CR. The role of insulin receptor-kinase domain autophosphorylation in receptor-mediated activities. *J Biol Chem* 1992;267:13719–13727

28. White MF, Shoelson SE, Keutmann H, Kahn CR. A cascade of autophosphorylation in the beta subunit activates phosphotransferase of the insulin receptor. *J Biol Chem* 1988;263:2969–2980

29. Tornqvist HE, Avruch J. Relationship of site-specific beta subunit tyrosine autophosphorylation to insulin activation of the insulin receptor (tyrosine) protein kinase activity. *J Biol Chem* 1988;263:4593–4601

30. Myers MG, White MF. Insulin signal transduction and the IRS proteins. *Annu Rev Pharmacol Toxicol* 1996;36:615–658

31. Paz K, Voliovitch H, Hadari YR, Roberts CT, LeRoith D, Zick Y. Interaction between the insulin receptor and its downstream effectors. *J Biol Chem* 1996;271: 6998–7003

32. Rhodes CJ, White MF. Molecular insights into insulin action and secretion. *Eur J Clin Invest* 2002;32(Suppl. 3):3–13

33. Petersen KF, Shulman GI. Etiology of insulin resistance. *Am J Med* 2006;119:S10–S16

34. LeRoith D, Zick Y. Recent advances in our understanding of insulin action and insulin resistance. *Diabetes Care* 2001;24:588–597

35. Kahn CR. Insulin action, diabetogenes, and the cause of type II diabetes. *Diabetes* 1994;43:1066–1084

36. Shepherd PR, Withers DJ, Siddle K. Phosphoinositide 3-kinase: the key switch mechanism in insulin signaling. *Biochem J* 1998;333:471–490

37. Yu J, Zhang Y, McIlroy J, Rordorf-Nikolic T, Orr GA, Backer JM. Regulation of the p85/p110 phosphatidylinositol 3'-kinase: stabilization and inhibition of the p110 alpha catalytic subunit by the p85 regulatory subunit. *Mol Cell Biol* 1998;18:1379–1387

38. Dhand R, Hara K, Hiles I, Bax B, Gout I, Panayotou G, Fry MJ, Yonezawa K, Kasuga M, Waterfield MD. PI 3-kinase: structural and functional analysis of inter-subunit interactions. *EMBO J* 1994;13:511–521

39. Klippel A, Escobedo JA, Hirano M, Williams LT. The interaction of small domains between the subunits of phosphatidylinositol 3-kinase determines enzyme activity. *Mol Cell Biol* 1994;14:2675–2685

40. Fu Z, Aronoff-Spencer E, Wu H, Gerfen GJ, Backer JM. The iSH2 domain of PI 3-kinase is a rigid tether for p110 and not a conformational switch. *Arch Biochem Biophys* 2004;432:244–251

41. Vivanco I, Sawyers CL. The phosphatidylinositol 3-kinase AKT pathway in human cancer. *Nat Rev Cancer* 2002;2:489–501

42. Qiao L, Goldberg JL, Russell JC, Sun XJ. Identification of enhanced serine kinase activity in insulin resistance. *J Biol Chem* 1999;274:10625–10632

43. Um SH, Frogerio F, Watanabe M, Picard F, Joaquin M, Sticker M, Fumagalli S, Allegrini PR, Kozma SC, Auwerx J, Thomas G. Absence of S6K1 protects against age- and diet-induced obesity while enhancing insulin sensitivity. *Nature* 2004;431:200–205

44. Patti ME, Kahn BB. Nutrient sensor links obesity with diabetes risk. *Nat Med* 2004;10:1049–1050

45. Qiao L, Zhande R, Jetton TL, Zhou G, Sun XJ. In vivo phosphorylation of insulin receptor substrate 1 at serine 789 by a novel serine kinase in insulin-resistant rodents. *J Biol Chem* 2002;277:26530–26539

46. Shah OJ, Wang Z, Hunter T. Inappropriate activation of the TSC/Rheb/mTOR/S6K cassette induces IRS1/2 depletion, insulin resistance, and cell survival deficiencies. *Curr Biol* 2004;14:1650–1656

47. Alessi DR, James SR, Downes CR, et al. Characterization of a 3-phosphoinositide-dependent protein kinase which phosphorylates and activates protein kinase B alpha. *Curr Biol.* 1997;7:261–269.

48. Kido Y, Burks DJ, Withers D, Bruning JC, Kahn RC, White MF, Accili D. Tissue-specific insulin resistance in mice with mutations in insulin receptor, IRS-1, and IRS-2. *J Clin Invest* 2000;105:199–205

49. Kadowaki T. Insights into insulin resistance and type 2 diabetes from knockout mouse models. *J Clin Invest* 2000;106:459–465

50. Taha C, Klip A. The insulin signaling pathway. *J Membr Biol* 1999;169:1–12

51. Egawa K, Sharma PM, Nakashima N, Huang Y, Huver E, Boss GR, Olefsky JM. Membrane-targeted phosphatidylinositol 3-kinase mimics insulin action and induces a state of cellular insulin resistance. *J Biol Chem* 1999;274:14306–14314

52. Whitehead JP, Clark SF, Urso B, James DE. Signalling through the insulin receptor. *Curr Opin Cell Biol* 2000;12:222–228

53. Copps KD, White MF. Regulation of insulin sensitivity by serine/threonine phosphorylation of insulin receptor substrate proteins IRS1 and IRS2. *Diabetologia* 2012;55:2565–2582

54. Guo S. Insulin signaling, resistance, and metabolic syndrome: insights from mouse models into disease mechanisms. *J Endocrinol* 2014;220:T1–T23

55. Sano H, Kane S, Sano E, et al. Insulin-stimulated phosphorylation of a Rab GTPase-activating protein regulates GLUT4 translocation. *J Biol Chem* 2003;278:14599–14602

56. Beurel E, Griego SF, Jope RS. Glycogen synthase kinase-3 (GSK3) regulation, action, and diseases. *Pharmacol Ther* 2015;148:114–131

57. Accili D, Arden KC. FoxOs at the crossroads of cellular metabolism, differentiation, and transformation. *Cell* 2004;117:421–426

58. Chakraborty A, Koldobskiy MA, Bello NT, et al. Inositol pyrophosphates inhibit Akt signaling, thereby regulating insulin sensitivity and weight gain. *Cell* 2010;143:897–910

59. Taylor SI. Lilly Lecture 1992: Molecular mechanisms of insulin resistance. *Diabetes* 1992;41:1473–1490

60. Semple RK, Savage DB, Cochran EK, Gorden P, O'Rahilly S. Genetic syndromes of severe insulin resistance. *Endocr Rev* 2011;32:498–514

61. Pende M, Kozma SC, Jaquet M, Oorshcot V, Burcelin R, Le Marchand-Brustel Y, Klumperman J, Thorens B, Thomas G. Hypoinsulinemia, glucose intolerance and diminished β-cell size in S6K1-deficient mice. *Nature* 2000;408:994–997

62. Tremblay F, Krebs M, Dombrowski L, Brehm A, Bernroider E, Roth E, Nowotny P, Waldhausl W, Marette A, Roden M. Overactivation of S6 kinase 1 as a cause of human insulin resistance during increased amino acid availability. *Diabetes* 2005;54:2674–2684

63. Tzatsos A, Kandor KV. Nutrients suppress phosphatidylinositol 3-kinase/Akt signaling via Raptor-dependent mTOR-mediated insulin receptor substrate 1 phosphorylation. *Mol Cell Biol* 2006;26:63–76

64. Hirosumi J, Tuncman G, Chang L, Gorzun CZ, Uysal KT, Maeda K, Karin M, Hotamisligil GS. A central role for JNK in obesity and insulin resistance. *Nature* 2002;420:333–336

65. Gao Z, Zhang X, Zuberi A, Hwang D, Quon MJ, Lefevre M, Ye J. Inhibition of insulin sensitivity by free fatty acids requires activation of multiple serine kinases in 3T3-L1 adipocytes. *Mol Endocrinol* 2004;18:2024–2034

66. Nguyen MTA, Satoh H, Favelyukis S, Babendure JL, Imamura T, Sbodio JI, Zalevsky J, Dahiyat B, Chi N-W, Olefsky JM. JNK and tumor necrosis factor-

alpha mediate free fatty acid-induced insulin resistance in 3T3-L1 adipocytes. *J Biol Chem* 2005;280:35361–35371

67. Bandyopadhyay GK, Yu JG, Ofrecio J, Olefsky JM. Increased p85/55/50 expression and decreased phosphatidylinositol 3-kinase activity in insulin-resistant human skeletal muscle. *Diabetes* 2005;54:2351–2359

68. Mussig K, Fiedler H, Staiger H, Weigert C, Lehmann R, Schleicher ED, Häring HU. Insulin-induced stimulation of JNK and the PI 3-kinase/mTOR pathway leads to phosphorylation of serine 318 of IRS-1 in C2C12 myotubes. *Biochem Biophys Res Commun* 2005;335:819–825

69. Hiratani K, Haruta T, Tani A, Kawahara J, Usui I, Kobayashi M. Roles of mTOR and JNK in serine phosphorylation, translocation, and degradation of IRS-1. *Biochem Biophys Res Commun* 2005;335:836–842

70. Yuan M, Konstantopoulos N, Lee J, Hansen L, Li ZW, Karin M, Shoelson SE. Reversal of obesity- and diet-induced insulin resistance with salicylates or targeted disruption of IKK-beta. *Science* 2001;293:1673–1677

71. Perseghin G, Petersen K, Shulman GI. Cellular mechanism of insulin resistance: potential links with inflammation. *Int J Obes Relat Metab Disord* 2003;27(Suppl. 3):S6–11

72. Gao Z, Hwang D, Bataille F, Lefevre, York D, Quon MJ, Ye J. Serine phosphorylation of insulin receptor substrate 1 by inhibitor kB kinase complex. *J Biol Chem* 2002;277:48115–48121

73. Kim JK, Kim Y-J, Fillmore JJ, Chen Y, Moore I, Lee J, Yuan M, Li ZW, Karin M, Perret P, Shoelson SE, Shulman GI. Prevention of fat-induced insulin resistance by salicylate. *J Clin Invest* 2001;108:437–446

74. Hundal RS, Petersen KF, Mayerson AB, Rahdhawa PS, Inzucchi S, Shoelson SE, Shulman GI. Mechanism by which high-dose aspirin improves glucose metabolism in type 2 diabetes. *J Clin Invest* 2002;109:1321–1326

75. Kim F, Tysseling KA, Rice J, Gallis B, Haji L, Giachelli CM, Raines EW, Corson MA, Schwartz MW. Activation of IKKβ by glucose is necessary and sufficient to impair insulin signaling and nitric oxide production in endothelial cells. *Mol Cell Cardiol* 2005;39:327–334

76. Hotamisligil GS, Peraldi P, Budavari A, Ellis R, White MF, Spiegelman BM. IRS-1-mediated inhibition of insulin receptor tyrosine kinase activity in TNF-alpha and obesity-induced insulin resistance. *Science* 1996;271:665–668

77. Li Y, Soos TJ, Li X, Wu J, Degennaro M, Sun X, Littman DR, Birnbaum MJ, Polakiewicz RD. Protein kinase C theta inhibits insulin signaling by phosphory-lating IRS1 at Ser(1101). *J Biol Chem* 2004;279:45304–45307

78. Bell KS, Shcmitz-Peiffer C, Lim-Fraser M, Biden TJ, Cooney GJ, Kraegen EW. Acute reversal of lipid-induced muscle insulin resistance is associated with rapid alteration in PKC-θ localization. *Am J Physiol Endocrinol Metab* 2000;279:E1196–E1201

79. Semple RK, Halberg NH, Burling K, et al. Paradoxical elevation of high-molecu-lar wright adiponectin in acquired extreme insulin resistance due to insulin recep-tor antibodies. *Diabetes* 2007;56:1712–1717

80. Antuna-Puente B, Boutet E, Vigouroux C, et al. Higher adiponectin levels in patients with Berardinelli-Seip congenital lipodystrophy due to seipin as com-pared with 1-acylglycerol-3-phosphate-o-acyltransferase-2 deficiency. *J Clin Endocrinol Metab* 2010;95:1463–1468

81. Hattori Y, Hirama N, Suzuli K, Hattori S, Kasai K. Elevated plasma adiponectin and leptin levels in sisters with genetically defective insulin receptors. *Diabetes Care* 2007;30:e109

82. Semple RK, Sleigh A, Murgatroyd PR, et al. Postreceptor insulin resistance contrib-utes to human dyslipidemia and hepatic steatosis. *J Clin Invest* 2009;119:315–322

83. Musso C, Cochran E, Moran SA, et al. Clinical course of genetic diseases of the insulin receptor (type A and Rabson-Mendenhall syndromes): a 30-year pro-spective. *Medicine (Baltimore)* 2004;83:209–222

84. Sasaoka T, Rose DW, Jhun BH, Saltiel AR, Draznin B, Olefsky JM. Evidence for a functional role of Shc proteins in mitogenic signaling induced by insulin, insulin-like growth factor-1, and epidermal growth factor. *J Biol Chem* 1994;269:13689–13694

85. Ish-Shalom D, Christoffersen CT, Vorwerk P, et al. Mitogenic properties of insulin and insulin analogs mediated by the insulin receptor. *Diabetologia* 1977;40(Suppl. 2): S25–S31

86. Leitner JW, Kline T, Carel K, Goalstone ML, Draznin B. Hyperinsulinemia potentiates activation of p21Ras by growth factors. *Endocrinology* 1997;138:2211–2214

87. Goalstone ML, Draznin B. Effect of insulin on farnesyltransferase activity in 3T3-L1 adipocytes. *J Biol Chem* 1996;271:27585–27589

88. Goalstone ML, Carel K, Leitner JW, Draznin B. Insulin stimulates the phosphorylation and activity of farnesyltransferase via the Ras-Map kinase pathway. *Endocrinology* 1997;138:5119–5124

89. Muntoni S, Muntoni S, Draznin B. Effects of chronic hyperinsulinemia in insulin-resistant patients. *Curr Diab Rep* 2008;8:233–238

90. Draznin B. Mitogenic action of insulin: friend, foe or 'frenemy'? *Diabetologia* 2010;53:229–233

91. Semple RK. EJE PRIZE 2015:How does insulin resistance arise, and how does it cause disease? Human genetic lessons. *Eur J Endocrinol* 2016;174:R209–R223

92. Flier JS, Kahn CR, Roth J, Bar RS. Antibodies that impair insulin receptor binding in an unusual diabetic syndrome with severe insulin resistance. *Science* 1975;190:63–65

93. Kahn CR, Flier JS, Bar RS, et al. The syndromes of insulin resistance and acanthosis nigricans. Insulin receptor disorders in man. *New Engl J Med* 1976;294:739–745

94. Barbieri RL, Ryan KJ. Hyperandrogenism, insulin resistance, and acanthosis nigricans syndrome: a common endocrinopathy with distinct pathophysiologic features. *Am J Obstet Gynecol* 1983;147:90–101

95. Rabson SM, Mendenhall EN. Familial hypertrophy of pineal body, hyperplasia of adrenal cortex and diabetes mellitus; report of 3 cases. *Am J Clin Pathol* 1956;26:283–290

96. Donohue WL, Uchida I. Leprechaunism: a euphemism for a rare familial disorder. *J Pediatr* 1954;45:505–519

97. Ogilvy-Stuart AL, Soos MA, Hands SJ, et al. Hypoglycemia and resistance to ketoacidosis in a subject without functional insulin receptors. *J Clin Endocrinol Metab* 2001;86:3319–3326

98. George S, Rochford JJ, Wolfrum C, et al. A family with severe insulin resistance and diabetes due to a mutation in Akt2. *Science* 2004;304:1325–1328

99. Dash S, Sano H, Rochford JJ, et al. A truncation mutation in TBC1D4 in a family with acanthosis nigricans and postprandial hyperinsulinemia. *Proc Natl Acad Sci U S A* 2009;106:9350–9355

100. Cochran E, Musso C, Gorden P. The use of U-500 in patients with extreme insulin resistance. *Diabetes Care* 2005;28:1240–1244

101. Lane WS. Use of U-500 regular insulin by continuous subcutaneous insulin infusion in patients with type 2 diabetes and severe insulin resistance. *Endocr Pract* 2006;12:251–256

102. Nakae J, Kato M, Murashita M, et al. Long-term effect of recombinant human insulin-like growth factor 1 on metabolic and growth control in a patient with leprechaunism. *J Clin Endocrinol Metab* 1998;83:542–549

103. Vestergaard H, Rossen M, Urhammer SA, Muller J, Pedersen O. Short- and long-term metabolic effects of recombinant human IGF-1 treatment in patients with severe insulin resistance and diabetes mellitus. *Eur J Endocrinol* 1997;136: 475–482

104. Kuzuya H, Matsuura N, Sakamoto M, et al. Trial of insulin-like growth factor 1 therapy for patients with extreme insulin resistance syndromes. *Diabetes* 1993;42:696–705

105. Zenobi PD, Glatz Y, Keller A, et al. Beneficial metabolic effects of insulin-like growth factor 1 in patients with severe insulin resistant diabetes type A. *Eur J Endocrinol* 1994;131:251–257

106. Weber DR, Stanescu DE, Semple R, et al. Continuous subcutaneous IGF-1 therapy via insulin pump in a patient with Donohue syndrome. *J Pediatr Endocrinol Metab* 2014;27:1237–1241

107. Moreira RO, Zagury RL, Nascimento TS, Zagury L. Multidrug therapy in a patient with Rabson-Mendenhall syndrome. *Diabetologia* 2010;53:2454–2455

3
The Lipodystrophy Syndromes: Clinical Features and Treatments

Megan Mattingly, RN, MPH;[1] Areli Valencia, BA;[1] Elaine Cochran, MSN, CRNP;[1] Rebecca J. Brown, MD, MHS;[1] and Phillip Gorden, MD[1]

The Lipodystrophies

The lipodystrophies are a heterogeneous group of conditions characterized by loss of adipose tissue and, usually, metabolic disturbance. They are subdivided into generalized and partial forms with further subdivision into congenital (gene mutations) or acquired (autoimmune) forms.[1-11]

Considerable progress has been made in describing new genetic abnormalities in both the generalized (GLD) and partial lipodystrophies (PLD). Historically, the genetic forms of GLD have been referred to as the Berardinelli-Seip syndrome, but are more appropriately characterized by their genetic etiology. There are several forms of PLD, appropriately referred to by their genetic etiology when known (Table 3.1). Patients with a familial inheritance pattern of PLD whose genes have yet to be identified are referred to as the Köbberling variety of familial partial lipodystrophy (FPL).

Patients with acquired lipodystrophy may have other autoimmune conditions (Table 3.2). The most definite association is with juvenile dermatomyositis.[29]

---

[1]Diabetes, Endocrinology and Obesity Branch, National Institute of Diabetes and Digestive and Kidney Diseases, National Institutes of Health, Bethesda, MD

DOI: 10.2337/9781580406666.03

Table 3.1—Genetic Forms of Lipodystrophy

Type of Lipodystrophy	Associated Genetic Mutations	Alternative Names	Inheritance Pattern	Reference
Congenital Generalized Lipodystrophy (CGL)	AGPAT2	CGL1, BSCL1	AR	12
	BSCL2	CGL2, BSCL2	AR	13
	CAV1	CGL3	AR (single case)	14
	PTRF	CGL4	AR	15
Familial Partial Lipodystrophy (FPL)	Unknown	FPL Type 1, Köbberling variety	Usually AD	16
	LMNA	FPL Type 2, Dunnigan variety	AD	17,18
	PPARγ	FPL Type 3	AD	19
	PLIN1	FPL Type 4	AD	20
	CIDEC	FPL Type 5	AR (single case)	21
	LIPE	FPL Type 6	AR	22,23
Atypical Progeria/ Mandibuloacral Dysplasia (MAD)	LMNA, ZMPSTE24, others	MAD Type A, MAD Type B, others	AD, AR, de novo	24,25
Uncommon Forms	PCYT1A	-	AR	26
	ADRA2A	-	AD	27
	AKT2	-	AD	14
	PI3K	SHORT syndrome	AD	28

AR, Autosomal recessive; AD, Autosomal dominant; BSCL, Berardinelli-Seip Congenital Lipodystrophy

Table 3.2—Autoimmune Conditions Associated with Acquired Forms of Lipodystrophy

Autoimmune thyroiditis or marker autoantibodies
Autoimmune hepatitis
Type 1 diabetes or marker autoantibodies (GAD, etc.)
Lymphoma[33]
Vitiligo
Renal disease[34]

However, features of lipodystrophy may also appear in conditions such as lupus.[30] Patients also frequently present with panniculitis; characteristically it starts in the distal extremities and progresses proximally. Thus, varying periods of times may elapse between the initial appearance of lipodystrophy and the complete generalized form. The Barraquer-Simons syndrome refers to a form of acquired PLD that usually is not associated with metabolic complications but is associated with nephritis, thrombocytopenia, and other forms of immune dysfunction.[30] PLD can also be associated with HIV infection. In this circumstance, the lipodystrophy results from specific protease inhibitors used to treat the viral condition.[31,32]

From our experience at the National Institutes of Health (NIH), over 95% of patients with congenital generalized lipodystrophies (CGLs) have mutations in 1-acylglycerol-3-phosphate O-acyltransferase 2 (AGPAT2) or Berardinelli-Seip congenital lipodystrophy 2 (BSCL2), and the other major types of GLD are the acquired forms. Other rare genetic causes of CGL include mutations in polymerase I and transcript release factor and CAV1.[14,15]

The most frequent genetic causes of FPL are mutations in LMNA (Dunnigan form) or PPARγ. Most other patients with FPL have the Köbberling variety, although rarer genetic causes are described, including mutations in PLIN1,[20] CIDEC,[21] LIPE,[23] and AKT2.[35]

Another example of lipodystrophy occurring within a syndrome of insulin resistance is the SHORT syndrome, an autosomal dominant disorder that has been associated with mutations in PI3-kinase.[36,37] There are also a number of lipodystrophy syndromes that fall under the category of progeroid diseases (Table 3.1).

In this chapter, we will emphasize: *1*) clinical features of various lipodystrophies, *2*) metabolic disturbances that characterize the lipodystrophies, *3*) nonmetabolic features that characterize lipodystrophies, and *4*) conventional, and especially, novel therapies for metabolic complications of lipodystrophy.

The lipodystrophy syndromes represent an extreme form of the obesity-related metabolic syndrome, but by contrast with obesity, lipodystrophy syndromes offer an opportunity to define an etiologic basis for metabolic disease, and therefore, pursue a precision form of therapy (Figure 3.1).[38] The similarity in the obesity-related metabolic syndrome and the lipodystrophies is striking. The most fundamental feature underlying insulin resistance and dyslipidemia in lipodystrophy and in the common obesity-associated metabolic syndrome is excess energy storage, result-

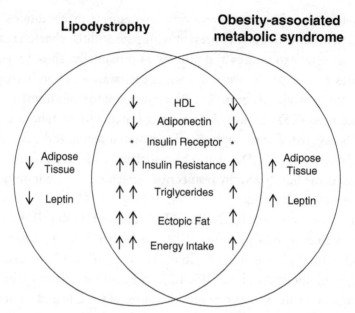

Figure 3.1 — Similarities and differences between lipodystrophy and obesity.

*Regulated insulin receptor gene expression such that high insulin levels results in low insulin receptor expression and vice-versa
Source: Bar RS et al.[40]

ing from excessive energy intake relative to expenditure. In the lipodystrophy syndromes, the cause of hyperphagia has a clear biological underpinning: leptin deficiency. In obesity, circulating leptin levels are high, but there appears to be a form of relative leptin resistance such that high circulating leptin levels do not appropriately limit nutrient intake. It is possible that there is a disorder of adipose tissue that diverts lipid stores to ectopic sites. This is certainly true in animal models and is a fruitful area for clinical investigation.[39]

The discovery of leptin provided the first genetic basis for hyperphagia, and most genes related to eating behavior are in this pathway. This includes the leptin receptor, proopiomelanocortin, and melanocortin-4.[41]

Clinical Features

Generalized

Most often the congenital generalized forms of lipodystrophy are diagnosed at birth or within the first year of life.[3] At the NIH, the majority (41 of

50) of patients with CGL presented as children or adolescents. Patients with acquired forms of lipodystrophy also usually present in childhood or adolescence, but loss of adipose tissue can appear at any age.

GLDs are characterized by near-total deficiency of subcutaneous body fat, including the face, body, and extremities. However, there are subtle differences in fat distribution based on genotype. For instance, in the BSCL2 mutations, there may be loss of mechanical fat in the hands and feet so that there is a marked reduction in the volume of the thenar and hypothenar eminence of the hands, and increased callouses in the feet with loss of the arch (Figure 3.2). In the AGPAT2 mutation, there is preservation of mechanical fat in the face, hands, and feet, with enlargement of the hands and feet leading to an acromegaloid appearance (Figure 3.3). However, in both forms there is a reduction in total body fat.

Additional physical features include umbilical prominence, splenomegaly, and hepatomegaly.[3] Hepatomegaly resulting from severe steatosis is common and may progress to steatohepatitis, cirrhosis, and liver failure.[3] Plain X-rays may demonstrate cysts in long bones (most common in AGPAT2 mutations but also may be seen in BSCL2 mutations).[42] Because of the loss of fat and muscle hypertrophy, lipodystrophy syndromes are usually distinguishable from

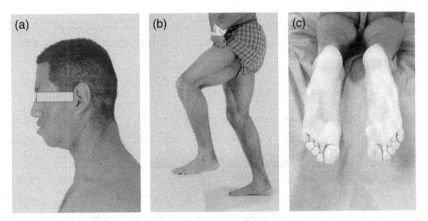

Figure 3.2—Phenotype of *BSCL2* mutation.

Physical phenotype of male with generalized lipodystrophy due to autosomal recessive *BSCL2* mutation (a/b). This mutation is associated with loss of mechanical fat in the thenar and hypothenar eminences of the hands and soles of the feet (c).

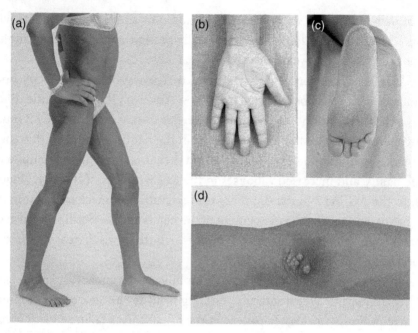

Figure 3.3—Phenotype of *AGPAT2* mutation.

Physical phenotype of female with generalized lipodystrophy due to autosomal recessive *AGPAT2* mutation. There is a reduction in total body fat (a), but this mutation is associated with an actual increase of fat in the hands (b) and feet (c). Due to hyperlipidemia, eruptive xanthomata may appear as shown in a patient's elbow (d).

other conditions such as various cachectic syndromes. Females with CGL may have irregular menstrual periods, polycystic ovaries, infertility, clitoromegaly, and hirsutism.[3,11]

Partial

In the partial forms of lipodystrophy, there is typically preservation of certain fat depots, particularly in the head, neck, and torso, with loss of fat in the extremities, resembling Cushing's syndrome.[10,11] The reason for this fat distribution is unknown. PLD patients sometimes come to medical attention because of abnormal fat distribution, but more often present with metabolic derangements. In some cases, patients with partial forms of lipodystrophy may present a diagnostic dilemma. For instance, some of these patients are actually obese with a BMI of 30 kg/m² or greater, and others are overweight (BMI 25–29). In the NIH cohort, 38% of PLD patients were overweight and 23%

had BMI >30. As mentioned above, there are other conditions that may simulate these partial forms of lipodystrophy, such as Cushing's syndrome, but also other obesity-related conditions where there appears to be a greater degree of central obesity than is seen in the extremities.[43] Patients with PLD, however, may be distinguished by the complete deficiency of subcutaneous fat in certain depots (most commonly the buttocks and legs), as opposed to simply a decreased amount of fat in these depots relative to the trunk and abdomen.

Other Distinguishing Features of the Lipodystrophy Syndromes

In both partial and generalized types of lipodystrophy, we can see the following additional clinical features: eruptive xanthomata, hirsutism, and acanthosis nigricans. These are all secondary features of hypertriglyceridemia and insulin resistance.

There is an important sexual dimorphism because female patients predominate in both the generalized and partial forms. Two recent natural history studies of GLD, done in Brazil and Turkey, reported about 61% female[44] and 54% female patients,[42] respectively. This is partially due to a referral bias, as females generally have a more severe metabolic derangement and requirement for treatment. In some instances where siblings of both sexes present, only the female sibling requires treatment. Further, it is more difficult to distinguish PLD in males, who might simply appear to have some degree of muscle hypertrophy. Female patients may also present at the time of puberty with signs or symptoms of hyperandrogenism and other features of polycystic ovarian syndrome.

Metabolic Features

The most common metabolic complications of both GLD and PLD are summarized in Figure 3.4.[45]

The primary physiologic abnormality in lipodystrophy is diminished subcutaneous adipose tissue. This deficiency leads to low levels of the adipocyte-derived hormones such as adiponectin and leptin (Figure 3.5).

Low leptin is sensed by the hypothalamus as a signal of starvation, resulting in hyperphagia. The excess energy consumed cannot be accommodated in adipose tissue, and therefore is accumulated as ectopic fat in liver and muscle tissue, which correlates strongly with insulin resistance. It is important to note

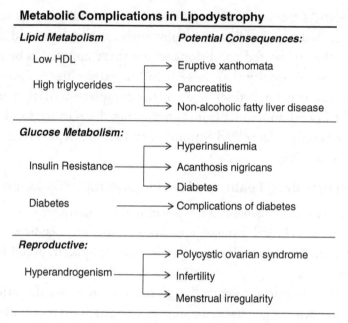

Figure 3.4—Metabolic complications of lipodystrophy.

that hyperphagia may not be recognized in these patients without a careful history because they do not become obese (especially in the generalized form).

Lipid Abnormalities

Hypertriglyceridemia associated with excessive ectopic fat accumulation is the most characteristic metabolic feature of the lipodystrophies. The other distinct lipid abnormality is a low concentration of high-density lipoprotein-cholesterol (HDL-c).[46] Other lipids such as total cholesterol may be moderately elevated, but are not particularly remarkable in this disorder. These features are all common to the obesity-associated metabolic syndrome, but are more extreme in the lipodystrophies (Figure 3.3).

Although elevated serum triglycerides are characteristic of the lipodystrophies, there is considerable heterogeneity from patient to patient, but the degree of abnormality is similar in the GLD and PLD patients.[45] Patients with the most extreme hypertriglyceridemia may have eruptive xanthomata appear on multiple sites. Pancreatitis and nonalcoholic fatty liver disease (NAFLD) are also frequently seen as consequences of hypertriglyceridemia.

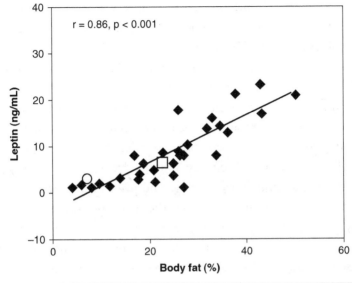

	Generalized Lipodystrophy ○ (n = 55)	Partial Lipodystrophy □ (n = 31)	P value
Body Fat (%)	9 ± 2	22 ± 4	< 0.001
Leptin (ng/mL)	1.13 ± 0.74	6.23 ± 3.96	< 0.001

Data are mean ± SD. Mean percent body fat and leptin levels for generalized and partial lipodystrophy are plotted in the graph above.

Figure 3.5—Leptin concentration correlates with percent body fat.

The bases for the disordered triglyceride metabolism, based on animal models, are abnormalities in transcription factors and enzymes that regulate triglyceride synthesis. More recently, however, other factors such as apolipoprotein CIII and the angiopoietin-like factors that regulate triglyceride breakdown via lipolysis have been identified.[47,48]

Glucose Abnormalities

Lipodystrophy patients are almost uniformly insulin resistant. The mechanism of insulin resistance in this class of diseases is not completely clear, but it correlates strongly with ectopic fat deposition in liver and muscle. We see a dichotomy in insulin action with the extreme insulin resistance in lipodystrophy.[49] Patients are resistant to the glucose regulatory effects of insulin, meaning they have impaired insulin-mediated suppression of hepatic glucose production and deficient uptake of glucose in muscle. Yet, insulin is fully active in stimulating lipid production/synthesis; consequently, we observe high serum triglycerides and accumulation of ectopic fat. The prevalence of diabetes in these patients is high as expected. However, as in all diabetic syndromes, the expression of hyperglycemia is a function of diminished insulin secretion. While in rodent models a form of lipotoxicity from ectopic lipid in the pancreas may impair insulin secretion, it is not clear that this is relevant to the human lipodystrophies.[50] These patients are susceptible to the microvascular complications of diabetes, and as in all diabetic patients, these microvascular complications are a function of the duration and severity of hyperglycemia. Since many patients come to medical attention at a young age and prior to the time they develop hyperglycemia, they have not developed these complications. We have seen retinopathy, neuropathy, nephropathy, and even extremity amputations in a few cases in the NIH cohort. Renal disease, discussed further below, may be seen in these patients, but the most common form is not diabetic nephropathy.

Reproductive Abnormalities

In GLD, there are two fundamental disorders of the reproductive system in women. The first is an abnormality of gonadotropin secretion, leading to partial hypogonadotropic hypogonadism. Women with GLD undergo normal pubertal development, but often have primary or secondary amenorrhea or oligomenorrhea.[51] The failure to develop menarche or regular cycles results from the absence of the normal ultradian rhythm of LH secretion due to leptin deficiency.[52,53] The second abnormality relates to the features of the polycystic ovary syndrome (PCOS), which is primarily due to insulin resistance and hyperinsulinemia.[54,55] Under these circumstances the ovary shifts sex steroid synthesis to the production of androgens, and this is associated with the polycystic enlargement of the ovary. Women with GLD are usually infertile with rare exceptions.[51,56] Following leptin therapy, ovulation and fertility can be restored and several pregnancies have resulted in the NIH cohort.[57] In contrast to the female patients, male patients appear to progress through the phases of puberty in a relatively normal manner, though their fertility is not clear.[51]

In PLD there may be subfertility analogous to the general population with PCOS, but because leptin levels are higher, they do not appear to have partial hypogonadotropic hypogonadism. In our experience, it is not uncommon for women to have one or more children.

Other Endocrine Features

Both the hypothalamic-pituitary-thyroid axis and the hypothalamic-pituitary-adrenal axis appear to function in a normal manner in patients with lipodystrophy.[52,58] Though there is no specific abnormality in the growth hormone – insulin-like growth factor-1 (IGF-1) axis in lipodystrophy patients, there is an increase in IGF-1 levels following leptin replacement therapy. This increase in IGF-1 appears to be a consequence of improved insulin sensitivity, as IGF-1 is lower in insulin-resistant states.[2,54]

Other Organ-specific Diseases

Other organ-specific diseases are summarized in Figure 3.6.

Liver

The most characteristic liver disease seen in GLD and PLD is NAFLD.[2,59] Over 80% of our patients with GLD and PLD have non-alcoholic steatohepatitis (NASH), which is a precursor to further liver disease, including cirrhosis and end-

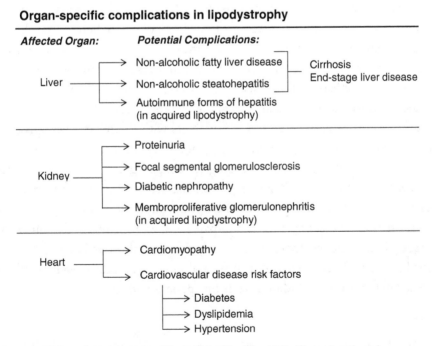

Figure 3.6—Organ-specific complications in lipodystrophy.

stage liver disease (ESLD). Patients with the BSCL2 mutation appear to be particularly prone to developing advanced liver disease at an early age. In fact, four of our 15 patients with BSCL2 mutation have died of ESLD. These patients came to our attention when they had already developed advanced liver disease, and an open question is whether this might have been prevented with leptin replacement. It is clear that the pathologic features of inflammation and oxidative stress can be ameliorated by leptin replacement.[59,60]

While NASH is the predominant form of liver disease in lipodystrophy, patients with acquired forms of lipodystrophy may also have autoimmune hepatitis (AIH) related to their general autoimmune condition.[59] It is important for clinicians to recognize that both NASH and AIH may be present simultaneously, as the therapies for these conditions are different. We have seen patients who appear to respond to therapy for NASH but who developed portal hypertension secondary to AIH. Other forms of liver disease, such as chronic viral hepatitis, may be seen in these patients as well.[2,59]

Kidney/Renal Disease

Renal disease is common in patients with GLD and the most common manifestation is proteinuria.[61] At least two-thirds of our patients have clinical grade proteinuria and upwards of one-third of patients may have nephrotic range proteinuria. In part, the severe proteinuria results from hyperfiltration that is characteristic of insulin resistance. This type of proteinuria may be ameliorated by those measures used to treat the metabolic disorder.

Renal biopsies performed in CGL patients with the most severe proteinuria have shown that the predominant pathology is focal segmental glomerular sclerosis. In patients with acquired generalized lipodystrophy (AGL), we have seen membrano-proliferative glomerular nephritis.[34,61] While diabetic nephropathy does occur in patients with lipodystrophy, it is not the most common form of renal disease. This may in part be due to the relatively young age of these patients; hence, there is a relatively short duration of diabetes. Kidney transplants have been carried out in several of our patients as well as others reported in literature, including at least one patient with PLD.[62,63]

Heart

Lipodystrophy patients have numerous risk factors for cardiovascular disease, including dyslipidemia, diabetes, and hypertension. It is likely that these patients have premature cardiovascular disease. However, the most striking cardiac manifestation of CGL is cardiomyopathy rather than vascular disease.[64,65] The lack of severe vascular disease in our CGL patients may relate to their relatively young age. Cardiomyopathy in CGL tends to be more severe in those patients with the BSCL2 mutation,[64] although one of our patients with the AGPAT2 mutation required cardiac transplantation. More severe forms of cardiomyopathy are also seen in patients with progeroid forms of lipodystrophy.[66,67]

Treatment

Conventional therapies are summarized in Table 3.3.

Standard therapies have been utilized in treating patients with GLD with modest effects. The fundamental treatment for patients with GLD centers on diet. An ideal diet for children over the age of two is comprised of 55% carbohydrate, 20% protein, and 25% fat (1/3 monounsaturated, 1/3 polyunsaturated, 1/3 saturated fats). Children need appropriate caloric intake to support growth. This must be done with caution because both excess fat and carbohydrate may promote hyperlipidemia. In addition, excess caloric intake will lead to increased triglyceride synthesis and potentially increase hepatic steatosis in these patients. The weight goals for growing children need to be tempered against the fact that children with GLD do not have adipose tissue, and their weight may therefore be lower than peers of the same age and sex. Typically,

Table 3.3—Standard Treatments for Lipodystrophy

Dysfunction	Specific Treatment	Overall Treatment
Diabetes	Metformin Insulin Thiazolidinediones (PLD only)	Diet Metreleptin (Leptin replacement therapy)
Hypertriglyceridemia	Fibrates Statins Omega-3 fatty acids	
Renal complications (Proteinuria)	Angiotensin-converting enzyme (ACE) inhibitors	

PLD, Partial Lipodystrophy

caloric needs in patients with GLD are 1,800–2,200 calories/day after peak growth has been achieved.[1]

Regarding diabetes therapy, metformin has been used effectively in children as early as 6 months of age, although its use is off-label in children under 10 years of age. Doses we employ are 40–60 mg/kg/day for children less than 30 kg. For children and adults greater than 30 kg, doses of 2 g daily are well tolerated after a gradual dose escalation. Thiazolidinediones have been used in patients with PLD but should not be used in GLD because of their potential to promote steatosis (demonstrated in rodent models).[68,69] Other hypoglycemic agents such as sulfonylureas, acarbose, or GLP-1 analogs have not been used extensively in lipodystrophy.

In cases where glycemic targets are not met with oral agents, exogenous insulin is indicated. Because of the patients' degree of insulin resistance, this form of diabetes often requires >3 units/kg/day. Thus, concentrated U-500 insulin is the most efficient and effective form of insulin in patients with lipodystrophy, and is especially useful in patients who lack subcutaneous tissue and require large volumes of insulin. Insulin glargine should be avoided in these patients since it requires formation of a crystal structure in adipose to provide its long-acting property.

Standard therapies to treat the severe hypertriglyceridemia of lipodystrophy include fibrates, statins, and omega-3 fatty acids.

Given the background of diabetes and proteinuria, medications such as ACE inhibitors are recommended to protect the kidneys.

In women with oligomenorrhea or amenorrhea, caution is recommended in the use of exogenous estrogen, particularly in oral formulations, as this may lead to a significant rise in triglycerides. In women needing contraception, barrier methods are best tolerated, but progesterone delivered through intrauterine devices has also been useful with minimal adverse effects on blood triglyceride levels.

Leptin Discovery and Pharmaceutical Development

In 1994 Dr. Jeffrey Friedman discovered leptin.[70] Leptin is produced and secreted by fat cells, and blood concentration is a function of the adipose tissue mass. While the existence of a circulating factor that regulates food intake had long been postulated by the work of Coleman in the *ob/ob* mouse,[71] the identity of the protein now allowed for its production and preparation of a pharmaceutical, metreleptin (Myalept).

Leptin Replacement in Generalized Lipodystrophy

Following the failure of metreleptin treatment in clinical trials of patients with obesity, in which circulating leptin levels are high due to the expanded fat mass,[72] the focus shifted to use of metreleptin in conditions with low circulating leptin levels. In extremely rare patients with congenital leptin deficiency due to leptin gene mutations, metreleptin treatment normalized hyperphagia, hypothalamic dysfunction, and body weight.[58,73] Lipodystrophy is another condition associated with low leptin levels, and because of our center for the study of syndromic forms of insulin resistance, we were positioned to examine metreleptin efficacy in this population.

From 2000 to 2014, 55 patients with GLD were treated with metreleptin at the NIH Clinical Center. Ultimately, this study led to the February 2014 FDA approval of metreleptin for the treatment of generalized forms of lipodystrophy. In the first seven patients treated at the NIH, and two additional patients treated at the University of Texas Southwestern Medical Center, it quickly became apparent that metreleptin was remarkably effective in controlling metabolic derangements that had not responded to conventional therapy.[74] This was further confirmed in subsequent studies.[45,75,76]

The overall responses to metreleptin are shown in Table 3.4. Patients reported a sense of satiety and satiation as an initial response to metreleptin

Table 3.4 — Summary of the Effects of Metreleptin Treatment on Generalized Lipodystrophy

Clinical Parameter	Major Effects
Appetite	Decreased
Body weight	Decreased
Insulin resistance	Decreased
Diabetes	Decreased A1C Decreased insulin doses
Hypertriglyceridemia	Decreased
Steatohepatitis	Improved
Reproduction (in females)	Normalized menstrual cycles Increased fertility Decrease to normalization of androgen production
Kidney disease	Decreased hyperfiltration Decreased protein excretion

therapy.[77] This may result in some weight loss over the first 4–6 months of therapy, with stabilization thereafter.[78] The next major effects of metreleptin treatment are improvement in the marked dyslipidemia, including extreme elevation of triglycerides in serum and ectopic tissues,[79] as well as in insulin resistance and diabetes. In addition, in young women, metreleptin decreases androgen production and normalizes gonadotropin secretion.[53,54] Metreleptin does not ameliorate the low HDL-C levels observed in patients with GLD. This is in contrast to treatments for the obesity-related metabolic syndromes, which increase HDL-C levels reciprocally with reductions in triglycerides.[46] As mentioned previously, NASH is common in patients with GLD, and metreleptin improves the NASH score and produces some degree of stabilization in patients with more advanced fibrosis.[59] Additionally, proteinuria may significantly improve with metreleptin therapy.[34,61]

Japanese investigators, using the NIH protocol, demonstrated the same favorable response of metreleptin in their lipodystrophy patients, and their studies led to approval of metreleptin therapy for all types of lipodystrophy in Japan.[80,81]

Metreleptin Administration

Prior to initiation of metreleptin therapy, conventional therapies should be optimized. Providers located in the United States who prescribe metreleptin therapy are required to enroll in the Myalept Injection Risk Evaluation and Mitigation Strategy (REMS) program. REMS is a strategy to manage known or potential serious risks associated with a drug product and is required by the FDA to ensure that the benefits of a drug outweigh its risks.

The greatest barrier to metraleptin efficacy in patients with GLD is patient/family nonadherence to the prescribed regimen. Although this nonadherence can occur at any age, it is most notable during the teenage years. To minimize nonadherence, providers must work closely with the patient/family on the dosing and regimen; use of an 8-mm injection needle is recommended to penetrate their thick epidermis but avoid an intramuscular injection. Although once-daily regimens are helpful when compliance is an issue, twice-daily regimens may be more effective in producing the desired physiologic effects of leptin replacement. Exogenous insulin therapy may be necessary when metreleptin therapy is initiated. U-500 insulin is the best form of insulin to administer to this group of patients as a 2–3 injection/day regimen. Some patients may be able to discontinue exogenous insulin therapy completely after metreleptin therapy is established.[45]

While metreleptin has not been approved for use in pregnant women, several pregnancies have occurred in patients receiving metreleptin. Metreleptin was continued at prepregnancy doses during pregnancy and lactation without obvious teratogenicity.[57]

Safety and Tolerability

Safety data submitted as part of the FDA approval of metreleptin were based on 100 patients with GLD or PLD treated with metreleptin at NIH and other sites, as well as safety data from clinical trials in over 500 obese patients.[72]

The most frequent treatment-related adverse events were weight loss, abdominal pain, hypoglycemia, fatigue, headache, decreased appetite, and injection site reactions (bruising and urticaria). In the instances of hypoglycemia, patients were on concomitant exogenous insulin therapy or insulin secretagogues. Dose adjustments or cessation of exogenous insulin therapy may be necessary. Such patients need to closely monitor their blood glucose with initiation of metreleptin therapy and/or any increases in metreleptin dose.

Hypersensitivity reactions (urticaria, rash, anaphylaxis) have been observed and need to be reported promptly to the provider. In our experience with cutaneous reactions, antihistamine medications were effective. Occasionally, temporary dose reductions in metreleptin may be needed. The provider needs to note that due to a lack of subcutaneous fat, metreleptin injection will normally cause a raised bleb under the skin, which slowly diminishes as the medication is absorbed. Worrisome injection site reactions have redness that persists for at least 6 hours (often more than 24 hours), itch, and recur with each injection.

The metreleptin U.S. label has two boxed warnings. The first is the risk of neutralizing antibodies. Anti-metreleptin antibodies with *in vitro* neutralizing activity have been identified in a small number of patients treated with metreleptin. These antibodies may lead to a loss of efficacy of metreleptin and carry a theoretical risk of inhibiting the activity of endogenous leptin. The latter effect could induce a phenotype similar to congenital leptin deficiency; however, it likely has little clinical relevance in patients with GLD, who have very low endogenous leptin. Severe infections (sepsis) were observed in two patients in the NIH study who developed *in vitro* neutralizing antibodies to leptin. However, both patients had risk factors for sepsis (advanced cirrhosis and poor dental hygiene), and thus it remains unclear if antibodies to leptin increase the risk of sepsis in patients without underlying risk factors. Risks of neutralizing antibodies to leptin should be weighed by the provider along with the benefits of therapy.[82]

T-cell lymphoma has been reported in patients with acquired GLD. Three cases of T-cell lymphoma occurred in patients receiving metreleptin therapy. One patient with a pretherapy cutaneous lesion progressed to T-cell lymphoma while on treatment. Lymphoma has also been reported in AGL patients who have not received metreleptin. Since this has been seen only in patients with other autoimmune features, it is most likely that lymphoma is a manifestation of autoimmunity and unrelated to metreleptin treatment.[33] However, given the uncertainty about metreleptin and lymphoma, providers should consider the risks and benefits of treatment in patients with acquired forms of lipodys-trophy, particularly in patients who have hematologic abnormalities prior to therapy. Leptin has also been proposed to be involved in the pathogenesis of obesity-associated cancers, such as breast and colon cancer; however, convinc-ing human data to support this are lacking.[83]

Progression or development of autoimmune disease, including both mem-branoproliferative glomerulonephritis[61] and autoimmune hepatitis,[59] have been reported during metreleptin treatment, but it is not clear that the drug played a role versus the natural history of underlying autoimmunity in these patients.

Conclusion

The lipodystrophies represent a group of syndromes that have a special place in the history of science and medicine. This begins with the first descrip-tion of the GLD syndromes by Berardinelli and Seip over 60 years ago.[84,85]

The next major advance came with the development of techniques to iden-tify the genetic mutations. This has led to the description of multiple different genes that form the etiologic basis of the syndromes, an effort that has been spearheaded in the U.S. by A. Garg, in Canada by R.A. Hegle, and in France by J. Magre. These genetic studies have focused on the lipid droplet and the basis of adipocyte development.

The next major event was the discovery of leptin by Jeffrey Friedman.[73] This is a seminal discovery because it first identified the adipocyte as the source of leptin and thus as an endocrine organ and second, provided the central mechanism for controlling energy balance.

While it is conceivable that metreleptin, possibly in combination with other drugs, may still provide a treatment for obesity, the major pharmaceutical role of metreleptin is restricted to leptin-deficient states. Rodent studies showed that leptin is effective in two different animal models: leptin gene mutations[70,71] and lipodystrophy.[86,87] Subsequently, leptin's effectiveness was replicated in patients with congenital leptin deficiency, as shown by Farooqi et al.,[73] and in patients with lipodystrophy syndromes, as studied in the Intramural program of the NIDDK/NIH and elsewhere.

Further, we have shown that the lipodystrophies are a model of the obesity-associated metabolic syndrome, which is epidemic worldwide. The knowledge gained in the study of lipodystrophy will hopefully provide guidance for treating metabolic syndrome with the type of precision medicine that is now possible for congenital leptin deficiency and lipodystrophy.

References

1.   Meehan CA, Cochran E, Kassai A, Brown RJ, Gorden P. Metreleptin for injection to treat the complications of leptin deficiency in patients with congenital or acquired generalized lipodystrophy. *Expert Rev Clin Pharmacol* 2016;9:59–68

2.   Brown RJ, Gorden P. Leptin therapy in patients with lipodystrophy and syndromic insulin resistance. In *Leptin: Regulation and Clinical Applications*. Dagogo-Jack S, Ed. Switzerland, Springer International Publishing, 2015, p. 225–236

3.   Handelsman Y, Oral EA, Bloomgarden ZT, Brown RJ, Chan JL, Einhorn D, et al. The clinical approach to the detection of lipodystrophy - an AACE consensus statement. *Endocr Pract* 2013;19:107–116

4.   Agarwal AK, Garg A. Genetic basis of lipodystrophies and management of metabolic complications. *Annu Rev Med* 2006;57:297–311

5.   NORD Physician Guide to the Lipodystrophy Disorders [Internet], 2013. Available from http://nordphysicianguides.org/lipodystrophies. Accessed 2 August 2016

6.   Congenital Generalized Lipodystrophy [Internet] 2015. Available from http://rarediseases.org/rare-diseases/congenital-generalized-lipodystrophy. Accessed 1 August 2016

7.   Familial Partial Lipodystrophy [Internet], 2015. Available from https://rarediseases.org/rare-diseases/familial-partial-lipodystrophy. Accessed 10 May 2017

8. Acquired Lipodystrophy [Internet], 2015. Available from: http://rarediseases. org/rare-diseases/acquired-lipodystrophy. Accessed 1 August 2016

9. Huang-Doran I, Sleigh A, Rochford JJ, O'Rahilly S, Savage DB. Lipodystrophy: metabolic insights from a rare disorder. *J Endocrinol* 2010;207:245–255

10. Garg A. Clinical review: lipodystrophies: genetic and acquired body fat disorders. *J Clin Endocrinol Metab* 2011;96:3313–3325

11. Garg A. Acquired and inherited lipodystrophies. *N Engl J Med* 2004;350:1220–1234

12. Agarwal AK, Arioglu E, de Almeida S, Akkoc N, Taylor SI, Bowcock AM, et al. AGPAT2 is mutated in congenital generalized lipodystrophy linked to chromosome 9q34. *Nat Genet* 2002;31:21–23

13. Magre J, Delepine M, Khallouf E, Gedde-Dahl T, Jr., Van Maldergem L, Sobel E, et al. Identification of the gene altered in Berardinelli-Seip congenital lipodystrophy on chromosome 11q13. *Nat Genet* 2001;28:365–370

14. Kim CA, Delepine M, Boutet E, El Mourabit H, Le Lay S, Meier M, et al. Association of a homozygous nonsense caveolin-1 mutation with Berardinelli-Seip congenital lipodystrophy. *J Clin Endocrinol Metab* 2008;93:1129–1234

15. Hayashi YK, Matsuda C, Ogawa M, Goto K, Tominaga K, Mitsuhashi S, et al. Human PTRF mutations cause secondary deficiency of caveolins resulting in muscular dystrophy with generalized lipodystrophy. *J Clin Invest* 2009;119:2623–2633

16. Herbst KL, Tannock LR, Deeb SS, Purnell JQ, Brunzell JD, Chait A. Köbberling type of familial partial lipodystrophy: an underrecognized syndrome. *Diabetes Care* 2003;26:1819–1824

17. Cao H, Hegele RA. Nuclear lamin A/C R482Q mutation in Canadian kindreds with Dunigan-type familial partial lipodystrophy. *Hum Mol Genet* 2000;9:109–112

18. Shackleton S, Lloyd DJ, Jackson SNJ, Evans R, Niermeijer MF, Singh BM, et al. LMNA, encoding lamin A/C, is mutated in partial lipodystrophy. *Nat Genet* 2000;24:153–156

19. Barroso I, Gurnell M, Crowley VE, Agostini M, Schwabe JW, Soos MA, et al. Dominant negative mutations in human PPARgamma associated with severe insulin resistance, diabetes mellitus and hypertension. *Nature* 1999;402:880–883

20. Gandotra S, Le Dour C, Bottomley W, Cervera P, Giral P, Reznik Y, et al. Perilipin deficiency and autosomal dominant partial lipodystrophy. *N Engl J Med* 2011;364:740–748

21. Rubio-Cabezas O, Puri V, Murano I, Saudek V, Semple RK, Dash S, et al. Partial lipodystrophy and insulin resistant diabetes in a patient with a homozygous nonsense mutation in CIDEC. *EMBO Mol Med* 2009;1:280–287

22. Albert JS, Yerges-Armstrong LM, Horenstein RB, Pollin TI, Sreenivasan UT, Chai S, et al. Null mutation in hormone-sensitive lipase gene and risk of type 2 diabetes. *N Engl J Med* 2014;370:2307–2315

23. Farhan SM, Robinson JF, McIntyre AD, Marrosu MG, Ticca AF, Loddo S, et al. A novel LIPE nonsense mutation found using exome sequencing in siblings with late-onset familial partial lipodystrophy. *Can J Cardiol* 2014;30:1649–1654

24. Novelli G, Muchir A, Sangiuolo F, Helbling-Leclerc A, D'Apice MR, Massart C, et al. Mandibuloacral dysplasia is caused by a mutation in LMNA-encoding lamin A/C. *Am J Hum Genet* 2002;71:426–431

25. Agarwal AK, Fryns JP, Auchus RJ, Garg A. Zinc metalloproteinase, ZMPSTE24, is mutated in mandibuloacral dysplasia. *Hum Mol Genet* 2003;12:1995–2001

26. Payne F, Lim K, Girousse A, Brown RJ, Kory N, Robbins A, et al. Mutations disrupting the Kennedy phosphatidylcholine pathway in humans with congenital lipodystrophy and fatty liver disease. *Proc Natl Acad Sci U S A* 2014;111:8901–8906

27. Garg A, Sankella S, Xing C, Agarwal AK. Whole-exome sequencing identifies ADRA2A mutation in atypical familial partial lipodystrophy. *JCI Insight* 2016;1:e86870

28. Thauvin-Robinet C, Auclair M, Duplomb L, Caron-Debarle M, Avila M, St-Onge J, et al. PIK3R1 mutations cause syndromic insulin resistance with lipoatrophy. *Am J Hum Genet* 2013;93:141–149

29. Bingham A, Mamyrova G, Rother KI, Oral E, Cochran E, Premkumar A, et al. Predictors of acquired lipodystrophy in juvenile-onset dermatomyositis and a gradient of severity. *Medicine (Baltimore)* 2008;87:70–86

30. Misra A, Peethambaram A, Garg A. Clinical features and metabolic and autoimmune derangements in acquired partial lipodystrophy: report of 35 cases and review of the literature. *Medicine (Baltimore)* 2004;83:18–34

31. Lee JH, Chan JL, Sourlas E, Raptopoulos V, Mantzoros CS. Recombinant methionyl human leptin therapy in replacement doses improves insulin resistance and metabolic profile in patients with lipoatrophy and metabolic syndrome induced by the highly active antiretroviral therapy. *J Clin Endocrinol Metab* 2006;91:2605–2611

32. Mulligan K, Khatami H, Schwarz JM, Sakkas GK, DePaoli AM, Tai VW, et al. The effects of recombinant human leptin on visceral fat, dyslipidemia, and insulin resistance in patients with human immunodeficiency virus-associated lipoatrophy and hypoleptinemia. *J Clin Endocrinol Metab* 2009;94:1137–1144

33. Brown RJ, Chan JL, Jaffe ES, Cochran E, DePaoli AM, Gautier JF, et al. Lymphoma in acquired generalized lipodystrophy. *Leuk Lymphoma* 2016;57:45–50

34. Musso C, Javor E, Cochran E, Balow JE, Gorden P. Spectrum of renal diseases associated with extreme forms of insulin resistance. *Clin J Am Soc Nephrol* 2006;1:616–622

35. George S, Rochford JJ, Wolfrum C, Gray SL, Schinner S, Wilson JC, et al. A family with severe insulin resistance and diabetes due to a mutation in AKT2. *Science* 2004;304:1325–1328

36. Winnay JN, Solheim MH, Dirice E, Sakaguchi M, Noh HL, Kang HJ, et al. PI3-kinase mutation linked to insulin and growth factor resistance in vivo. *J Clin Invest* 2016;126:1401–1412

37. Avila M, Dyment DA, Sagen JV, St-Onge J, Moog U, Chung BH, et al. Clinical reappraisal of SHORT syndrome with PIK3R1 mutations: towards recommendation for molecular testing and management. *Clin Genet.* 24 October 2015 [Epub ahead of print]

38. Gorden P, Lupsa BC, Chong AY, Lungu AO. Is there a human model for the 'metabolic syndrome' with a defined aetiology? *Diabetologia* 2010;53:1534–1536

39. Wang MY, Grayburn P, Chen S, Ravazzola M, Orci L, Unger RH. Adipogenic capacity and the susceptibility to type 2 diabetes and metabolic syndrome. *Proc Natl Acad Sci U S A* 2008;105:6139–6144

40. Bar RS, Gorden P, Roth J, Kahn CR, De Meyts P. Fluctuations in the affinity and concentration of insulin receptors on circulating monocytes of obese patients: effects of starvation, refeeding, and dieting. *J Clin Invest* 1976;58:1123–1135

41. Farooqi IS, O'Rahilly S. Leptin: a pivotal regulator of human energy homeostasis. *Am J Clin Nutr* 2009;89:980S–984S

42. Akinci B, Onay H, Demir T, Ozen S, Kayserili H, Akinci G, et al. Natural history of congenital generalized lipodystrophy: a nationwide study from Turkey. *J Clin Endocrinol Metab* 2016;101:2759–2767

43. Strickland LR, Guo F, Lok K, Garvey WT. Type 2 diabetes with partial lipodystrophy of the limbs: a new lipodystrophy phenotype. *Diabetes Care* 2013;36:2247–2253

44. Lima JG, Nobrega LH, de Lima NN, do Nascimento Santos MG, Baracho MF, Jeronimo SM. Clinical and laboratory data of a large series of patients with congenital generalized lipodystrophy. *Diabetol Metab Syndr* 2016;8:23

45. Diker-Cohen T, Cochran E, Gorden P, Brown RJ. Partial and generalized lipodystrophy: comparison of baseline characteristics and response to metreleptin. *J Clin Endocrinol Metab* 2015;100:1802–1810

46. Joseph J, Shamburek RD, Cochran EK, Gorden P, Brown RJ. Lipid regulation in lipodystrophy versus the obesity-associated metabolic syndrome: the dissociation of HDL-C and triglycerides. *J Clin Endocrinol Metab* 2014;99:E1676–1680

47. Kassai A, Muniyappa R, Levenson AE, Walter MF, Abel BS, Ring M, et al. Effect of leptin administration on circulating apolipoprotein CIII levels in patients with lipodystrophy. *J Clin Endocrinol Metab* 2016;101:1790–1797

48. Asthana A, Abel BS, Skarulis MC, Gorden P, Brown RJ, Muniyappa R. Effects of recombinant human leptin (metreleptin) therapy on plasma angiopoietin-like proteins 3 and 4 in lipodystrophy patients. Late-breaking abstract presented at the Endocrine Society's 97th Annual Meeting and Expo, 5–8 March 2015, at the San Diego Endocrine Society, Seattle, WA

49. Brown MS, Goldstein JL. Selective versus total insulin resistance: a pathogenic paradox. *Cell Metab* 2008;7:95–96

50. Unger RH, Zhou YT. Lipotoxicity of beta-cells in obesity and in other causes of fatty acid spillover. *Diabetes* 2001;50(Suppl. 1):S118–S121

51. Musso C, Cochran E, Javor E, Young J, Depaoli AM, Gorden P. The long-term effect of recombinant methionyl human leptin therapy on hyperandrogenism and menstrual function in female and pituitary function in male and female hypoleptinemic lipodystrophic patients. *Metabolism* 2005;54:255–263

52. Oral EA, Ruiz E, Andewelt A, Sebring N, Wagner AJ, Depaoli AM, et al. Effect of leptin replacement on pituitary hormone regulation in patients with severe lipodystrophy. *J Clin Endocrinol Metab* 2002;87:3110–3117

53. Abel BS, Muniyappa R, Stratton P, Skarulis MC, Gorden P, Brown RJ. Effects of recombinant human leptin (metreleptin) on nocturnal luteinizing hormone secretion in lipodystrophy patients. *Neuroendocrinology* 2016;103:402–407

54. Lungu AO, Zadeh ES, Goodling A, Cochran E, Gorden P. Insulin resistance is a sufficient basis for hyperandrogenism in lipodystrophic women with polycystic ovarian syndrome. *J Clin Endocrinol Metab* 2012;97:563–567

55. Musso C, Shawker T, Cochran E, Javor ED, Young J, Gorden P. Clinical evidence that hyperinsulinaemia independent of gonadotropins stimulates ovarian growth. *Clin Endocrinol (Oxf)* 2005;63:73–78

56. Cortes VA, Smalley SV, Goldenberg D, Lagos CF, Hodgson MI, Santos JL. Divergent metabolic phenotype between two sisters with congenital generalized lipodystrophy due to double AGPAT2 homozygous mutations. a clinical, genetic and In Silico study. *PLoS One* 2014;9:e87173

57. Maguire M, Lungu A, Gorden P, Cochran E, Stratton P. Pregnancy in a woman with congenital generalized lipodystrophy: leptin's vital role in reproduction. *Obstet Gynecol* 2012;119:452–455

58. Paz-Filho G, Delibasi T, Erol HK, Wong ML, Licinio J. Congenital leptin deficiency and thyroid function. *Thyroid Res* 2009;2:11

59. Safar Zadeh E, Lungu AO, Cochran EK, Brown RJ, Ghany MG, Heller T, et al. The liver diseases of lipodystrophy: the long-term effect of leptin treatment. *J Hepatol* 2013;59:131–137

60. Javor ED, Ghany MG, Cochran EK, Oral EA, DePaoli AM, Premkumar A, et al. Leptin reverses nonalcoholic steatohepatitis in patients with severe lipodystrophy. *Hepatology* 2005;41:753–760

61. Javor ED, Moran SA, Young JR, Cochran EK, DePaoli AM, Oral EA, et al. Proteinuric nephropathy in acquired and congenital generalized lipodystrophy: baseline characteristics and course during recombinant leptin therapy. *J Clin Endocrinol Metab* 2004;89:3199–3207

62. McNally M, Mannon RB, Javor ED, Swanson SJ, Hale DA, Gorden P, et al. Successful renal transplantation in a patient with congenital generalized lipodystrophy: a case report. *Am J Transplant* 2004;4:447–449

63. Casali RE, Resnick J, Goetz F, Simmons RL, Najarian JS, Kjellstrand C. Renal transplantation in a patient with lipoatrophic diabetes. a case report. *Transplantation* 1978;26:174–177

64. Lupsa BC, Sachdev V, Lungu AO, Rosing DR, Gorden P. Cardiomyopathy in congenital and acquired generalized lipodystrophy: a clinical assessment. *Medicine (Baltimore)* 2010;89:245–250

65. Khalife WI, Mourtada MC, Khalil J. Dilated cardiomyopathy and myocardial infarction secondary to congenital generalized lipodystrophy. *Tex Heart Inst J* 2008;35:196–199

66. Guo X, Ling C, Liu Y, Zhang X, Zhang S. A case of novel Lamin A/C mutation manifesting as atypical progeroid syndrome and cardiomyopathy. *Can J Cardiol* 2015;32:e29–31

67. Ambrosi P, Kreitmann B, Lepidi H, Habib G, Levy N, Philip N, et al. A novel overlapping phenotype characterized by lipodystrophy, mandibular dysplasia, and dilated cardiomyopathy associated with a new mutation in the LMNA gene. *Int J Cardiol* 2016;209:317–318

68. Arioglu E, Duncan-Morin J, Sebring N, Rother KI, Gottlieb N, Lieberman J, et al. Efficacy and safety of troglitazone in the treatment of lipodystrophy syndromes. *Ann Intern Med* 2000;133:263–274

69. Gavrilova O, Haluzik M, Matsusue K, Cutson JJ, Johnson L, Dietz KR, et al. Liver peroxisome proliferator-activated receptor gamma contributes to hepatic steatosis, triglyceride clearance, and regulation of body fat mass. *J Biol Chem* 2003;278:34268–34276

70. Zhang Y, Proenca R, Maffei M, Barone M, Leopold L, Friedman JM. Positional cloning of the mouse obese gene and its human homologue. *Nature* 1994;372:425–432

71. Coleman DL. A historical perspective on leptin. *Nat Med* 2010;16:1097–1099

72. Heymsfield SB, Greenberg AS, Fujioka K, Dixon RM, Kushner R, Hunt T, et al. Recombinant leptin for weight loss in obese and lean adults: a randomized, controlled, dose-escalation trial. *JAMA* 1999;282:1568–1575

73. Farooqi IS, Matarese G, Lord GM, Keogh JM, Lawrence E, Agwu C, et al. Beneficial effects of leptin on obesity, T cell hyporesponsiveness, and neuroendocrine/metabolic dysfunction of human congenital leptin deficiency. *J Clin Invest* 2002;110:1093–1103

74. Oral EA, Simha V, Ruiz E, Andewelt A, Premkumar A, Snell P, et al. Leptin-replacement therapy for lipodystrophy. *N Engl J Med* 2002;346:570–578

75. Chong AY, Lupsa BC, Cochran EK, Gorden P. Efficacy of leptin therapy in the different forms of human lipodystrophy. *Diabetologia* 2010;53:27–35

76. Javor ED, Cochran EK, Musso C, Young JR, Depaoli AM, Gorden P. Long-term efficacy of leptin replacement in patients with generalized lipodystrophy. *Diabetes* 2005;54:1994–2002

77. McDuffie JR, Riggs PA, Calis KA, Freedman RJ, Oral EA, DePaoli AM, et al. Effects of exogenous leptin on satiety and satiation in patients with lipodystrophy and leptin insufficiency. *J Clin Endocrinol Metab* 2004;89:4258–4263

78. Moran SA, Patten N, Young JR, Cochran E, Sebring N, Reynolds J, et al. Changes in body composition in patients with severe lipodystrophy after leptin replacement therapy. *Metabolism* 2004;53:513–519

79. Petersen KF, Oral EA, Dufour S, Befroy D, Ariyan C, Yu C, et al. Leptin reverses insulin resistance and hepatic steatosis in patients with severe lipodystrophy. *J Clin Invest* 2002;109:1345–1350

80. Ebihara K, Kusakabe T, Hirata M, Masuzaki H, Miyanaga F, Kobayashi N, et al. Efficacy and safety of leptin-replacement therapy and possible mechanisms of leptin actions in patients with generalized lipodystrophy. *J Clin Endocrinol Metab* 2007;92:532–541

81. Ebihara K, Masuzaki H, Nakao K. Long-term leptin-replacement therapy for lipoatrophic diabetes. *N Engl J Med* 2004;351:615–616

82. Chan JL, Koda J, Heilig JS, Cochran EK, Gorden P, Oral EA, et al. Immunogenicity associated with metreleptin treatment in patients with obesity or lipodystrophy. *Clin Endocrinol (Oxf)* 2016;85:137–149

83. Strong AL, Ohlstein JF, Biagas BA, Rhodes LV, Pei DT, Tucker HA, et al. Leptin produced by obese adipose stromal/stem cells enhances proliferation and metastasis of estrogen receptor positive breast cancers. *Breast Cancer Res* 2015;17:112

84. Berardinelli W. An undiagnosed endocrinometabolic syndrome: report of 2 cases. *J Clin Endocrinol Metab* 1954;14:193–204

85. Seip M, Trygstad O. Generalized lipodystrophy. *Arch Dis Child* 1963;38:447–453

86. Shimomura I, Hammer RE, Ikemoto S, Brown MS, Goldstein JL. Leptin reverses insulin resistance and diabetes mellitus in mice with congenital lipodystrophy. *Nature* 1999;401:73–76

87. Reitman ML, Arioglu E, Gavrilova O, Taylor SI. Lipoatrophy revisited. *Trends Endocrinol Metab* 2000;11:410–416

4
Diabetes in Diseases of the Exocrine Pancreas

Jessica Abramowitz, MD;[1] Uma Gunasekaran, MD;[1] Xanthia F. Samaropoulos, MD, MPH;[1] Anna Tumyan, MD;[1] and Ildiko Lingvay, MD, MPH, MSCS[1,2]

Introduction

Diabetes that is caused by or occurs in the setting of an exocrine pancreas abnormality is classified as a distinct form of diabetes by the American Diabetes Association as well as by the World Health Organization. These forms of diabetes have distinct pathophysiologic features, which highlight the close interaction between the exocrine and endocrine pancreas. The distinction of this form of diabetes from the classical type 2 diabetes or type 1 diabetes is important as it has direct clinical implications regarding therapy, long-term outcomes, and patient counseling.

The prevalence of diabetes related to exocrine disorders varies around the globe. In India, for example, it can represent as much as 15–20% of all cases of diabetes due to the high prevalence of "tropical diabetes" (an entity associated with malnutrition and sometimes pancreatitis), while in the Western world the prevalence is estimated at 5–10%. Within this category of diabetes, by far the

[1]Division of Endocrinology/Department of Internal Medicine, University of Texas Southwestern Medical Center, Dallas, TX

[2]Department of Clinical Sciences, University of Texas Southwestern Medical Center, Dallas, TX

DOI: 10.2337/9781580406666.04

Table 4.1—Estimates of Diabetes Occurrence in Various Diseases of the Exocrine Pancreas

Disease of the Exocrine Pancreas	Diabetes Occurrence (%)
Pancreatitis	
Acute (diagnosis within 12 months of event)	5–15%[1]
Chronic	20–80%[2]
Fibrocalculous Pancreatopathy	90%[3]
Pancreatic Cancer	50%[4]
Pancreatectomy - total	100%
Pancreatectomy - partial	
Distal	<20%
40–80%	19–48%
80–90%	58–100%[2]
Cystic Fibrosis	40–50%[5]
Hemochromatosis	20–60%[6,7]

most common condition is chronic pancreatitis (approximately 80%), followed by pancreatic cancer (approximately 8%). Table 4.1 shows the estimates of diabetes occurrence in the respective exocrine pancreas diseases.

This chapter will review diseases of the exocrine pancreas that cause or are associated with diabetes, specifically acute and chronic pancreatitis, fibrocalculous pancreatopathy, pancreatic cancer, pancreatic trauma and pancreatectomy, and genetic conditions like cystic fibrosis, hemochromatosis, and certain forms of maturity-onset diabetes of the young (MODY). We focus on the pathophysiology of diabetes in these conditions as well as the clinical presentation, therapeutic management, and other patient-related considerations.

Exocrine–Endocrine Pancreas Relationship

While the exocrine and endocrine pancreas are traditionally regarded as two separate organ systems, a strong interrelationship between these exists, both anatomically and physiologically. The pancreatic circulatory system is unique as it has an intra-organ portal system that allows the exocrine pancreas to receive a large part of its blood supply through the islets. As a consequence, the exocrine pancreas is exposed to high concentrations of islet hormones that modulate its function and growth.

Diabetes is commonly associated with exocrine pancreatic abnormalities, both structural and functional. Patients with diabetes have reduction in pancreatic size, changes in the pancreatic duct system, acinar atrophy, fibrosis, and fatty degeneration. Functional alterations are also common and include reduced serum and fecal pancreatic enzyme levels, reduced secretagogue-stimulated secretion, and reduced enzyme content in the pancreas. Several hypotheses have been postulated to explain these clinical correlations. A prevalent view implicates the lack of the trophic hormone insulin, coupled with high levels of inhibitory hormones like glucagon and somatostatin, an effect that is likely hastened by the development of atherosclerosis-induced decrease in the exocrine pancreas perfusion. This hypothesis is indirectly supported by data showing a correlation between the severity of diabetes and the degree of exocrine pancreatic dysfunction in humans, and animal data showing an increase in amylase output in rats with insulin-producing tumors (reversible on resection).[8,9]

The relationship between the exocrine and endocrine pancreas is bidirectional as evidenced not just by a high prevalence of exocrine abnormalities in patients with diabetes, but also by a high incidence of diabetes in patients with exocrine diseases, particularly pancreatitis and cancer. These conditions will be further detailed in this chapter. Lastly, a common underlying pathology can lead to the occurrence of both exocrine and endocrine pancreatic abnormalities, as in cases of autoimmune-mediated inflammation (not covered in this chapter) or certain genetic defects (discussed further in this chapter).

Acute Pancreatitis

Acute pancreatitis is the most common pancreatic disease, with an annual incidence of 4.9–35 cases per 100,000 population.[10] It is an acute inflammatory process of the pancreas that is self-limiting in the vast majority of cases, but recurrent episodes of acute pancreatitis may lead to chronic pancreatitis in about 10% of cases. Acute and chronic pancreatitis can have numerous underlying etiologies ranging from structural (obstructive or congenital malformations) to toxic, metabolic, drug-induced, infection, trauma, genetic, and autoimmune, although a cause cannot always be identified.

Patients with acute pancreatitis may present with concurrent hyperglycemia or develop diabetes after the acute event is resolved. Hyperglycemia has been reported in up to 50% of cases of acute pancreatitis. It usually develops in the early phase of the disease and mainly in patients with severe disease;

therefore, it is used as one of the markers for predicting the severity of pancreatitis. Hyperglycemia is usually transient, resolving once the acute process reverses; however, permanent diabetes may result from severe necrotizing pancreatitis in about 5% of cases. The risk of diabetes increases by at least twofold after an episode of acute pancreatitis, with 15% of patients developing newly diagnosed diabetes within 1 year and 40% within 5 years after the first episode of acute pancreatitis.[1] Furthermore, repeated episodes of acute pancreatitis can further increase the risk of subsequent development of diabetes.

In acute pancreatitis, hyperglycemia is primarily caused by the acute inflammatory response to pancreatic injury. In this condition, the pancreatic islets are relatively spared. In contrast, in severe necrotizing pancreatitis, most of the exocrine tissue is lost along with islets. Hyperglycemia in acute pancreatitis is usually transient and a result of several factors: hyperglucagonemia due to stress, elevated levels of other stress hormones such as catecholamines and cortisol, increased insulin resistance due to systemic inflammation, and relative hypoinsulinemia due to β-cell dysfunction.

Initial management of patients with acute pancreatitis consists of removal of precipitating causes (if identifiable) and supportive care including fluid resuscitation, pain control, and nutritional support. Patients with hyperglycemia should be treated with intravenous insulin therapy initially. When oral intake is reestablished, the intravenous insulin therapy should be transitioned to subcutaneous insulin administration until hyperglycemia resolves. Hypoglycemic agents other than insulin have no role in the treatment of hyperglycemia associated with the acute pancreatitis episode.

Chronic Pancreatitis

Chronic pancreatitis is a progressive inflammatory process that leads to fibrosis with calcification and results in permanent structural damage of the exocrine and endocrine pancreatic tissue. The prevalence of chronic pancreatitis is estimated at 50 cases per 100,000 persons; it is more common in men and ages 30–40 years. Chronic pancreatitis is the most common disease of the exocrine pancreas associated with the development of diabetes. Diabetes has been observed in 20–80% of patients with chronic pancreatitis with the majority of patients developing diabetes several years after the diagnosis of chronic pancreatitis.[2] The risk factors for development of diabetes in chronic pancreatitis include longer duration of disease, prior partial distal pancreatectomy or significant pancreatic resection, and early onset of calcific disease.[2] Diabetes is also more likely to occur in patients with a family history of type 1 and type 2 diabetes.

Diabetes in chronic pancreatitis occurs as a result of decreased insulin secretion caused by both a reduction in the number of islets and their functional capacity. These changes occur from chronic inflammation leading to extensive fibrosis and progressive scarring of pancreatic parenchyma with subsequent loss of vascularity and ischemic injury. Islet damage in chronic pancreatitis leads to the loss not only of insulin-secreting pancreatic β-cells, but also of glucagon-secreting alpha cells and pancreatic polypeptide (PP)-secreting gamma cells. PP deficiency usually occurs early in the course of disease and may be an early marker for the development of endocrine dysfunction in patients with exocrine insufficiency due to chronic pancreatitis.[11] Impaired glucagon secretion usually occurs late in the course of the disease and may predispose patients to frequent episodes of hypoglycemia. Furthermore, maldigestion and malabsorption of nutrients due to pancreatic exocrine insufficiency leads to impaired secretion of incretin hormones such as glucagon-like peptide-1 (GLP-1) and gastric inhibitory polypeptide and diminished glucose-dependent insulin secretion, further contributing to postprandial hyperglycemia. In comparison with type 2 diabetes, peripheral tissue sensitivity to insulin is not commonly impaired in patients with chronic pancreatitis.[12]

Diabetes in this setting is often diagnosed late and misclassified as type 1 or type 2 diabetes. Screening for diabetes should occur at the time of the diagnosis of chronic pancreatitis and annually thereafter, using current diagnostic tests and criteria. Diabetes due to pancreatitis should also be suspected in patients with diabetes who have clinical, biochemical, or radiographic evidence of pancreatitis in the absence of typical features suggestive of either type 1 diabetes (absence of autoantibodies to islet cell, glutamic acid decarboxylase, insulinoma antigen-2, or insulin) or type 2 diabetes (no clinical or biochemical evidence of insulin resistance such as acanthosis nigricans or hyperinsulinemia). Measurement of PP response to insulin-induced hypoglycemia, secretin infusion, or mixed-nutrition ingestion may also help to differentiate diabetes due to pancreatitis from other types of diabetes.[11] An absent PP response to mixed-nutrient ingestion is a specific indicator of diabetes due to pancreatitis, whereas PP levels may be normal or decreased in type 1 diabetes and elevated in type 2 diabetes. The diagnostic evaluation of suspected cases without previous diagnosis of pancreatitis should include testing for evidence of exocrine pancreatic insufficiency (measurement of fecal elastase-1 or direct function testing) and imaging modalities such as endoscopic ultrasound, magnetic resonance imaging, or computer tomography to evaluate for evidence of pancreatic pathology.[13]

Hyperglycemia in the setting of chronic pancreatitis can range in severity from a milder form of only intermittent glucose intolerance during periods of stress or illness (usually in the early stages) to the frank form of overt insulin-dependent diabetes. There are no specific guidelines available for treatment of diabetes due to pancreatitis, and therapy should be dictated by patient phenotype and by the degree of residual β-cell function. In cases of mild persistent hyperglycemia, use of oral hypoglycemic agents may be considered. Metformin may be beneficial especially if there is concomitant insulin resistance; however, use is limited by gastrointestinal side effects. Short-acting insulin secretagogues (sulfonylureas and glinides) may also be cautiously considered, keeping in mind the already high risk of hypoglycemia in this population. Sodium-glucose cotransporter 2 (SGLT2) inhibitors may also be helpful based on their mechanism of action that is independent of insulin secretion, but no studies are yet available in this setting. In all other cases insulin is the preferred treatment agent since the principal defect is insulin deficiency. Incretin-based therapies (DPP-IV inhibitors and GLP-1 receptor agonists) should be avoided; in fact, patients with a history of acute or chronic pancreatitis have been actively excluded from all studies using incretin mimetics due to concerns of drug-induced pancreatitis.

Treatment of the more advanced cases can be very challenging. First, concomitant loss of both insulin and counterregulatory glucagon secretion leads to wide glycemic excursions and frequent hypoglycemia, both treatment-related and spontaneous. Second, the coexistence of pancreatic exocrine insufficiency leading to maldigestion and malabsorption, coupled with the underlying symptoms of chronic pancreatitis that include frequent nausea, vomiting, and inconsistent oral intake due to abdominal pain, leads to unpredictable insulin dose and timing requirements and further increases the risk of hypo- and hyperglycemia. However, since the β-cell deficit is seldom absolute, diabetic ketoacidosis is rare, unlike in patients with type 1 diabetes. Such patients are best treated with either basal-bolus or pump-delivered insulin therapy in order to maximize the flexibility of insulin delivery and minimize glucose excursions.

Oral pancreatic enzyme replacement helps to improve fat digestion and absorption, control steatorrhea, and prevent deficiencies of fat-soluble vitamins. These are also important for maintaining incretin hormone secretion, which can lead to improvement of postprandial glucose tolerance.[14] Vitamin D replacement—a fat-soluble vitamin—is important to prevent development of metabolic bone disease.

Total pancreatectomy with islet autotransplantation (TPIAT) is a definitive treatment of recurrent acute or chronic pancreatitis with the primary indication of providing pain relief. Islet autotransplantation is done in the setting of total pancreatectomy to prevent or ameliorate surgical diabetes. TPIAT—a radical and risky procedure—should not be performed solely as a treatment for chronic pancreatitis–associated diabetes.[15]

Although data are limited, previous reports suggest that patients with diabetes due to chronic pancreatitis are at increased risk for microvascular complications and, therefore, should be monitored for the development of complications using the guidelines available for patients with type 1 and type 2 diabetes.[16]

Fibrocalculous Pancreatopathy (Tropical Diabetes)

Fibrocalculous pancreatic diabetes (FCPD), also known as tropical pancreatitis, is a rare form of secondary diabetes that occurs as a result of non-alcoholic chronic calcific pancreatitis of unknown etiology. It predominantly affects young and malnourished individuals and is found in tropical developing countries.

The hallmarks of the disease are the occurrence of chronic, recurrent abdominal pain starting in childhood followed by the development of pancreatic calculi associated with pancreatic duct dilatation and extensive pancreatic fibrosis later in adolescence. Subsequent exocrine and endocrine pancreatic insufficiency lead to development of malnutrition, steatorrhea, and insulin-dependent, ketosis-resistant diabetes, which may be difficult to control due to wide glycemic variations and frequent hypoglycemia. The term tropical calcific pancreatitis is used to describe patients with this condition prior to the onset of diabetes.[17]

The first cases of FCPD were described by Zuidema in 1959 from Indonesia.[18] Since the initial publication, cases of FCPD have been reported from many tropical countries including in Africa (Nigeria, Uganda), Asia (India,

Bangladesh, Sri Lanka), and South America (Brazil); however, the highest prevalence at present is found in southwestern India.

Earlier studies from India (from 1991–1995) demonstrated a prevalence of FCPD of 1.6% in the general population. In more recent reports (from 2006–2010), the prevalence of FCPD decreased to 0.2%, whereas the mean BMI of the patients had significantly increased. While the exact reasons for these changes are not clear, improvements in socioeconomic status and nutrition have been postulated as important contributing factors.

The pathogenesis of FCPD is thought to be multifactorial, yet the exact mechanism of pancreatic injury remains unknown. Many factors have been associated with FCPD, including: 1) malnutrition, though this may be an effect rather than the cause of the disease; 2) a toxic effect of cyanide derived from frequent ingestion of cassava plant (*Manioc esculenta*), which is extensively cultivated in many tropical and subtropical countries.[19-21] Cassava contains cyanogenic glycosides linamarin and lotustralin, which may lead to pancreatic injury in the setting of impaired detoxification associated with malnourishment. However, this hypothesis was not supported by several epidemiologic studies.[22,23] 3) Familial aggregation and genetic factors might also contribute as up to 8% of cases of FCPD occurred in members of the same family with both horizontal and vertical transmission of the disease. Recent studies confirmed an association between SPINK 1 mutations and FCPD.[24] 4) Lastly, increased oxidant stress from Vitamin C and A deficiency might also contribute to the development of FCPD.[25]

The pathologic process starts from the head of the pancreas and subsequently extends to the body and tail regions. By the time diabetes develops, the pancreas is usually atrophic and appears firm and nodular on palpation. Pancreatic stones are usually detected a decade after onset of abdominal pain and are predominantly located in the large pancreatic ducts and may be associated with ductal dilatation. They may vary in size, reaching up to 4.5 cm in length, and consist predominantly of calcium carbonate.

As the disease progresses, widespread destruction and acinar loss are seen. It is hypothesized that islets are destroyed due to surrounding fibrosis and disruption of vasculature, as evidenced by a paucity of alpha and β-cells, reduced islet number in some cases, and hyperplasia in others. Nesidioblastosis has been also described. There is no evidence of "insulinitis." Significant loss of β-cells mass and defects in insulin secretion are major contributors to diabetes in chronic calcific pancreatitis. There is also evidence to suggest that insulin resistance may play a role in these cases.[26]

The classic presentation of FCPD consists of recurrent abdominal pain, pancreatic calcification, steatorrhea, and diabetes. Most patients are young and lean, with a low BMI reported in 72% of patients presenting with insulin-dependent diabetes. Severe recurrent abdominal pain is usually the first presenting symptom and may occur even in childhood. Maldigestion and steatorrhea are usually late manifestations of the disease and may occur a decade or two after the first episode of abdominal pain. Overt steatorrhea has been reported in only 30% of patients, possibly due to low dietary fat intake.

Diabetes occurs in up to 90% of cases, usually 10–20 years after the onset of abdominal pain and is diagnosed between the ages of 20–35 years. The diabetes in FCPD is usually severe, insulin dependent, and may be difficult to control due to frequent hypoglycemia due to concomitant glucagon deficiency. However, β-cells continue to function and ketosis is rare. Other factors contributing to ketosis resistance in FCPD include decreased glucagon reserve and reduced supply of nonesterified fatty acid (NEFA), the substrate needed for ketogenesis, due to malnutrition and decreased adipose tissue mass.[3]

The occurrence of long-term microvascular complications including advanced retinopathy, nephropathy, and neuropathy in patients with FCPD is common and similar to that found in patients who have type 2 diabetes. In contrast, macrovascular complications are rare, possibly due to young age of onset, low BMI, and low cholesterol levels.

Patients with FCPD may also develop complications due to chronic pancreatitis including pseudocysts, pseudoaneurysms, pancreatic abscess, and obstructive jaundice, which can be due to common bile duct obstruction or associated with pancreatic carcinoma. Patients with FCPD are at 100-fold higher risk of pancreatic malignancy compared to the general population and should be evaluated promptly in cases of concerning symptoms.[27]

Diagnosis of FCPD is based on the evidence of non-alcoholic chronic calcific pancreatitis in patients with the typical clinical features described above (Table 4.2). Interestingly, features like malnutrition, young age at onset, and absence of ketosis are useful but not essential for diagnosis.

The classic plain radiographic feature of FCPD is the presence of coarse pancreatic calcifications with the typical "bag of stones" appearance described

Table 4.2—Proposed Criteria for the Diagnosis of FCPD

Diagnostic criteria for fibrocalculous pancreatic diabetes:
Occurrence in a "tropical" country
Diabetes by WHO Study Group criteria

Evidence of chronic pancreatitis: pancreatic calculi on X-ray or at least three of the following:
  a) Abnormal pancreatic morphology by ultrasonography
  b) Chronic abdominal pain since childhood
  c) Steatorrhea
  d) Abnormal pancreatic function test

Absence of other causes of chronic pancreatitis

Source: Adapted from Mohan et al.[17]

in the severe cases (Figure 4.1 and Figure 4.2). Other useful imaging modalities include abdominal ultrasound, computer tomography, endoscopic retrograde cholangiopancreatography, and endoscopic ultrasonography.

Management of patients with FCPD is complex and frequently complicated by their poor socioeconomic status and lack of education. More than 80% of patients with FCPD require insulin for the control of hyperglycemia and to ensure appropriate weight gain. A basal-bolus insulin regimen is usually the treatment of choice. Oral hypoglycemic agents (usually sulfonylureas) may be used with caution in a minority of patients with less advanced disease and preserved β-cell function. Oral pancreatic enzymes are useful for the treatment of steatorrhea along with macro and micronutrient deficiency; however, the cost may be prohibitive.[19] The general principles of dietary management in these situations place an emphasis on extra caloric and protein intake due to concomitant malnutrition and exocrine pancreatic insufficiency.

Surgery is performed for severe intractable and recurrent abdominal pain. Surgical options include drainage procedures, sphincteroplasty, pancreatic necrosectomy, partial or subtotal pancreatectomy, and nerve ablation procedures (celiac plexus block).[30]

Pancreatic Cancer

Pancreatic cancer is the fourth leading cause of cancer-related death in the United States.[31] There is a bidirectional relationship between pancreatic cancer and diabetes where type 2 diabetes is considered a risk factor for pancreatic

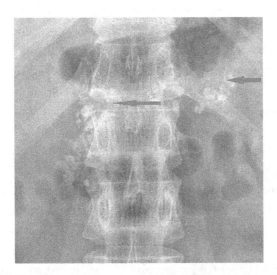

Figure 4.1—X-Ray of abdomen showing the classic radio-opaque pancreatic calcifications (arrows).

Source: Dasgupta R, Naik D, Thomas N.[29]

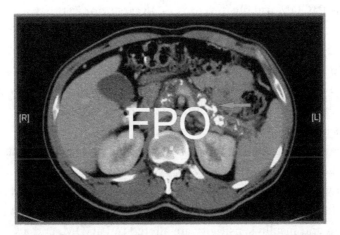

Figure 4.2—Contrast-enhanced computed tomography scan of the abdomen showing the large, ductal calcification (arrows) with ductal dilatation predominantly involving the main pancreatic duct in a patient with fibrocalcific pancreatic diabetes.

Source: Dasgupta R, Naik D, Thomas N.[29]

cancer, but also pancreatic cancer can induce diabetes. The latter, called pancreatic cancer–associated diabetes (PaCDM), usually precedes the diagnosis of cancer by several years. The relationship between pancreatic cancer and diabetes has long been recognized, with the first case reported in 1833.[32]

There is a noted increase in the prevalence of diabetes diagnosed 24 to 36 months prior to a diagnosis of pancreatic cancer.[33] In a study of 232 patients with stage 1 or 2 pancreatic cancer, 50% of patients had diabetes.[4] Therefore, new-onset diabetes may highlight patients at high risk for pancreatic cancer but may also be a marker of early pancreatic cancer.

There are several hypotheses regarding the mechanisms responsible for the development of PaCDM. One theory suggests that pancreatic cancer may create a state of stress akin to pregnancy, weight gain, or steroid therapy, which can precipitate hyperglycemia in a susceptible host. Pancreatic cancer and diabetes have common risk factors (older age, obesity, family history), and thus the high frequency of new-onset diabetes in pancreatic cancer may indicate that pancreatic cancer is a specific stressor that precipitates the progression to diabetes in an individual already at risk. Another hypothesis is related to the cachexia associated with pancreatic cancer, but the temporal relationship does not support this view as PaCDM usually develops 2–3 years prior to the diagnosis of cancer while cachexia-associated symptoms occur only about 2 months before the diagnosis of pancreatic cancer. An additional proposed mechanism implicates tumor-induced pancreatic destruction. Several factors make this hypothesis unlikely: 1) PaCDM may be present even prior to a radiologically detectable tumor; 2) PaCDM is associated with high insulin levels and insulin resistance; 3) diabetes improves after tumor resection.[34]

An emerging hypothesis suggests that PaCDM is a "paraneoplastic" manifestation of pancreatic cancer caused by diabetogenic tumor-secreted products. This hypothesis is supported by the observation that PaCDM resolves in more than half of the cases following surgical removal of the tumor. Both insulin secretion and insulin sensitivity are altered in PaCDM, and a schematic of proposed mechanistic contributors is presented in Figure 4.3. Adrenomedullin, a 52–amino acid pluripotent hormone, appears to play an important role as its secretion is upregulated in pancreatic cancer lines and inhibits glucose-stimulated insulin secretion from β-cells. Plasma levels of adrenomedullin are higher in patients with pancreatic cancer compared with patients with diabetes or controls. Furthermore, levels of adrenomedullin are higher in patients with

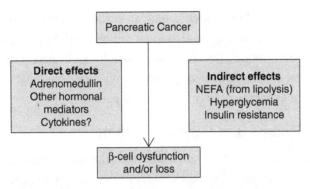

Figure 4.3—Proposed mechanisms of β-cell dysfunction/loss in pancreatic cancer.

Source: Sah RP et al.[34]

pancreatic cancer who developed diabetes compared to those who did not, findings supporting the possible role of this molecule in the pathophysiology of PaCDM.

PaCDM and type 2 diabetes are often hard to distinguish as the clinical presentation of hyperglycemia, underlying metabolic abnormalities, and patient phenotype (age, gender distribution, BMI, family history of diabetes) are very similar. One distinctive feature between the two entities is the weight trajectory. Type 2 diabetes is typically associated with weight gain except when the presentation is acute or the diagnosis is delayed, in which case weight loss may occur due to the effect of severe hyperglycemia and the ensuing catabolic state, but weight is usually regained upon initiation of appropriate treatment. In contrast, weight loss is a common presentation of pancreatic cancer. A case control study comparing patients with new-onset type 2 diabetes and PaCDM reported that at the onset of diabetes there was a significant difference in weight loss with 59% of PaCDM patients who lost weight compared to 30% with type 2 diabetes.[35] Also weight loss associated with pancreatic cancer causes a paradoxical worsening of hyperglycemia.

The best treatment for PaCDM is resection of the pancreatic tumor.[4,36] Glycemic control has also been shown to improve following neoadjuvant chemotherapy for pancreatic cancer.[37] Metformin and peroxisome proliferator–activated receptor gamma agonists have been suggested to improve survival of pancreatic cancer based on epidemiological studies, but no definitive prospective studies exist.[38,39] While these therapies can be tried if no contraindications exist and they are tolerated by the patient, insulin is ultimately the most effective and safest treatment option, targeted to a glycemic goal that is commensurate with the life expectancy of the respective patient.

Pancreatic Trauma and Pancreatectomy

Processes that cause severe pancreatic damage, like pancreatic trauma and pancreatectomy, may cause diabetes.[40] Occurrence of pancreatic injury in the setting of trauma is rare, though associated with high morbidity and mortality, and data are limited regarding endocrine function outcome. In contrast, more evidence is emerging regarding the effects of pancreatic surgery on endocrine function as these operations have increased in frequency, especially distal pancreatectomies for benign pancreatic lesions or chronic pancreatitis.

Pancreatic injury can occur following trauma to the upper abdomen and is more frequent in penetrating abdominal injuries compared to blunt trauma. Blunt injury to the pancreas occurs frequently with upper abdominal trauma, such as in motor vehicle accidents or bicycle injuries where the pancreas is compressed against the vertebral bodies. Penetrating pancreatic trauma may occur with stabbing or gunshot wounds.[41]

Pancreatic trauma is difficult to diagnose clinically due to the retroperitoneal location of the pancreas and therefore is more accurately assessed intraoperatively during surgical treatment of abdominal trauma. Serum markers of pancreatic activity, such as amylase or lipase, are an unreliable measure of pancreatic injury after abdominal trauma, and there is minimal evidence or consensus regarding their use. Computed tomography is the most common imaging modality used to assess for pancreatic injury, and endoscopic retrograde cholangiopancreatography can be performed to assess the integrity of the pancreatic duct. Magnetic resonance imaging may add additional information in the diagnosis of pancreatic injury.[42] Pancreatectomy (usually partial) is often required in severe pancreatic injuries. In a small retrospective surgical case series, 3 of 19 patients with pancreatic trauma reported development of diabetes over a five-year follow-up period, suggesting a relatively low rate of endocrine pancreas dysfunction following pancreatic trauma. Of the three patients with reported diabetes, one patient had a distal pancreatectomy due to blunt abdominal trauma; the other two had penetrating abdominal injuries and one was managed with surgical debridement while the other was managed conservatively.[43] Other small studies showed no increased risk of endocrine dysfunction following either surgical or conservative management of acute pancreatic trauma in children.[44–46]

Pancreatectomy performed for nontraumatic causes is also associated with the development of diabetes, with the risk depending on islet cell reserve, extent of resection, and type of surgery that is performed.

Distal pancreatectomy involves the resection of the tail and body of the pancreas and is considered the standard of care for patients with benign lesions or potentially malignant lesions. It has been used more frequently recently as higher-resolution imaging techniques identify more benign lesions, such as intrapancreatic mucinous neoplasms. Other indications for distal pancreatectomy include chronic pancreatitis or ductal disease in the body or tail of the pancreas. In a retrospective study that followed 235 patients in a single institution who underwent distal pancreatectomy for different indications (including pancreatitis and pancreatic masses), the rate of new onset insulin dependent diabetes was 8%.[47] A smaller study of 125 patients found a postoperative diabetes rate of 9%, while in a study comparing splenic preservation in pancreatectomy for low-grade malignant disease, 5% of patients developed diabetes postoperatively.[48,49] This suggests a low rate of diabetes following distal pancreatectomy in patients with normal pancreatic tissue. The rates of diabetes following pancreatectomy for chronic pancreatitis are higher; a study of 90 patients found an overall risk of 46% over 2 years[50] and a study of 224 patients found a postoperative rate of diabetes of 37%.[51]

Central pancreatectomy involves the removal of the body of the pancreas, usually reserved for small, benign lesions. This procedure is rarely performed due to its high risk of surgical complications. One such complication is pancreatic fistula formation, which may cause inflammation-induced islet cell destruction, but studies overall have shown good endocrine pancreatic function postoperatively.[52]

In a *proximal pancreatic resection*, the head of the pancreas is resected and when performed as a pancreatoduododenectomy, the duodenum, gallbladder, and bile duct are resected as well. When proximal pancreatectomy is performed for chronic pancreatitis, diabetes occurs in 15–48% of patients, with lower rates observed if the procedure spares the duodenum with its intestinal enzymes and a smaller amount of pancreatic tissue is resected.[53–56] Although data are limited regarding proximal resection for benign and malignant tumors, when performed for pancreatic cancer it often leads to resolution of diabetes as discussed above (see section on pancreatic cancer).

Total pancreatectomy may be performed for benign or metastatic tumors or chronic pancreatitis. A total pancreatectomy always leads to insulin-dependent diabetes.

Islet cells are located throughout the pancreas with similar density present in the head and body and the highest density (more than twofold higher) in the pancreatic tail.[57] Partial resection of the pancreas will cause a commensurate decrease in islet cell and resulting absolute deficiency in both β- and α-cell function. The ultimate extent of insulin deficiency depends on the type and extent of resection, as well as the function of the residual β-cell.[52]

In mild postpancreatectomy diabetes, dietary modification, exercise, and/or any noninsulin antidiabetic agents may be sufficient for management. Following total pancreatectomy, insulin is required for survival as absolute insulinopenia ensues after surgery. General treatment principles in this setting follow those of type 1 diabetes, though the glycemic excursions could be more pronounced as there is a complete lack of insulin as well as other islet hormones, such as glucagon. Autologous islet cell transplantation has been successfully used in some centers to treat the resulting diabetes after total pancreatectomy for benign conditions.[58]

Genetic Conditions

Cystic Fibrosis

Cystic fibrosis–related diabetes (CFRD) is a distinct type of diabetes caused by the genetic condition cystic fibrosis (CF). CFRD shares features of both type 1 and type 2 diabetes as there is both insulin deficiency caused by pancreatic islet cell destruction and insulin resistance that is multifactorial in causation.[59] The incidence of diabetes in patients with CF has increased as innovations in the treatment of CF-related complications and advancements in the field of lung transplantation have led to increased longevity. Furthermore, there is evidence that CFRD might adversely affect CF morbidity and mortality rates as malnutrition and decline of pulmonary function have been reported to occur up to four years before the development of diabetes.[59]

CFRD is now considered to be the most common nonpulmonary comorbidity of CF, occurring in approximately 20% of adolescents and 40–50% of adults, as prevalence of CFRD increases significantly with age.[5] The increase in prevalence of CFRD is thought to be multifactorial and increased awareness, improvements in screening practices, and longer life spans of CF patients have all contributed.[5] Several risk factors for the development of CFRD have been identified based on large-scale observational studies: increased age, female gender, exocrine pancreatic insufficiency, severe CF genotype, lung function, poor nutritional status, and liver disease.[60] Furthermore, because genotype is highly predictive of pancreatic status in CF and the ΔF508 homozygous genotype is known to be associated with pancreatic insufficiency in nearly all CF patients, patients with this genotype have a higher prevalence of CFRD as compared to compound heterozygotes and other genotype groups.[60] Interestingly, the prevalence of CFRD is found to be higher in patients with more severe pulmonary disease, worse pulmonary function, more pulmonary exacerbations treated with antibiotics and glucocorticoids, and higher prevalence of pulmonary infections with *Pseudomonas aeruginosa*, *Burkholderia cepacia*, *Stenotrophomonas maltophilia*, *Candida*, and *Aspergillus*.[60]

Although CFRD shares features of both type 1 and type 2 diabetes (Table 4.3), there are distinct differences that place this clinical entity in a separate category.[61]

Although the hallmark feature of CFRD is a reduction in β-cell mass due to islet cell destruction leading to insulin deficiency, the etiology of CFRD is intricate and the mechanisms leading to the development of CFRD have not been fully elucidated at present.[61] It is believed that pancreatic damage arises from changes in the composition of pancreatic secretions secondary to the mutation in the cystic fibrosis transmembrane regulator (CFTR) protein with resulting thick, viscous secretions blocking the pancreatic ducts, causing interstitial edema, impairing blood flow, and thus leading to both pancreatic endocrine and exocrine damage (Figure 4.4).[62] The initial stage of insulin deficiency is later followed by a component of insulin resistance thought to be related to increased counterregulatory hormones and inflammatory cytokines during acute CF exacerbations as well as the use of exogenous glucocorticoids and other immunosuppressant therapies used to treat certain pulmonary infections and following lung transplantation.[61]

There are several complications of diabetes in CF that may directly impact morbidity and/or mortality. Patients with CFRD appear to be immune to the traditional diabetes-related macrovascular complications as no patient with

Table 4.3—Clinical Characteristics of CFRD Compared with Type 1 and Type 2 Diabetes

	CFRD	Type 1 Diabetes	Type 2 Diabetes
Prevalence in population	35%	0.2%	11%
Peak age of onset	20–24 years	Childhood, adolescence	Mid to late adulthood
Usual body habitus	Normal to underweight	Normal	Obese
Insulin deficiency	Severe but not complete	Complete	Partial, variable
Insulin resistance	Modest, waxes and wanes with infection	Usually modest	Severe
Autoimmune etiology	No	Yes	No
Ketones	Rare	Yes	Rare
Glycated hemoglobin (HbA1c)	Unpredictable relation to mean blood glucose	Related to mean blood glucose	Related to mean blood glucose
Usual treatment	Insulin	Insulin	Oral agents, insulin
Microvascular complications	Yes	Yes	Yes
Macrovascular complications	No	Yes	Yes
Metabolic syndrome features	No	No	Yes
Cause of death	Lung disease	Cardiovascular	Cardiovascular

Source: Reprinted with permission from Moran A et al.[61]

CF has been reported to have died from atherosclerotic cardiovascular disease. However, microvascular complications do occur, including diabetic polyneuropathy, nephropathy, and retinopathy, and are related to the duration of CFRD and glycemic control.[61] Most important is the impact of diabetes on survival in CF as patients with CFRD, particularly females, have a significantly higher mortality rate (greater than sixfold) than patients with CF without diabetes.[62] The presence of CFRD (both insulin deficiency and hyperglycemia) negatively impacts CF pulmonary disease. In fact, nutritional status and pulmonary function have been shown to progressively decline in CF patients with

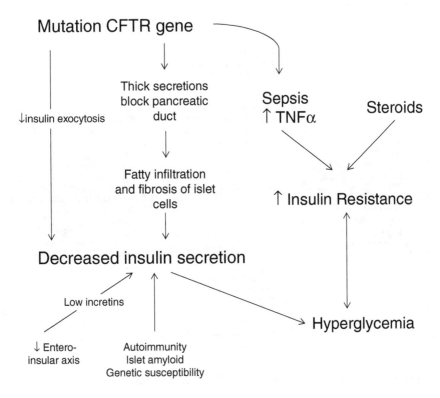

Figure 4.4—Proposed pathophysiologic events leading to CFRD.

Source: Brennan AL, Beynon J.[62]

evidence of impaired glucose tolerance up to four years before the actual diagnosis of CFRD is made.[61] Insulin deficiency affects nutritional status by creating a catabolic state with excessive protein and fat breakdown with multiple studies demonstrating that the anabolic effects of insulin replacement improve not only nutrition and pulmonary function but also lead to decreased morbidity and mortality from CF-related pulmonary infections.[61]

CFRD is frequently clinically silent; therefore, annual screening for CFRD is recommended starting at age 10 years in all patients with CF.[63] Testing should be performed during a period of stable baseline health, in the absence of any concomitant illnesses or infections, and any abnormal test should be confirmed with a repeat measurement on a separate date, unless unequivocal symptoms of hyperglycemia are present (Figure 4.5). The current gold standard for screening is the 2-hour 75-gram oral glucose tolerance test, as

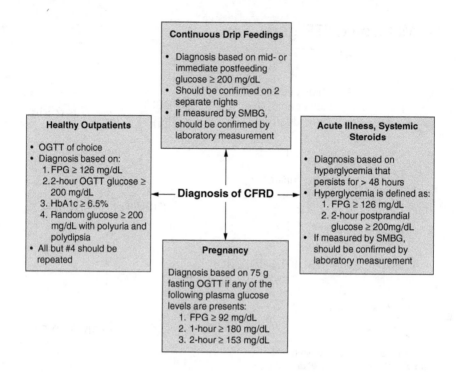

Figure 4.5—Criteria for the diagnosis of CFRD.

Source: Reprinted with permission from Moran A et al.[63]

hemoglobin A1C, fructosamine, urine glucose, and random glucose have all been shown to have low sensitivity and poor predictive ability in detecting diabetes in the CF population.[63] Although continuous glucose monitoring is currently not the standard of care for CFRD screening purposes, there are a few early studies that suggest that continuous glucose monitoring may identify early abnormalities in glucose tolerance not detected by the oral glucose tolerance test.[64] The diagnosis of CFRD is made using the standard American Diabetes Association criteria.[63]

Patients with CFRD should preferably be managed by a specialized multidisciplinary team with expertise in diabetes and CF.[63] The mainstay of therapy is insulin; other antidiabetic agents are not recommended as they have not been shown to be efficacious in improving the nutritional and metabolic outcomes in contrast to the anabolic effects of insulin.[63] Blood glucose goals, hemoglobin A1C goals, and screening for both microvascular and macrovascular

Table 4.4—Comparison between Nutrition Recommendations for Type 1/Type 2 Diabetes and CFRD

	Type 1/Type 2 Diabetes	CFRD
Calories	Calculated for maintenance, growth, or reduction diets	120–150% RDA Calories never restricted
Carbohydrate	Individualized	Total intake unrestricted
Fat	Individualized <10% calorie intake from saturated fats Dietary cholesterol intake <300 mg/d	High fat intake (35–40% of total calories)
Protein	Protein reduction in presence of diabetic nephropathy (0.8 g/kg)	Protein reduction may not be appropriate
Sodium	Salt restriction to reduce macrovascular complications (<2,400 mg/d)	High-sodium diet essential (>4,000 mg/d)

Source: Brennan AL, Beynon J.[62]

complications for CFRD patients are the same as for all patients with diabetes. However, nutritional goals and guidelines for patients with CFRD are very different as adequate caloric intake to maintain BMI is critical to their health and survival (Table 4.4).[63]

The prevalence of CFRD has risen dramatically over the past 20 years as survival has increased with improved treatments including lung transplantation for CF patients. CFRD is a unique condition that is different from type 1 and type 2 diabetes, including its pathophysiology, diagnosis, and management. It is essential for clinicians to recognize these differences to adequately treat this condition. Obtaining glycemic control and recognizing its importance in patients with CFRD is especially significant because glycemic control is correlated with lung function and overall survival. Future research questions to be addressed include development of improved screening tests, evaluation of the potential utility of other antidiabetic agents that increase insulin release and reduce insulin resistance, and the study of the development and management of chronic complications related to CFRD.

Hemochromatosis

Hemochromatosis is an inherited condition in which iron deposition occurs in multiple tissues. This can subsequently lead to hypogonadism, diabetes, liver disease, cardiomyopathy, and arthritis, as well as damage to the pancreas, pituitary, skin, and joints.[6,7] Hereditary hemochromatosis is classified into three types. Type 1 is defined by a mutation in the HFE gene, the gene encoding the hereditary hemochromatosis protein, and constitutes 80% of cases.[6] Type 2 (also known as juvenile hemochromatosis) is further subclassified as Type 2a, associated with a mutation in hemojuvelin, and Type 2b, associated with a mutation in hepcidin. Type 3 is characterized by mutations in the transferrin receptor 2.[65]

The population prevalence of hemochromatosis is thought to be 0.06–0.4%, with most patients being 40–50 years of age at the time of presentation. A higher prevalence of the HFE mutation is seen in persons of Northern European descent. The frequency of diabetes in all patients with HFE mutation is estimated to be between 20–50%.[7]

Two major mutations in HFE have been identified: Cys282Tyr and His63Asp. Homozygosity for the Cys282Tyr mutation accounts for 80–90% of clinical iron overload cases. Compounded heterozygosity of Cys282Tyr and His63Asp account for 7–8% of cases. HFE mutations are inherited in an autosomal recessive pattern with high phenotypic penetrance. Other mutations include Ser65Cys HFE, genes encoding transferrin receptor 2, hemojuvelin, hepcidin, and ferroportin. Another iron disorder associated with diabetes is hereditary aceruloplasminemia.[7]

Hemochromatosis is defined by the triad of hepatomegaly, diabetes, and hyperpigmented (or "bronze") skin,[7] but with more screening and earlier diagnosis, fewer patients exhibit this classic triad. In one study of 56 families and 93 individuals, only 7% of patients with familial hereditary hemochromatosis showed signs of the triad.[66] The diagnosis of hemochromatosis should be considered in patients with a transferrin saturation >45% and serum ferritin >300 ug/L. Transferrin saturation is more specific for Cys282Tyr mutation as ferritin levels are commonly elevated in other conditions. HFE gene mutation testing is commonly available and can be used to screen family members if needed. In non–HFE-related iron overload disorders, liver biopsy or magnetic resonance imaging can be utilized for diagnosis. Screening is suggested in patients with iron overload and individuals who are greater than 20 years of age with a first-degree relative with hereditary hemochromatosis. Screening would include serum transferrin saturation, ferritin levels, and HFE mutation testing.[7]

In healthy individuals, hepcidin binds to ferroportin, an iron transporter responsible for the export of iron from cells, which subsequently causes

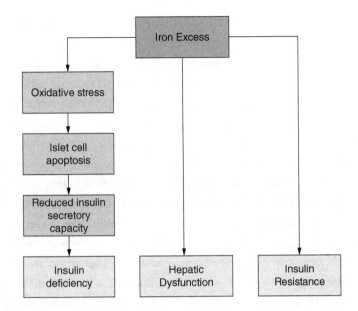

Figure 4.6—Mechanisms for the development of diabetes in hemochromatosis. Diabetes can be caused by insulin deficiency, hepatic dysfunction, or insulin resistance alone or in combination.

Source: Swaminathan S et al.[6]

degradation. In patients with hemochromatosis, hepcidin levels are inappropriately low even with iron sufficiency, so there is no regulation of iron deposition.[7] There are three mechanisms by which hemochromatosis is thought to cause diabetes: insulin deficiency, hepatic dysfunction, and insulin resistance (Figure 4.6).

The commonly reported clinical features of hemochromatosis include fatigue, liver disease, and arthritis in patients with ferritin levels >1,000 ug/L. Additional symptoms can include abdominal pain and loss of libido.[6]

There are other iron overload disorders that can impair glucose metabolism. Hereditary aceruloplasmenia, when there is no synthesis of ceruloplasmin, can cause progressive iron deposition in tissues and similar development of diabetes as in hemochromatosis. Transfusional iron overload can cause impaired glucose tolerance and type 2 diabetes, and this condition is associated with high serum ferritin levels. When treated with chelation therapy, glucose tolerance can improve in up to one-third of patients. Porphyria cutanea tarda has been associated with glucose intolerance. Friedreich's ataxia is associated with mitochondrial iron accumulation and a high incidence of type 2 diabetes. High dietary intake of iron, such as in meat, has also been associated with diabetes.[6]

Common diabetes complications include nephropathy, retinopathy, neuropathy, and cardiovascular disease, but information on these conditions in patients with hemochromatosis is limited. In hemochromatosis, with increased iron deposition causing subsequent oxidative stress that then increases intracellular iron, this cycle can cause renal damage. Iron-deficient diets and chelation therapy have been shown to prevent progression of nephropathy.[6] The Cys282Tyr mutation has been associated with proliferative diabetic retinopathy.[67] In one cohort of 46 patients, idiopathic neuropathy was seen in 26% of patients while only 6% had diabetic neuropathy.[68] This study was limited by inadequate information on the number of patients who had diabetes in the cohort. Studies have shown an increased incidence of cardiovascular disease in iron overload disorders with chelation therapy improving cardiovascular outcomes. Increased heme intake and iron stores have also been associated with cardiovascular events, but there have also been conflicting studies showing no association between iron overload and cardiovascular disease.[6]

The mainstay of treatment for hemochromatosis is repeated phlebotomy with a goal of reducing serum ferritin level to < 50 ug/L. In two studies, it was found that patients who had diabetes did not have a reduction in insulin doses after treatment with phlebotomy.[6] Phlebotomy is only useful in the prevention of secondary organ damage and not for the treatment of diabetes. There are no specific guidelines for the treatment of secondary diabetes due to hemochromatosis, and so it should be treated like any other form of diabetes though one would expect that in later stages of hemochromatosis insulin would be needed due to decreased islet cell insulin secretion.

Patients with hereditary hemochromatosis who develop diabetes have a lower survival compared to their counterparts who do not develop diabetes or liver cirrhosis, whereas individuals who do not develop diabetes have survival rates similar to the general population.[69] This is postulated because patients do not develop secondary conditions from tissue damage from iron deposition. Therefore, early diagnosis and treatment of hemochromatosis is critical to reduce the development of comorbidities including the development of diabetes.

MODYs

MODY is the designation for a group of monogenic disorders with hetero-genic manifestations, which share key features: autosomal inheritance (strong family history), early onset of diabetes (generally before age 25), no signs of autoimmunity or insulin resistance, and preserved endogenous insulin secre-tion. The clinical features overlap greatly with the more common type 1 and type 2 diabetes, which is the reason why these conditions are misclassified in more than 80% of cases.[70] It is estimated that the prevalence of MODY among all forms of diabetes could be up to 5%. To date 13 different MODYs have been named and it is likely that more will be identified in the future.[71] The clinical characteristics are heterogeneous even among those who carry the same muta-tion; therefore, the clinical presentation is not a reliable predictor of the under-lying pathogenesis. Diagnosis of MODY is made by performing genetic testing by direct sequencing of the gene.

In this chapter, we review only three of the less common MODY forms—MODY 4, MODY 5, and MODY 8, as these have associated exocrine pancre-atic findings. Exocrine pancreatic dysfunction has been reported in patients with the most common form of MODY (MODY 3, due to mutation in the HNF1α gene), but the prevalence (13%) appears to be similar to that noted in patients with type 1 diabetes (19%), although much higher than in the general population without diabetes (4%).[72] Therefore the exocrine pancreatic abnor-mality in this condition is perhaps related to hyperglycemia rather than directly to the specific mutation.

MODY 4 (IPF1)

MODY 4 is caused by a mutation in the Insulin Promoter Factor 1 (IPF1) gene, located on chromosome 13q12. This gene encodes the protein IPF1 (also known as *PDX1* [pancreatic and duodenal homeobox 1]), which is a transcrip-tion factor that plays a critical role in pancreatic development, including β-cell maturation and duodenal differentiation in the embryo. In adults, this gene continues to play a role in the regulation and expression of genes for insulin, GLUT2, glucokinase, and somatostatin.

MODY 4 is very rare (<1% of all MODYs); in fact, only one family is well characterized.[73,74] A child with the homozygous IPF1 mutations was born with pancreatic agenesis; yet a number of older relatives who were heterozygous had mild hyperglycemia or diabetes. None of the heterozygous mutation carriers were severely insulin-deficient and all were controlled with either diet or oral hypoglycemic agents.

MODY 5 (HNF1ZB)

MODY 5 is caused by a mutation in the hepatic nuclear factor 1B (HNF1B) gene, located on chromosome 17q12. The gene product, HNF1B (also known as transcription factor) is involved in early stages of embryonic development of several organs, including the pancreas, where it contributes to differentiation of pancreatic endocrine progenitors from nonendocrine embryonic duct cells. It is estimated that mutations in this gene are responsible for approximately 5% of all MODY cases. Interestingly, 30–60% of HNF1B mutations and deletions are spontaneous; therefore, a family history of renal disease or diabetes is not essential to prompt a screen for this disorder.[75]

HNF1B-MODY is a multisystem disorder, with abnormalities ranging from the pancreas and kidney to the reproductive system. A wide variation in phenotypes has been noted even within a single pedigree; hence, affected individuals with identical mutations may display different combinations and severities of organ involvement.

The degree of insulin deficiency resulting from mutations in this gene is variable. Half of all HNF1B mutation carriers develop early-onset diabetes, yet they tend to be more insulin resistant than patients with the more common forms of MODY (specifically MODY 3 and MODY 1). Diabetes can develop from infancy through middle adult life, and some family members who carry the gene remain free of diabetes into later adult life. Most of those who develop diabetes show atrophy of the entire pancreas, with mild or subclinical deficiency of exocrine as well as endocrine function. Birth weight is reduced as a result of reduced insulin secretion in utero.[76]

Because of the coexisting pancreatic atrophy and insulin resistance, HNF1B diabetes is not sensitive to sulfonylureas (unlike MODY 3 and MODY 1), and early insulin therapy is required.

Renal disease is the predominant phenotype but is very variable in nature with phenotypes that include renal cysts (most frequent), renal dysplasia, renal tract malformations, and/or familial hypoplastic glomerulocystic kidney disease. Renal abnormalities begin with structural alterations (small kidneys, renal cysts, anomalies of the renal pelvis, and calices), but many develop progressive renal failure associated with chronic cystic disease of the kidneys. In some cases, renal cysts may be detected in utero. Kidney disease may develop before or after hyperglycemia, and a significant number of people with MODY 5 are discovered in renal clinics.[77]

Various minor or major anomalies of the reproductive system have also been described and occur regardless of the presence or absence of renal involvement. Male defects include epididymal cysts, agenesis of the vas deferens, or infertility due to abnormal spermatozoa. Affected women have vaginal agenesis, hypoplastic, or bicornuate uterus.

Other metabolic abnormalities associated with MODY 5 include gout and hyperuricemia, as well as elevated liver enzymes (without clinically significant liver disease).

MODY 8 (CEL)

MODY 8 has an autosomal dominant inheritance and is caused by a mutation in the noncoding region of the carboxyl ester lipase (CEL) gene located on chromosome 9q34.[78] This gene is mainly expressed in the pancreatic acinar tissue and mammary gland, and not in the pancreatic β-cells; therefore, β-cell dysfunction is an unexplained phenotype. The gene product is CEL (also known as bile salt–stimulated lipase), a glycoprotein secreted from the pancreas into the digestive tract and from the breast tissue into human milk. This protein is activated in the intestine by bile salts and helps the hydrolysis and absorption of cholesterol and fat-soluble vitamins. The pathophysiology of diabetes in this condition is not fully understood, but an upregulation in mitogen-activated protein kinase (MAPK) signaling in the pancreatic secretome is thought to be contributing.[79]

Mutations in the CEL gene are found in <1% of all patients with MODY, and only two Norwegian families harboring mutations in this gene have been identified to date.[78]

Patients first present in childhood with symptoms suggestive of pancreatic exocrine insufficiency (abdominal pain and fatty stools). Diabetes is usually diagnosed later, during early adulthood. Interestingly, a common associated feature is pancreatic cysts, which are noted before the development of diabetes.[79] A study evaluating nine patients with this condition noted that a demyelinating neuropathy is very prevalent.[70] Given the limited clinical experience with this entity, specific treatment recommendations for management of hyperglycemia cannot be made; treatment with pancreatic enzymes improves the symptoms of exocrine pancreatic deficiency and increases fat-soluble vitamin levels.[70]

Conclusion

In this chapter, we reviewed important and often misdiagnosed causes of diabetes related to diseases of the exocrine pancreas. While these clinical entities represent only about 10% of all cases of diabetes, physicians should *1)* maintain an appropriate index of suspicion in cases that do not fully fit the common presentation of type 1 or type 2 diabetes, *2)* be knowledgeable about the various conditions that can lead to diabetes to appropriately direct the diagnostic workup, *3)* be familiar with the diagnostic workup necessary to screen for diabetes in patients with these conditions, and *4)* when a diagnosis is made, apply physiology-based treatment for each individual case.

References

1. Das SL, Singh PP, Phillips AR, Murphy R, Windsor JA, Petrov MS. Newly diagnosed diabetes mellitus after acute pancreatitis: a systematic review and meta-analysis. *Gut* 2014;63:818–831

2. Malka D, Hammel P, Sauvanet A, Rufat P, O'Toole D, Bardet P, et al. Risk factors for diabetes mellitus in chronic pancreatitis. *Gastroenterology* 2000;119:1324–1332

3. Barman KK, Premalatha G, Mohan V. Tropical chronic pancreatitis. *Postgrad Med J* 2003;79:606–615

4. Pannala R, Leirness JB, Bamlet WR, Basu A, Petersen GM, Chari ST. Prevalence and clinical profile of pancreatic cancer-associated diabetes mellitus. *Gastroenterology* 2008;134:981–987

5. Moran A, Dunitz J, Nathan B, Saeed A, Holme B, Thomas W. Cystic fibrosis-related diabetes: current trends in prevalence, incidence, and mortality. *Diabetes Care* 2009;32:1626–1631

6. Swaminathan S, Fonseca VA, Alam MG, Shah SV. The role of iron in diabetes and its complications. *Diabetes Care* 2007;30:1926–1933

7. Utzschneider KM, Kowdley KV. Hereditary hemochromatosis and diabetes mellitus: implications for clinical practice. *Nat Rev Endocrinol* 2010;6:26–33

8. Okabayashi Y, Ohki A, Sakamoto C, Otsuki M. Relationship between the severity of diabetes mellitus and pancreatic exocrine dysfunction in rats. *Diabetes Res Clin Pract* 1985;1:21–30

9. Sakamoto C, Otsuki M, Ohki A, Kazumi T, Yamasaki T, Yuu H, et al. Exocrine and endocrine secretion from isolated perfused rat pancreas with islet cell tumors induced by streptozotocin and nicotinamide. *Dig Dis Sci* 1984;29:443–447

10. Talley NJ, Locke GR, Saito YA. *GI Epidemiology*. Malden, MA, Blackwell Publishing, 2007, p. 221–225

11. Rickels MR, Bellin M, Toledo FG, Robertson RP, Andersen DK, Chari ST, et al. Detection, evaluation and treatment of diabetes mellitus in chronic pancreatitis: recommendations from PancreasFest 2012. *Pancreatology* 2013;13:336–342

12. Yasuda H, Harano Y, Ohgaku S, Kosugi K, Suzuki M, Hidaka H, et al. Insulin sensitivity in pancreatitis, liver diseases, steroid treatment and hyperthyroidism assessed by glucose, insulin and somatostatin infusion. *Horm Metab Res* 1984;16:3–6

13. Ewald N, Bretzel RG. Diabetes mellitus secondary to pancreatic diseases (Type 3c)—are we neglecting an important disease? *Eur J Intern Med* 2013;24: 203–206

14. Ebert R, Creutzfeldt W. Reversal of impaired GIP and insulin secretion in patients with pancreatogenic steatorrhea following enzyme substitution. *Diabetologia* 1980;19:198–204

15. Bellin MD, Freeman ML, Gelrud A, Slivka A, Clavel A, Humar A, et al. Total pancreatectomy and islet autotransplantation in chronic pancreatitis: recommendations from PancreasFest. *Pancreatology* 2014;14:27–35

16. Couet C, Genton P, Pointel JP, Louis J, Gross P, Saudax E, et al. The prevalence of retinopathy is similar in diabetes mellitus secondary to chronic pancreatitis with or without pancreatectomy and in idiopathic diabetes mellitus. *Diabetes Care* 1985;8:323–328

17. Mohan V, Premalatha G, Pitchumoni CS. Tropical chronic pancreatitis: an update. *J Clin Gastroenterol* 2003;36:337–346

18. Zuidema PJ. Cirrhosis and disseminated calcification of the pancreas in patients with malnutrition. *Trop Geogr Med* 1959;11:70–74

19. Yajnik CS. Diabetes secondary to tropical calcific pancreatitis. *Baillieres Clin Endocrinol Metab* 1992;6:777–796

20. Sathiaraj E, Gupta S, Chutke M, Mahurkar S, Mansard MJ, Rao GV, et al. Malnutrition is not an etiological factor in the development of tropical pancreatitis—a case-control study of southern Indian patients. *Trop Gastroenterol* 2010;31:169–174

21. McMillan DE, Geevarghese PJ. Dietary cyanide and tropical malnutrition diabetes. *Diabetes Care* 1979;2:202–208

22. Swai AB, McLarty DG, Mtinangi BL, Tatala S, Kitange HM, Mlingi N, et al. Diabetes is not caused by cassava toxicity. A study in a Tanzanian community. *Diabetes Care* 1992;15:1378–1385

23. Girish BN, Rajesh G, Vaidyanathan K, Balakrishnan V. Assessment of cassava toxicity in patients with tropical chronic pancreatitis. *Trop Gastroenterol* 2011;32: 112–116

24. Schneider A, Suman A, Rossi L, Barmada MM, Beglinger C, Parvin S, et al. SPINK1/PSTI mutations are associated with tropical pancreatitis and type II diabetes mellitus in Bangladesh. *Gastroenterology* 2002;123:1026–1030

25. Braganza JM, Schofield D, Snehalatha C, Mohan V. Micronutrient antioxidant status in tropical compared with temperate-zone chronic pancreatitis. *Scand J Gastroenterol* 1993;28:1098–2104

26. Chari ST, Mohan V, Pitchumoni CS, Viswanathan M, Madanagopalan N, Lowenfels AB. Risk of pancreatic carcinoma in tropical calcifying pancreatitis: an epidemiologic study. *Pancreas* 1994;9:62–66

27. Zargar AH, Laway BA, Masoodi SR, Shah NA, Shah JA. Fibricalculous pancreatic diabetes from the Kashmir Valley. *Ann Saudi Med* 1996;16:144–147

28. Tiengo A. Diabetes secondary to pancreatopathy. In *Proceedings of the Post EASD International Symposium on Diabetes Secondary to Pancreatopathy, Padova, Italy, 1987.* Amsterdam, Excerpta Medica, 1988

29. Dasgupta R, Naik D, Thomas N. Emerging concepts in the pathogenesis of diabetes in FCPD (fibrocalculous pancreatic diabetes). *J Diabetes* 2015;7:754–761

30. Unnikrishnan R, Mohan V. Fibrocalculous pancreatic diabetes (FCPD). *Acta Diabetol* 2015;52:1–9

31. Jemal A, Murray T, Ward E, Samuels A, Tiwari RC, Ghafoor A, et al. Cancer statistics, 2005. *CA Cancer J Clin* 2005;55:10–30

32. Bright R. Cases and observations connected with disease of the pancreas and duodenum. *Med Chir Trans* 1833;18:1–56

33. Chari ST, Leibson CL, Rabe KG, Timmons LJ, Ransom J, de Andrade M, et al. Pancreatic cancer-associated diabetes mellitus: prevalence and temporal association with diagnosis of cancer. *Gastroenterology* 2008;134:95–101

34. Sah RP, Nagpal SJ, Mukhopadhyay D, Chari ST. New insights into pancreatic cancer-induced paraneoplastic diabetes. *Nat Rev Gastroenterol Hepatol* 2013;10: 423–433

35. Hart PA, Kamada P, Rabe KG, Srinivasan S, Basu A, Aggarwal G, et al. Weight loss precedes cancer-specific symptoms in pancreatic cancer-associated diabetes mellitus. *Pancreas* 2011;40:768–772

36. Permert J, Ihse I, Jorfeldt L, von Schenck H, Arnquist HJ, Larsson J. Improved glucose metabolism after subtotal pancreatectomy for pancreatic cancer. *Br J Surg* 1993;80:1047–1050

37. Gardner TB, Hessami N, Smith KD, Ripple GH, Barth RJ, Klibansky DA, et al. The effect of neoadjuvant chemoradiation on pancreatic cancer-associated diabetes mellitus. *Pancreas* 2014;43:1018–1021

38. Polvani S, Tarocchi M, Tempesti S, Bencini L, Galli A. Peroxisome proliferator activated receptors at the crossroad of obesity, diabetes, and pancreatic cancer. *World J Gastroenterol* 2016;22:2441–2459

39. Ambe CM, Mahipal A, Fulp J, Chen L, Malafa MP. Effect of metformin use on survival in resectable pancreatic cancer: a single-institution experience and review of the literature. *PLoS One* 2016;11:e0151632

40. American Diabetes Association. Standards of medical care in diabetes—2013. *Diabetes Care* 2013;36(Suppl. 1):S11–S66

41. Boffard KD, Brooks AJ. Pancreatic trauma—injuries to the pancreas and pancreatic duct. *Eur J Surg* 2000;166:4–12

42. Panda A, Kumar A, Gamanagatti S, Bhalla AS, Sharma R, Kumar S, et al. Evaluation of diagnostic utility of multidetector computed tomography and magnetic resonance imaging in blunt pancreatic trauma: a prospective study. *Acta Radiol* 2015;56:387–396

43. Al-Ahmadi K, Ahmed N. Outcomes after pancreatic trauma: experience at a single institution. *Can J Surg* 2008;51:118–124

44. de Blaauw I, Winkelhorst JT, Rieu PN, van der Staak FH, Wijnen MH, Severijnen RS, et al. Pancreatic injury in children: good outcome of nonoperative treatment. *J Pediatr Surg* 2008;43:1640–1643

45. Wales PW, Shuckett B, Kim PC. Long-term outcome after nonoperative management of complete traumatic pancreatic transection in children. *J Pediatr Surg* 2001;36:823–827

46. Snajdauf J, Rygl M, Kalousova J, Kucera A, Petru O, Pycha K, et al. Surgical management of major pancreatic injury in children. *Eur J Pediatr Surg* 2007;17:317–321

47. Lillemoe KD, Kaushal S, Cameron JL, Sohn TA, Pitt HA, Yeo CJ. Distal pancreatectomy: indications and outcomes in 235 patients. *Ann Surg* 1999;229: 693–698; discussion 698–700

48. King J, Kazanjian K, Matsumoto J, Reber HA, Yeh MW, Hines OJ, et al. Distal pancreatectomy: incidence of postoperative diabetes. *J Gastrointest Surg* 2008; 12:1548–1553

49. Shoup M, Brennan MF, McWhite K, Leung DH, Klimstra D, Conlon KC. The value of splenic preservation with distal pancreatectomy. *Arch Surg* 2002; 137:164–168

50. Hutchins RR, Hart RS, Pacifico M, Bradley NJ, Williamson RC. Long-term results of distal pancreatectomy for chronic pancreatitis in 90 patients. *Ann Surg* 2002;236:612–618

51. Riediger H, Adam U, Fischer E, Keck T, Pfeffer F, et al. Long-term outcome after resection for chronic pancreatitis in 224 patients. *J Gastrointest Surg* 2007; 11:949–959; discussion 959–960

52. Maeda H, Hanazaki K. Pancreatogenic diabetes after pancreatic resection. *Pancreatology* 2011;11:268–276

53. Beger HG, Schlosser W, Friess HM, Buchler MW. Duodenum-preserving head resection in chronic pancreatitis changes the natural course of the disease: a single-center 26-year experience. *Ann Surg* 1999;230:512–519; discussion 519–523

54. Keck T, Wellner UF, Riediger H, Adam U, Sick O, et al. Long-term outcome after 92 duodenum-preserving pancreatic head resections for chronic pancreatitis: comparison of Beger and Frey procedures. *J Gastrointest Surg* 2010;14:549–556

55. Traverso LW, Kozarek RA. Pancreatoduodenectomy for chronic pancreatitis: anatomic selection criteria and subsequent long-term outcome analysis. *Ann Surg* 1997;226:429–438

56. Sakorafas GH, Farnell MB, Nagorney DM, Sarr MG, Rowland CM. Pancreatoduodenectomy for chronic pancreatitis: long-term results in 105 patients. *Arch Surg* 2000;135:517–523; discussion 523–524

57. Wang X, Misawa R, Zielinski MC, Cowen P, Jo J, Periwal V, et al. Regional differences in islet distribution in the human pancreas—preferential beta-cell loss in the head region in patients with type 2 diabetes. *PLoS One* 2013;8:e67454

58. Balzano G, Maffi P, Nano R, Mercalli A, Melzi R, Aleotti F, et al. Autologous islet transplantation in patients requiring pancreatectomy: a broader spectrum of indications beyond chronic pancreatitis. *Am J Transplant* 2016;16:1812–1826

59. Moran A, Doherty L, Wang X, Thomas W. Abnormal glucose metabolism in cystic fibrosis. *J Pediatr* 1998;133:10–17

60. Marshall BC, Butler SM, Stoddard M, Moran AM, Liou TG, Morgan WJ. Epidemiology of cystic fibrosis-related diabetes. *J Pediatr* 2005;146:681–687

61. Moran A, Becker D, Casella SJ, Gottlieb PA, Kirkman MS, Marshall BC, et al. Epidemiology, pathophysiology, and prognostic implications of cystic fibrosis-related diabetes: a technical review. *Diabetes Care* 2010;33:2677–2683

62. Brennan AL, Beynon J. Clinical updates in cystic fibrosis-related diabetes. *Semin Respir Crit Care Med* 2015;36:236–250

63. Moran A, Brunzell C, Cohen RC, Katz M, Marshall BC, Onady G, et al. Clinical care guidelines for cystic fibrosis-related diabetes: a position statement of the American Diabetes Association and a clinical practice guideline of the Cystic Fibrosis Foundation, endorsed by the Pediatric Endocrine Society. *Diabetes Care* 2010;33:2697–2708

64. O'Riordan SM, Hindmarsh P, Hill NR, Matthews DR, George S, Greally P, et al. Validation of continuous glucose monitoring in children and adolescents with cystic fibrosis: a prospective cohort study. *Diabetes Care* 2009;32:1020–1022

65. Crawford DHG. Hereditary hemochromatosis types 1, 2, and 3. *Clin Liver Dis* 2014;3:96–97

66. Adams PC, Kertesz AE, Valberg LS. Clinical presentation of hemochromatosis: a changing scene. *Am J Med* 1991;90:445–449

67. Peterlin B, Globocnik Petrovic M, Makuc J, Hawlina M, Petrovic D. A hemochromatosis-causing mutation C282Y is a risk factor for proliferative diabetic retinopathy in Caucasians with type 2 diabetes. *J Hum Genet* 2003;48:646–649

68. Wouthuis SF, van Deursen CT, te Lintelo MP, Rozeman CA, Beekman R. Neuromuscular manifestations in hereditary haemochromatosis. *J Neurol* 2010;257:1465–1472

69. Niederau C, Fischer R, Sonnenberg A, Stremmel W, Trampisch HJ, Strohmeyer G. Survival and causes of death in cirrhotic and in noncirrhotic patients with primary hemochromatosis. *N Engl J Med* 1985;313:1256–1262

70. Vesterhus M, Raeder H, Aurlien H, Gjesdal CG, Bredrup C, Holm PI, et al. Neurological features and enzyme therapy in patients with endocrine and exocrine pancreas dysfunction due to CEL mutations. *Diabetes Care* 2008; 31:1738–1740

71. Anik A, Catli G, Abaci A, Bober E. Maturity-onset diabetes of the young (MODY): an update. *J Pediatr Endocrinol Metab* 2015;28:251–263

72. Vesterhus M, Raeder H, Johansson S, Molven A, Njolstad PR. Pancreatic exocrine dysfunction in maturity-onset diabetes of the young type 3. *Diabetes Care* 2008;31:306–310

73. Stoffers DA, Ferrer J, Clarke WL, Habener JF. Early-onset type-II diabetes mellitus (MODY4) linked to IPF1. *Nat Genet* 1997;17:138–139

74. Stoffers DA, Zinkin NT, Stanojevic V, Clarke WL, Habener JF. Pancreatic agenesis attributable to a single nucleotide deletion in the human IPF1 gene coding sequence. *Nat Genet* 1997;15:106–110

75. Ulinski T, Lescure S, Beaufils S, Guigonis V, Decramer S, Morin D, et al. Renal phenotypes related to hepatocyte nuclear factor-1beta (TCF2) mutations in a pediatric cohort. *J Am Soc Nephrol* 2006;17:497–503

76. Edghill EL, Bingham C, Slingerland AS, Minton JA, Noordam C, et al. Hepatocyte nuclear factor-1 beta mutations cause neonatal diabetes and intrauterine growth retardation: support for a critical role of HNF-1beta in human pancreatic development. *Diabet Med* 2006;23:1301–1306

77. Bingham C, Hattersley AT. Renal cysts and diabetes syndrome resulting from mutations in hepatocyte nuclear factor-1beta. *Nephrol Dial Transplant* 2004;19:2703–2708

78. Raeder H, Johansson S, Holm PI, Haldorsen IS, Mas E, Sbarra V, et al. Mutations in the CEL VNTR cause a syndrome of diabetes and pancreatic exocrine dysfunction. *Nat Genet* 2006;38:54–62

79. Raeder H, McAllister FE, Tjora E, Bhatt S, Haldorsen I, Hu J, et al. Carboxyl-ester lipase maturity-onset diabetes of the young is associated with development of pancreatic cysts and upregulated MAPK signaling in secretin-stimulated duodenal fluid. *Diabetes* 2014;63:259–269

Part II
Case Studies

Introduction

The following 21 cases present important examples of diabetes arising as a consequence of insulin resistance, genetic defects in insulin action, and diseases of exocrine pancreas. Genetic syndromes of insulin resistance are rare, but when encountered they present challenging diagnostic and therapeutic dilemmas. Cases 23–25 illustrate mutations in the insulin receptor gene. These mutations are usually autosomal recessive in nature and are characterized by the presence of extreme insulin resistance. Cases of lipodystrophy (Cases 26–30) occur with somewhat greater frequency but are still reasonably rare and certainly equally challenging, particularly in aspects of therapy. Pancreatogenic diabetes follows the destruction of exocrine and endocrine pancreas by disease processes usually initiated in the exocrine part of this important organ or after surgical removal of the pancreas due to either pancreatitis or oncological problems (Cases 31–34). Diabetes develops in many patients with cystic fibrosis who nowadays have much improved life expectancy (Case 37). Patients with hemochromatosis and liver diseases may develop diabetes (Cases 34–36) as do those treated with certain medications that interfere with either insulin secretion or insulin action, thus promoting hyperglycemia. The preceding chapters in Part II of this volume (Chapters 2–4) outline and discuss all these possibilities in more detail and in greater depth.

Case 23:
Type A Insulin Resistance

Anna Stears, MBBS, DM;[1] and Robert K. Semple, MB, PhD[2,3]

Case History

A 13-year-old female was referred to an endocrinologist for evaluation of excess facial hair growth and darkening of the skin in her neck, axillae, and groin. Facial hair growth in a male pattern had first been noticed around the age of 10 years and had gradually worsened over the next three years. Her mother reported noticing a distinctive body odor from around three years old, the appearance of pubic hair at around the age of six years, and development of diffuse fine hair growth on the back at five or six years of age. She had never been overweight and reported no menstrual bleeds.

On examination, she had pronounced acanthosis nigricans in her axillae and in the nuchal region and multiple skin tags in the axillae (Figure C23.1). She also had moderate to severe hirsutism, particularly in the sideburn area. Pubertal development was nearly complete. Acanthosis nigricans and hirsutism in a lean female led to the clinical suspicion of severe insulin resistance, and this was confirmed by biochemical assessment. The

[1]National Severe Insulin Resistance Service, Wolfson Diabetes & Endocrine Clinic, Cambridge University Hospitals NHS Foundation Trust, Cambridge Biomedical Campus, Cambridge, U.K.
[2]The University of Cambridge Metabolic Research Laboratories, Wellcome Trust-MRC Institute of Metabolic Science, Cambridge, U.K.
[3]The National Institute for Health Research Cambridge Biochemical Research Centre, Cambridge, U.K.

biochemical profile at first assessment and over the subsequent five years of follow-up is shown in Table C23.1. Nonfasting plasma insulin was severely elevated with normal blood glucose, and the insulin to C-peptide molar ratio was markedly raised, suggesting impaired insulin clearance. The lipid profile was normal, leptin was commensurate with overall adiposity, and blood concentration of adiponectin, a fat cell–derived protein normally inversely related to plasma insulin concentrations, was preserved. Estradiol concentration was normal for the follicular phase of the menstrual cycle, but testosterone was severely elevated to the bottom end of the normal range for males. Leutinizing hormone (LH) was mildly elevated, and follicle-stimulating hormone (FSH) was normal. Ovarian ultrasonography revealed polycystic ovaries. A clinical diagnosis of Type A insulin resistance was made, and advice about healthy diet and exercise was given. Pharmacological treatment was begun with metformin 1,000 mg twice daily, an anti-androgenic combined oral contraceptive pill, topical eflornithine, and spironolactone after counselling about the critical importance of reliable contraception.

The normal fasting lipid profile and relatively preserved adiponectin level in a lean patient with severe insulin resistance raised the possibil-

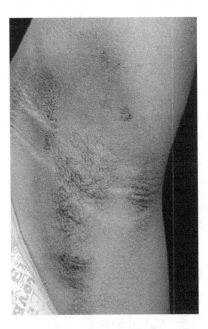

Figure C23.1—Axillary acanthosis in the patient described at 15 years old.

Table C23.1—Biochemical Profile of Patient Described Over Five Years of Follow-Up

Fasting/non-fasting	Non-fasting	Non-fasting	Fasting	Fasting	Fasting	Reference Range/Comment
Age, years	13	14	15	17	18	
BMI (kg/m²)	22.7	25.0	25.4	24.9	27.7	
BMI SDS	+1.05	+1.31	+1.29	+1.05	+1.34	
HbA$_{1c}$ (mmol/mol)	50	73	66	67	79	Target <53
%	6.7	8.8	8.2	8.3	9.4	<7
Glucose (mg/dL)	85	126	88	90	158	63–100 (f)
Insulin (pmol/L)	6620	2780	601	554	nd	0–60 (f)
C-peptide (pmol/L)	5759	3161	709	681	nd	174–960 (f)
Insulin: C-peptide molar ratio	1.1	0.9	0.8	0.8	nd	0.1–0.2
Adiponectin (mg/L)	8.9	12.5	9.5	7.1	nd	>8 in severe insulin resistance predicts INSR defect
Leptin (ug/L)	28.3	24.0	23.4	27.6	nd	2.2–24.4* 8.6–38.9#
Triglyceride (mg/dL)	71	62	44	88	62	<151
HDL-Chol (mg/dL)	66	62	50	47	50	>42
LH (units/L)	10.3	11.2	10.2	18.6	8.9	1.3–8.4
FSH (units/L)	4.9	5.4	3.7	2.7	4.4	2.9–8.4
Estradiol (pmol/L)	220	207	218	292	214	100–750
Testosterone (nmol/L)	12.9	13.5	14.1	18.3	10.4	0–1.8

nd, not determined; (f), fasting; *, range for BMI 20–25; #, range for BMI 25–30

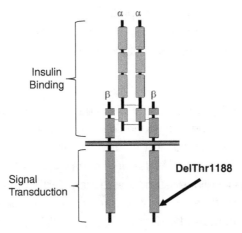

α   α

Insulin
Binding

β   β

DelThr1188

Signal
Transduction

Figure C23.2—Schematic of the insulin receptor, showing location of the deleted amino acid in the intracellular domain.

ity of a genetic insulin receptor defect. Screening of the insulin receptor (INSR) gene revealed a rare heterozygous mutation deleting a single amino acid from the intracellular portion of the insulin receptor, which is critically involved in transmitting insulin binding at the cell surface into cellular metabolic responses (p.delThr1188 in the mature receptor) (Figure C23.2). Her mother, who also had acanthosis nigricans and insulin resistance, proved to have the same mutation.

On reassessment at 14 years of age, primary amenorrhea and severe hirsutism persisted. Random blood testing in the late morning revealed an HbA$_{1c}$ of 8.8% (73 mmol/mol), and diabetes was diagnosed. Testosterone remained severely elevated, and gonadotrophins were unsuppressed. Further inquiry suggested low mood and poor compliance with all medications, including the contraceptive pill. Sporadic poor compliance persisted over ensuing years, and antiandrogenic therapy was stopped in view of concerns about teratogenicity. Metformin was also discontinued due to gastrointestinal side effects. At 17 years of age, laser depilation was begun with good effect, although facial hirsutism remained the patient's main concern. Progesterone courses were recommended to induce withdrawal bleeding at least three times yearly in the face of prolonged amenorrhea since discontinuing the oral contraceptive, and intensive support was offered to encourage weight loss and increased exercise. Throughout five years of follow-up, extreme hyperinsulinemia with variable but subop-timal glycemic control, normal lipid profile and adiponectin, and severely elevated testosterone persisted (Table C23.1).

Discussion

This case is a typical example of "Type A" insulin resistance, a term coined in the 1970s to denote young, lean women with severe insulin resis-tance but without evidence of a circulating insulin blocking antibody, or "Type B" insulin resistance.[1,2] The first mutations in the insulin receptor underlying Type A insulin resistance were identified in 1988, and since then a large number of different causative mutations have been reported, most commonly in the intracellular domain of the insulin receptor. These confer autosomal dominant severe insulin resistance, which affects both males and females, although it commonly remains undetected in men until tar-geted testing or until diabetes is diagnosed in adult life.

The biochemical profile of insulin resistance associated with acquired or inherited insulin receptor defects is distinct from severe insulin resis-tance caused by obesity or lipodystrophy, with characteristically normal lipid profile, absence of fatty liver, and usually preserved plasma adipo-nectin concentrations. These features in a lean patient with severe insu-lin resistance should prompt consideration of genetic testing of the INSR gene.[3,4]

Although diabetes is common in Type A insulin resistance, it commonly occurs with primary or secondary amenorrhea and/or features of hyperan-drogenism, in a pattern consistent with severe polycystic ovary syndrome. This is often the dominant concern of affected patients. Hyperandrogen-emia is common to all forms of severe insulin resistance in postpuber-tal girls, and may be severe, with testosterone levels sometimes reach-ing the normal male range, as in this case. Careful evaluation for sinister features suggesting an androgen-secreting tumor is important, but onset is characteristically gradual and tracks metabolic state when hyperan-drogenemia is driven by insulin resistance. Hyperandrogenism and oligo-menorrhea appear to be driven by high levels of insulin synergizing with gonadotrophins, and both improve if either insulin or gonadotrophins are suppressed. Where there is diagnostic doubt, evaluation of adrenal andro-gens and/or use of GnRH suppression testing may be used to support a diagnosis of insulin resistance-driven ovarian hyperandrogenism, and in some cases suppression of gonadotropins in patients with severe insulin resistance may be used therapeutically as well as diagnostically, though "add back" hormone replacement may often be necessary.[5] Use of an anti-androgenic oral contraceptive pill or use of intermittent progesterone to induce withdrawal bleeds remains a far more common strategy, however. If reliable contraception is in place, then off-label antiandrogenic therapy may have some efficacy in reducing hirsutism as in other forms of clinical hyperandrogenism.

The genetic defect in insulin signaling interacts very sensitively with other environmental factors, so encouraging exercise and preventing weight gain is a critical element of management. Pubertal insulin resistance also interacts with the genetic defect, and control of glycemia commonly improves somewhat as patients move into their third decade. Metformin is of value in both delaying and treating diabetes. In many patients with Type A insulin resistance extreme levels of hyperinsulinemia can be sustained for many years, suggesting robust β-cell function that is only relatively deficient in overcoming the severe insulin resistance.

In this patient, compliance with prescribed therapies was poor, to a significant degree due to mood disturbances driven by distress at the cosmetic consequences of hyperandrogenism. The central elements of her future management will be continued encouragement to lose weight and exercise, targeting of hyperandrogenism, possibly using GnRH agonist therapy, and encouragement to reintroduce insulin-sensitizing therapies, which, in the absence of specific data in Type A insulin resistance, will be guided empirically by clinical and biochemical response. Prognosis will be determined in large part by glycemic control. It is not clear at present whether the characteristic benign lipid profile seen in insulin receptor defects confers a lower long-term risk of atherosclerosis compared to other forms of severe insulin resistance.

References

1. Semple RK, Savage DB, Cochran EK, Gorden P, O'Rahilly S. Genetic syndromes of severe insulin resistance. *Endocr Rev* 2011;32:498–514

2. Musso C, Cochran E, Moran SA, Skarulis MC, Oral EA, Taylor S, Gorden P. Clinical course of genetic diseases of the insulin receptor (type A and Rabson-Mendenhall syndromes): a 30-year prospective. *Medicine (Baltimore)* 2004;83:209–222

3. Semple RK, Sleigh A, Murgatroyd PR, Adams CA, Bluck L, Jackson S, Vottero A, Kanabar D, Charlton-Menys V, Durrington P, Soos MA, Carpenter TA, Lomas

DJ, Cochran EK, Gorden P, O'Rahilly S, Savage DB. Postreceptor insulin resistance contributes to human dyslipidemia and hepatic steatosis. *J Clin Invest* 2009;119:315–322

4.   Semple RK, Cochran EK, Soos MA, Burling KA, Savage DB, Gorden P, O'Rahilly S. Plasma adiponectin as a marker of insulin receptor dysfunction: clinical utility in severe insulin resistance. *Diabetes Care* 2008;31:977–979

5.   Brown RJ, Joseph J, Cochran E, Gewert C, Semple R, Gorden P. Type B insulin resistance masquerading as ovarian hyperthecosis. *J Clin Endocrinol Metab* 102;2017:1789–1791.

Case 24:
Donohue Syndrome
(Leprechaunism)

Catherine Peters, MD;[1] and Robert K. Semple, MB, PhD[2,3]

Case History

The patient was a male infant, the first child of parents who were first cousins. He was born at term by elective caesarean section due to concern about intrauterine growth restriction (IUGR) and maternal gestational diabetes. His birth weight was 1.23 kg (–5.6 SDS), and he required hospital neonatal care for 2 months due to difficulty in establishing feeding, with poor weight gain despite large volumes of high-energy feeds. Blood glucose concentrations on intermittent testing were in the range of 900–1,350 mg/dL (50–75 mmol/L). Relative macrocephaly and abdominal distension led to magnetic resonance imaging of head and abdomen at 2 months old, but both were said to be normal. A clinical geneticist then noted that as well as impaired linear growth and poor weight gain, the infant had overgrowth of many soft tissues, with thick skin, thick lips, large ears, a large phallus, and rectal prolapse. A clinical diagnosis of Donohue syndrome (formerly known as leprechaunism) was made based on these dysmorphic features, and referral to a specialist unit was arranged.

---

[1]Department of Endocrinology, Great Ormond Street Hospital, London, U.K.

[2]The University of Cambridge Metabolic Research Laboratories, Wellcome Trust-MRC Institute of Metabolic Science, Cambridge, U.K.

[3]The National Institute for Health Research Cambridge Biochemical Research Centre, Cambridge, U.K.

DOI: 10.2337/9781580406666.04

Examination on referral confirmed the clinical appearance of Donohue syndrome, including triangular, coarse facies, enlarged lips, and a small, broad nose, with marked hypertrichosis and dry skin. Genitalia, hands, and feet appeared disproportionately enlarged. The diagnosis was supported biochemically by demonstration of extreme elevation of plasma insulin concentrations to above 300 mU/L (reference range <10). Further evaluation (Table C.24.1) demonstrated erratic glycemic control, featuring both hyperglycemia in the fed state and recurrent fasting hypoglycemia, mitigated by continuous feeding. IGF-1 and IGFBP3 were persistently undetectable, but pituitary function tests were normal. Plasma electrolyte concentrations were serially within the normal range, although the serum creatinine was persistently below 12 umol/L or 0.14 mg/dL (reference range 16–33 umol/L). Urinary albumin and calcium excretion was raised and bilateral medullary nephrocalcinosis was first noted at 5 months old, with a marked increase in urinary amino acids consistent with proximal renal tubular dysfunction.

Table C24.1 — Representative Laboratory Abnormalities in Patient Described

Analyte	Value	Reference Range	Age, months	Comment
Glucose (mg/dL)	214	63–110	3	
Insulin (mU/L)	>300	<10	3	Levels as high as 10,000 mU/L may be seen in Donohue syndrome (DS)
IGF-1 (ng/ml)	Undetectable	55–327	Many occasions	Commonly reported in DS
IGFBP3 (mg/L)	Undetectable	0.7–3.6	Many occasions	Commonly reported in DS
Growth hormone (mg/L)	2.3	n/a	3	
SHBG (nmol/L)	315	15–48	3	High, reflecting failure of insulin to suppress liver SHBG expression
Prothrombin time (seconds)	20.2	9.6–11.8	6	
APTT (seconds)	62	26–38	6	

(Continued)

Table C24.1—(Continued)

Thrombin time (seconds)	16	9.2–15	6	
Fibrinogen (g/L)	1.3	1.7–4.0	6	
Factor VII assay (IU/dL)	26	50–150		
Factor VIII (IU/dL)	161.7	50–150		
Factor IX assay (IU/dL)	31.1	50–150		
Factor XI assay (IU/dL)	44	50–150		Factor II,V,X normal

Genetic analysis of the insulin receptor (INSR) gene, encoding the insulin receptor, revealed the homozygous p.Gly111Glu mutation, replacing a neutral glycine with a negatively charged glutamate residue at amino acid 111 of the insulin proreceptor (amino acid 84 of the fully functional processed receptor) (Figure C24.1). Both parents were heterozygous for the mutation. This mutation had not been described before because it was not found in large control populations. As it makes a major change to a highly conserved amino acid, it was deemed to be the cause of the extreme insulin resistance. The mutation falls in the extracellular part of the insulin receptor that binds insulin, and is highly likely to impair insulin binding, to impair synthesis of the receptor and its routing to the cell surface, or both.

At 6 months of age, intubation that was started for the purpose of central venous catheter insertion provoked cardiopulmonary arrest, requiring epinephrine, cardiac compressions, and 24 hours of mechanical ventilation. Echocardiography revealed severe biventricular hypertrophy with left ventricular outlet obstruction. In view of continuing failure to thrive and poor metabolic control, a trial of recombinant human IGF-1 treatment was commenced at a dose of 33 mcg/kg/day administered subcutaneously. This did not observably improve any metabolic parameters, however, and in the face of declining clinical state was discontinued after 12 weeks.

Over the ensuing months poor metabolic control persisted, with development of further additional problems. Abdominal distension, initially noted at birth, progressively became more severe, with concomitant constipation, and worsening of an inguinal hernia and rectal prolapse. Feeding was poorly tolerated, and attempts to introduce dairy-, soya-, and wheat-free

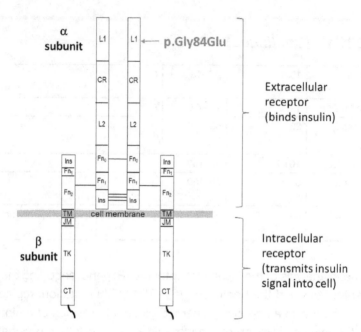

Figure C24.1 — Schematic of the insulin receptor, showing functional domains and position of the p.Gly84Glu mutation.

L1 and L2 = Epidermal Growth Factor-like domains; CR = Cysteine-rich region; Fn = fibronectin-like domain; Ins = insert region; TM = transmembrane domain; JM = juxtamembrane domain; TK = tyrosine kinase domain; CT = C terminal region

feeds led to further abdominal distension and ascites, ultimately leading to commencement of total parenteral nutrition. Low levels of vitamins D and K were corrected. Hepatosplenomegaly developed with raised serum alkaline phosphatase and gamma glutamyl transferase. Coagulopathy characterized by raised activated partial thromboplastin, prothrombin and thrombin times, and low concentrations of clotting factors including factor XI as well as vitamin K-dependent factors II, VII, IX, and X were observed. Albumin infusions were used to give clinical relief from marked ascites. Liver ultrasonography showed a normal liver echotexture with no evidence of portal hypertension, and investigation at a national pediatric liver unit failed to identify a cause for the hepatopathy. Liver biopsy was precluded by high procedure-related risks.

Blood glucose concentrations over the following months continued to fluctuate with feeding, ranging from prefeed hypoglycemia and to postfeed hyperglycemia up to 360 mg/dL (20 mmol/L). These large oscillations in glucose concentration were attenuated but not eliminated by parenteral nutrition. Accurate HbA$_{1c}$ calculations were not possible due to persisting high levels of fetal hemoglobin. Growth remained poor (persistently around –8 SDS for both height and weight).

Between 6 and 16 months of age, there were multiple episodes of pyrexia with no identifiable focus, and no organisms were cultured from blood. Acute, severe respiratory distress developed at the age of 16 months due to respiratory syncytial virus infection and ventilation was commenced. Response to conventional ventilation was poor, however, and in the face of escalating ventilatory and inotropic requirements, a decision to withdraw care was made by the family and medical team.

Discussion

Donohue syndrome, or "leprechaunism" (a synonym still often used, but which we disfavor), describes the extreme end of the spectrum of genetic defects of the insulin receptor.[1,2] It is invariably recessive, and features complete, or near complete, loss of receptor function. Its appearance is characteristic, but diagnosis may be delayed, as in this case, by failure to appreciate the significance of the combination of severe IUGR, postnatal impairment of linear growth, adipose and muscle development, contrasting with exuberant overgrowth of many other tissues, including skin (acanthosis nigricans or skin thickening), hair (hypertrichosis), gonads (especially in females, where ovarian overgrowth may be progressive and severe), sex hormone–dependent tissues (external genitalia and nipples), and viscera (nonfatty hepatomegaly, often with cholestasis, nephromegaly, often with nephrocalcinosis, left ventricular hypertrophy, and colonic mucosal overgrowth).

These features should immediately prompt measurement of blood glucose and insulin, though in many cases preprandial hypoglycemia and/or hyperglycemia are noted neonatally. Hyperinsulinemia is usually extreme, ranging from one to three orders of magnitude higher than normal. It is most likely that overgrowth is driven by enormously elevated insulin levels acting on the IGF-1 receptor. IGF-1 and IGFBP3 themselves are commonly suppressed, which may be a consequence of hyperinsulinemia feeding back erroneously to the hypothalamus via IGF-1 receptors, and loss of growth hormone receptor expression in the liver, which is positively regulated by the insulin receptor. It is not clear whether the additional hepatopathy and coagulopathy seen in this case are related to the underlying insulin receptor defect, and these possible aspects of the syndrome warrant study in other patients.

Despite near complete loss of insulin receptor function, infants with Donohue syndrome do not develop ketoacidosis, although in the milder Rabson-Mendenhall syndrome this can start to appear later in childhood.[3] The reason for this is not fully established, but important contributors have been suggested to be lack of adipose tissue, depriving the liver of free fatty acids as ketogenic substrate, deficiency of growth hormone, and/or persistence of IGF-1 receptor expression in an "immature" liver, allowing severe hyperinsulinemia to exert some direct hepatic effects.[4]

Management, as in this case, is extremely challenging, and the prognosis is almost invariably poor. Simple maneuvers such as continuous rather than bolus feeding may reduce fluctuations between hypoglycemia and hyperglycemia, and overall calorie content of feed needs to balance the competing needs to encourage growth and to reduce hyperglycemia. Insulin, even at extremely high doses, often has little effect, and so a variety of other alternative or adjunctive therapies have been reported, with little clear evidence of efficacy in most cases. As discussed also in Case 25, recombinant human IGF-1 is often employed, based on case reports and case series over the past 20 years suggesting efficacy both acutely, and in some cases chronically.[5] Nevertheless, gathering reliable data is extremely challenging in the face of genetic heterogeneity, and variable natural history of different INSR mutations. Uncertainties remain about the optimal mode of delivery and dosing schedule, long-term efficacy and therapeutic window, and the published literature may be skewed in favor of positive outcomes. In this case, there was no clear evidence of clinical benefit. Systematic prospective collection of data relating to rhIGF-1 therapy in Donohue syndrome is urgently required.

References

1. Taylor SI, Cama A, Accili D, Barbetti F, Quon MJ, de la Luz Sierra M, Suzuki Y, Koller E, Levy-Toledano R, Wertheimer E, et al. Mutations in the insulin receptor gene. *Endocr Rev* 1992;13:566–595

2. Semple RK, Savage DB, Cochran EK, Gorden P, O'Rahilly S. Genetic syndromes of severe insulin resistance. *Endocr Rev* 2011;32:498–514

3. Musso C, Cochran E, Moran SA, Skarulis MC, Oral EA, Taylor S, Gorden P. Clinical course of genetic diseases of the insulin receptor (type A and Rabson-

Mendenhall syndromes): a 30-year prospective. *Medicine (Baltimore)* 2004;83:209–222

4. Ogilvy-Stuart AL, Soos MA, Hands SJ, Anthony MY, Dunger DB, O'Rahilly S. Hypoglycemia and resistance to ketoacidosis in a subject without functional insulin receptors. *J Clin Endocrinol Metab* 2001;86:3319–3326

5. McDonald A, Williams RM, Regan FM, Semple RK, Dunger DB. IGF-I treatment of insulin resistance. *Eur J Endocrinol* 2007;157(Suppl. 1):S51–S56

Case 25:
Rabson-Mendenhall Syndrome

Rachel Williams, MD;[1] and Robert K. Semple, MB, PhD[2,3]

Case History

A female infant was born at term with a weight of 2.1 kg (z score −2.4) following a normal pregnancy. Clitoromegaly, hypertrichosis, and mild hyperpigmentation were noted at birth, and weight gain was slow postnatally. Hyperglycemia was detected incidentally and clinical suspicion of an insulin resistance syndrome led to assay of plasma insulin, which proved extremely elevated at >1,600 pmol/L (normal range <60), with C-peptide commensurately elevated. Hyperglycemia was exacerbated by high-energy feeding, with evidence of osmotic diuresis, and exogenous insulin was introduced. Blood glucose concentrations remained high despite rapid intravenous insulin dose titration to 10 units/kg/day, and despite subsequent intravenous bolus of 5 units/kg intravenous insulin. After rehydrating and moderating caloric intake, infusion of 3.6 units/kg/day insulin using a combination of continuous subcutaneous and intravenous delivery reduced glucose levels to 180–270 mg/dL (10–15 mmol/L). At 2 months

[1]The University of Cambridge Department of Paediatrics, Box 116, Level 8, Cambridge Biomedical Campus, Cambridge, U.K.

[2]The University of Cambridge Metabolic Research Laboratories, Wellcome Trust-MRC Institute of Metabolic Science, Cambridge, U.K.

[3]The National Institute for Health Research Cambridge Biochemical Research Centre, Cambridge, U.K.

of age, the infant weighed 3.6 kg, and had developed some subcutaneous adipose tissue despite continuing hyperglycemia. After discussion with the family, 0.5 mg rosiglitazone was introduced daily in an attempt at insulin sensitization.

Genetic analysis of the insulin receptor (INSR) gene revealed a novel homozygous mutation that replaces a highly conserved, positively charged arginine for non-polar, aromatic tryptophan at position 114 of the mature insulin receptor, in the insulin binding domain of the protein (Figure C25.1). Both parents were heterozygous for the mutation. Although the mutation had not been reported before, it was not found in control populations, and studies of the mutant protein in cell culture showed that the mutant receptor had a severely reduced ability to bind insulin (Figure C25.2).

At 4 months of age, blood glucose concentrations ranged between 140–320 mg/dL on 24 units of insulin delivered by continuous subcutaneous infusion and 0.5 mg rosiglitazone daily. HbA_{1c} was 11%. Moderate left ventricular hypertrophy was found on echocardiography, but after discussion with the family rosiglitazone was continued. At 6 months of age, weight was 7.1 kg and developmental milestones had been reached normally. At 7 months of age, fasting capillary blood glucose concentrations of

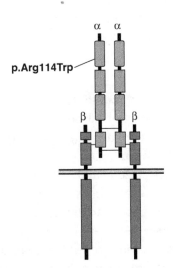

Figure C25.1—p.Arg114Trp (R114W) mutation in INSR. Schematic of the insulin receptor protein showing the location of the mutation in the extracellular, ligand-binding domain of the receptor.

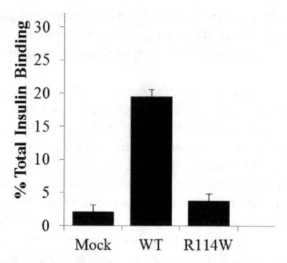

Figure C25.2—Impaired insulin binding by the mutant receptor compared to wild type receptor, assessed in artificially created receptors overexpressed in Chinese hamster ovary cells. "Mock" refers to cells to which no receptor was added and represents the baseline coming from hamster insulin receptors in the cells. Note that the numbering of the mutation is given according to the mature receptor sequence.

72 mg/dL (4 mmol/L) were recorded at home, and insulin infusion was stopped. Off insulin treatment, but still on rosiglitazone 0.5 mg daily, fasting blood glucoses were in the normal range, but postprandial concentrations were 180–270 mg/dL (10–15 mmol/L). By 1 year of age, the HbA$_{1c}$ had fallen to 7.1%, still on rosiglitazone at 0.5 mg daily. Rosiglitazone was later stopped around the age of 3 years on withdrawal of its regulatory approval in Europe due to concerns about cardiovascular risks in adults.

At the age of 5 years, the patient was referred to a specialist with a severe insulin resistance service for further evaluation. On examination, she showed normal linear growth, with height SD score –1.59, in keeping with her family, and weight SD score –0.56. She had moderate acanthosis nigricans in the nuchal area and in both axillae with some gingival hypertrophy. She was lean but not lipodystrophic, and she was prepubertal with no clinical hyperandrogenism. General examination was otherwise normal.

Biochemical investigations are shown in Table C25.1. These findings demonstrated diabetes with extremely elevated insulin concentrations, an elevated molar ratio of insulin to C-peptide, and suppressed serum IGF-1. Leptin was low, consistent with low whole-body adipose tissue, while adiponectin, a fat cell–derived protein that is severely suppressed in the face of most forms of severe and extreme insulin resistance, was preserved. The lipid profile, which is characteristically severely deranged in insulin resistance related to obesity or lipodystrophy, was normal. Echocardiography was now normal.

Adjunctive therapy with rhIGF-I was commenced at a dose initially of 0.1 mg/kg/day, increasing at monthly intervals to a total daily dose of 0.4 mg/kg/day. On reevaluation at 16 months of therapy, a marginal improvement in HbA_{1c} (from 67–70 mmol/L or 8.3–8.6%) and glucose and insulin excursions during oral glucose tolerance testing were noted, with restitution of serum IGF-1 concentration. Therapy was well tolerated with no reported side effects, and retinal photography and echocardiography have remained normal during rhIGF-1 therapy (Table C25.2).

Discussion

This patient has autosomal recessive extreme insulin resistance due to a homozygous mutation in the gene for the insulin receptor that severely impairs insulin binding. Although novel at the time of detection, subsequently the mutation has been described in another patient from the same

Table C25.1—Fasting Biochemical Profile of Patient Described at 5 Years of Age Prior to rhIGF-1 Therapy

	Baseline	Units	Reference
Total Cholesterol	174	mg/dL	<200 mg/dL
HDL Cholesterol	64	mg/dL	40–60 mg/dL
LDL Cholesterol	94	mg/dL	<100 mg/dL
IGF-I baseline	<3.3	nmol/L	5.1–32.75 nmol/L
Leptin	1.1	mcg/L	2.4–24.4
Adiponectin	7.2	mg/L	Levels >5 in face of severe insulin resistance suggestive of INSR defect
HbA_{1c}	70 (8.5)	mmol/mol (%)	

Table C25.2—Oral Glucose Tolerance Testing Results before rhIGF1 at Age 5 Years and at Age 6.5 Years after 12 Months of rhIGF1 Therapy

Time (min)	Glucose (mg/dL)		Insulin (pmol/L) (Fasting reference <60 pmol/L)		C-peptide (pmol/L)		Insulin: C-peptide molar ratio (reference 0.1–0.2)	
	Baseline	On IGF-I	Baseline	On IGF-I	Baseline	On IGF-I	Baseline	On IGF-I
0	256	167	3,910	1,590	3,303	1,466	1.2	1.1
30	394	313	4,410	2,750	5,263	3,058	0.8	0.9
60	401	385	4,160	4,280	5,561	4,667	0.7	0.9
90	405	374	5,360	3,640	4,270	3,542	1.3	1.0
120	347	343	5,110	3,370	6,157	3,005	0.8	1.1

geographical area, suggesting a possible geographical founder effect in the region of the Arabian Gulf.[1] Historical clinical descriptions have classified children with recessive insulin receptor defects as having either Donohue syndrome ("leprechaunism") or Rabson-Mendenhall syndrome (RMS); however, these designations are somewhat imprecisely applied. Both original descriptions were reported many years before identification of the underlying molecular defect, and rather than being discrete entities, they denote different points on the same disease spectrum.[2] Donohue syndrome is best used to describe patients with the most extreme presentations, who have little or no residual insulin receptor function. It is very rare for these patients to survive beyond infancy, with demise often caused by intercurrent infection (see Case 24). In this case, although extreme insulin resistance was identified neonatally, survival beyond infancy, and only modestly impaired growth, albeit allied to poorly controlled diabetes at five years old, make RMS an appropriate diagnosis. In most cases of RMS, linear growth impairment is more marked than in this case and, as in Donohue syndrome, this contrasts with many overgrowth features including hypertrichosis, acanthosis nigricans, gingival hypertrophy, and premature tooth eruption. Pineal hyperplasia was prominent in early reports, but this is likely another form of soft tissue overgrowth secondary to extreme hyperinsulinemia rather than being functionally important.

The biochemical profile seen in this case is typical of RMS, with extremely insulin resistant diabetes, elevated insulin to C-peptide molar ratio (indicative of impaired receptor-mediated insulin clearance in the liver with preserved renal C-peptide clearance), a normal lipid profile and liver function, low leptin, and relatively normal adiponectin concentrations. These findings discriminate patients with insulin receptor defects from those with obesity or lipodystrophy-driven severe insulin resistance, where severe dyslipidemia, fatty liver, and suppressed adiponectin concentration are the norm.

The management of diabetes and impaired growth in RMS is challenging and the natural history of the condition, while variable, usually features metabolic decompensation to produce intractable hyperglycemia at some point in the first or second decade of life. Demise due to hyperglycemic complications or ketoacidosis in the second or third decade has historically been common. Therapy is guided at present only by clinical experience and by small case series.[3] Exogenous insulin often adds little to the severe endogenous hyperinsulinemia, and so metformin is commonly used instead as first-line therapy.[4] It is used on an unlicensed basis in children younger than 12 years but is well tolerated. Scattered reports of other agents, such as thiazolidinediones and gliptins, exist, often in complex multidrug regimens, and few conclusions can be drawn about their efficacy from the individual cases described. An unusual feature of this case was the use of rosiglitazone in the first three years of life. It did not cause any discernible harm, and its use correlated with early improvement in glycemic control. However, as with all rare genetic receptoropathies, it is not possible to conclude that it was beneficial, especially as the natural history of patients with different novel mutations in the INSR gene is unclear.

There is evidence that subcutaneous leptin replacement in RMS may have metabolic benefits, probably driven by reduced BMI; however, this remains on an experimental basis and is not easily accessible.[5] There is a somewhat larger case literature describing use of rhIGF-1 in patients with insulin resistance secondary to insulin signaling defects.[6] Published data suggest that rhIGF1 is able, in some patients, to exert beneficial acute and longer term effects on glycemia, with doses of up to 0.4 mg/kg/day well tolerated with minimal side effects; however, all published reports were uncontrolled. The mechanism underlying the effect is uncertain. The intracellular signaling pathways for the insulin and IGF-1 receptors have many common elements, and stimulating IGF-1 receptors may prime common signaling intermediates to enhance insulin sensitivity. Formal proof of this hypothesis is lacking, however. Concerns have centered on potential adverse effects of rhIGF1 in promoting pathological tissue growth, especially in the retinal vessels, heart, and upper airway. While existing published data are relatively reassuring in this regard, the possibility exists of publication bias toward successful outcomes, and there is a pressing unmet need for more systematic international data gathering and curation, and for more rigorous studies of different therapeutic algorithms in RMS. At present, management of this very rare syndrome should be undertaken in collaboration with a specialized center with experience of the condition.

References

1.   Bastaki F, Nair P, Mohamed M, Khadora MM, Saif F, Tawfiq N, et al. Identification of a novel homozygous INSR variant in a patient with Rabson-Mendenhall syndrome from the United Arab Emirates. *Horm Res Paediatr* 2016;87:64–68

2.   Semple RK, Savage DB, Cochran EK, Gorden P, O'Rahilly S. Genetic syndromes of severe insulin resistance. *Endocr Rev* 2011;32:498–514

3.   Semple RK, Williams RM, Dunger DB. What is the best management strategy for patients with severe insulin resistance? *Clin Endocrinol (Oxf)* 2010;73:286–290

4.   Musso C, Cochran E, Moran SA, Skarulis MC, Oral EA, et al. Clinical course of genetic diseases of the insulin receptor (type A and Rabson-Mendenhall syndromes): a 30-year prospective. *Medicine (Baltimore)* 2004;83:209–222

5.   Brown RJ, Cochran E, Gorden P. Metreleptin improves blood glucose in patients with insulin receptor mutations. *J Clin Endocrinol Metab* 2013;98:E1749–E1756

6.   Regan FM, Williams RM, McDonald A, Umpleby AM, Acerini CL, O'Rahilly S, et al. Treatment with recombinant human insulin-like growth factor (rhIGF)-I/rhIGF binding protein-3 complex improves metabolic control in subjects with severe insulin resistance. *J Clin Endocrinol Metab* 2010;95:2113–2122

Case 26:
Familial Partial Lipodystrophy II (Dunnigan's Syndrome)

Peminda K. Cabandugama, MD;[1] Stephen A. Brietzke, MD;[1] Michael J. Gardner, MD;[1] and James R. Sowers, MD[1-3]

Case

A 35-year-old female with past medical history of diabetes (unknown type) diagnosed 13 years previously came in for diabetes management due to excessive insulin needs. Patient was diagnosed with diabetes when she was pregnant with her second child. At her clinic visit, the patient was noted to have a BMI of 25 kg/m² and body status as per Figures C26.1 and C26.2. Patient's insulin requirement was a total daily dose of approximately 260 units. Significant laboratory data at the time of presentation included glycated hemoglobin of 9.6%, a triglyceride level of 1,064 mg/dL, serum hepatic transaminases that were not measurable due to lipemia, and a low leptin level of 1.7 ng/mL.

The patient also provided a history of her mother, having the same body habitus as her but no medical evaluation, and a maternal aunt, with

[1]Department of Internal Medicine, Diabetes and Cardiovascular Center, University of Missouri, Columbia, MO

[2]Department of Physiology and Pharmacology, Diabetes and Cardiovascular Center, University of Missouri, Columbia, MO

[3]Harry S. Truman VA Hospital, D109 HSC Diabetes Center, Columbia, MO

DOI: 10.2337/9781580406666.04

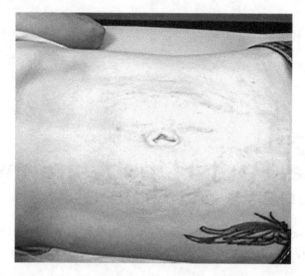

Figure C26.1—Patient's abdomen at time of clinic visit.

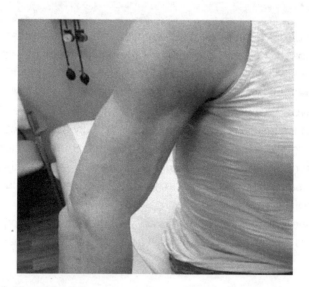

Figure C26.2—Patient's arm at time of clinic visit.

hypertriglyceridemia with the same body habitus who underwent three coronary artery bypass graft surgeries (first one at 32 years).

The patient is currently being managed conservatively on a basal/bolus insulin regimen and metformin. For her abnormal lipid panel, the patient is treated with omega-3 capsules (due to an intolerance of fibrates). Patient was also to be started on a statin but wishes to consider pregnancy in the future and would prefer not to take a statin currently.

The patient is currently being considered for metreleptin therapy while her mother will be brought in for genetic testing.

Discussion

Lipodystrophic syndromes are a conglomerate of genetic and acquired disorders that are characterized by metabolic derangements and a paucity or complete lack of adipose tissue. These patients are usually noted to have severe abnormalities including extreme insulin resistance, severe hypertriglyceridemia, progressive liver disease, and an increased metabolic rate. The type of lipodystrophy occurring is usually characterized by the area of fat loss on the patient.

Familial partial lipodystrophy II (FPLD2), also known as Dunnigan's syndrome, is a subset of lipodystrophic syndromes with the same metabolic derangements, but where the loss of subcutaneous fat is noted mainly in the extremities and from the abdomen and thorax. These patients may also have excessive fat deposition in the face and the neck, but this does not always have to be present. Fat losses on these patients are noted to occur with the onset of puberty and may also involve signs and symptoms of ovarian hyperandrogenism.[1] Studies have shown that affected women have a similar pattern of loss of subcutaneous fat from the extremities and the trunk but are more severely affected by the metabolic complications of insulin resistance than men.[2]

FPLD2 syndromes are noted to involve missense mutations of the LMNA gene and are currently thought to be an X-linked dominant trait, but very rarely they have also been found as autosomal dominant in some families. The locus for the autosomal dominant trait has been isolated to ch.1q21-22.[3]

Current standard of treatment is conservative with insulin and lipid-lowering agents along with a low-fat diet. Novel treatments like metreleptin[4] are now available on the market to treat leptin deficiencies associated with this condition but continue to remain untested on a large scale due to the rarity of the disorder.

References

1. Jackson SN, Howlett TA, McNally PG, et al. Dunnigan-Köbberling syndrome: an autosomal dominant form of partial lipodystrophy. *QJM* 1997;90:27–36

2. Garg A. Gender differences in the prevalence of metabolic complications in familial partial lipodystrophy (Dunnigan variety). *J Clin Endocrinol Metab* 2000; 85:1776–1782

3. Peters JM, Barnes R, Bennett L, et al. Localization of the gene for familial partial lipodystrophy (Dunnigan variety) to chromosome 1q21-22. *Nat Genet* 1998; 18:292–295

4. Rodriguez AJ, Mastronardi CA, Paz-Filho GJ. New advances in the treatment of generalized lipodystrophy: role of metreleptin. *Ther Clin Risk Manag* 2015;11:1391–1400

Case 27:
Familial Partial Lipodystrophy

Kathryn Evans Kreider, DNP, APRN, FNP-BC;[1] and Mark N. Feinglos, MD[1]

Case

TL, a 17-year-old white female, initially presented to a local hospital complaining of severe dark, thick skin in the axillae, base of the neck, and inguinal and perineal areas. She was concerned about the deepening of her voice and a 30-pound weight gain over the last year. Her menstrual periods had become very irregular, occurring once every 3–6 months. Her family history included a father with type 2 diabetes (T2D) and fatal myocardial infarction (MI) at age 49, paternal uncle with fatal MI at age 39, and multiple other family members with T2D. She was hospitalized for an initial workup, and the only positive findings were hypertension (160/105 mmHg, no previous history) and an abnormal glucose tolerance test. Physical exam findings included a cervical-dorsal fat pad, thick, dark hyperkeratotic skin in the areas described above, and supraclavicular fat accumulation. Testing for Cushing's syndrome, congenital adrenal hyperplasia, adrenogenital syndromes, growth hormone abnormalities, and other endocrinopathies was negative. Skull films, pelvic ultrasound, and electrocardiogram were normal.

[1]Duke University Medical Center, Durham, NC

DOI: 10.2337/9781580406666.04

The patient was lost to follow-up until she was 28 years old and was referred to an endocrinologist for uncontrolled diabetes despite insulin usage approaching 200 units per day. At that time, her hypertension, elevated triglycerides, significant insulin resistance, and lack of adipose tissue except above the clavicle, with bulky musculature in the periphery, led the endocrinology team to do a further workup including computerized tomography (CT) scan and a punch biopsy of her right back and right forearm. The biopsy results suggested "replacement of subcutaneous tissue by fibrous connective tissue, consistent with lipodystrophy," and the CT scan showed absence of adipose tissue except in the mediastinum.

Discussion

Familial partial lipodystrophy (FPLD) is a rare autosomal dominant disorder characterized by a loss of subcutaneous adipose tissue in the extremities with marked increases in dorsal, facial, and visceral adipose tissue.[1] The onset typically occurs during puberty and is associated with several chronic diseases including type 2 diabetes, hyperlipidemia, polycystic ovary syndrome, and premature cardiovascular disease.[2] Clinical features of FPLD are summarized in Table C27.1. FPLD is one of the two most common types of lipodystrophy syndromes with congenital generalized lipodystrophy being another most common form.[2] The diagnosis of FPLD is primarily dependent on the characteristic physical features. Lipodystrophy is often more readily apparent in women who have more adipose tissue at baseline, which often leads to more profound metabolic dysregulation and hyperandrogenism.[3] The measurement of adipose tissue loss or distribution can be done through anthrometry or ultrasound.[4] More accurate measures such as MRI, CT, or dual-energy X-ray absorptiometry are not readily used due to cost.[4] Several genetic tests are available for confirmation including lamin A (LMNA), peroxisome proliferator-activated receptor gamma (PPARG), and zinc metallopeptidase (ZMPSTE24). These genetic tests have low sensitivity; thus clinical diagnosis remains important. The most common type of inherited partial lipodystrophy is FPLD2, also known as Dunnigan's syndrome. FPLD2 has been reported in 200 patients with a prevalence of approximately 1 in every 15 million individuals.[4] Lipodystrophy syndromes should be considered in patients who present with extreme insulin resistance, significant dyslipidemia, and fatty liver disease.[3]

Table C27.1—Characteristic Features of Familial Partial Lipodystrophy

Physical Exam Findings	Comorbid Conditions
Generalized or partial absence of adipose tissue	Insulin resistance
Acanthosis nigricans	Fatty liver disease/NASH
Hyperandrogenism findings	Polycystic ovary syndrome (women)
Hepatomegaly/Organomegaly	Dyslipidemia
	Hypertension
	Cardiovascular disease

Source: Adapted from Fiorenza CG, Chou SH, Mantzoros CS.[4]

The treatment of FPLD includes diet, lifestyle, medication therapy, and management of associated diseases. Because individuals with FPLD are at high risk for diabetes and cardiovascular disease, diet recommendations include adherence to an American Heart Association diet including a low-fat (<30% calories), moderate-carbohydrate (<60% calories) diet with adequate fiber. Resistance training may prove more beneficial than aerobic exercise, as it may increase total lean body mass and decrease unwanted adipose deposits.[4] Regardless, any type of consistent exercise regimen is potentially beneficial for FPLD.

FPLD is characterized by decreased amounts of leptin and adiponectin, two hormones generated from adipose tissue. Individuals with Dunnigan's syndrome have a range of leptin levels from severe hypoleptinemia to normal levels. As such, one of the primary treatments for FPLD is leptin therapy, which has been shown to decrease triglycerides and hepatic steatosis and may help improve insulin sensitivity in those who have reduced leptin.[5] Other treatments should be directed at improving glycemic control and hypertriglyceridemia. Metformin and thiazolidinediones (TZDs) are particularly helpful therapies for diabetes as they target insulin resistance, though TZDs have fallen out of favor clinically. Insulin therapy is common for FPLD patients with diabetes, though doses may be high and difficult to tolerate due to loss of subcutaneous fat. Hypertriglyceridemia is commonly treated with fibrates, occasionally in combination with statins for optimal cardiovascular protection.[2]

Beginning in 2006, the patient participated in an NIH clinical trial confirming her diagnosis of FPLD2. The trial was designed to evaluate the

Table 27.2—Current Management of Patient TL

Comorbidities	Medications	Lab Results/Measurements
Coronary Artery Disease (age 48) Status post 4 stents to right coronary artery	Atorvastatin 80 mg Coreg 6.25 mg b.i.d. Plavix 75 mg Enalapril 10 mg Fenofibrate 145 mg Omega 3 fatty acids, 2 tabs/day	BP: 140/60 (HR 82) BMI: 31 kg/m^2 Lipid Profile: TC: 149, HDL: 26, TG: 467 (fibrate re-initiated)
Type 2 Diabetes	Glargine insuline (U-300), 80 units once daily Aspart insulin, 75 units TID before meals Metformin 2 grams daily	A1C 7.2%
Right Breast Cancer (age 50), mastectomy, in remission	–	–

effects of leptin treatment on patients with lipodystrophy and hypoleptinemia. Throughout the course of the trial, she received leptin subcutaneously twice daily at 100–200% of replacement dose (0.04 or 0.08 mg/kg). During her participation in the trial, TL's insulin requirement dropped significantly from over 350 to around 200 units/day. She maintained improved glucose control (HbA$_{1c}$ <7.5%). In addition, her triglycerides on a fibrate and statin decreased to <250 mg/dL. Unfortunately, TL developed breast cancer and had to stop the trial prematurely due to the potential exacerbation of cancer by leptin therapy.

The patient, now in her early 50s, has variable control of her T2D and her HbA$_{1c}$ has fluctuated between 5.7 and 8.6% over the years. Despite optimal medical therapy, she developed early-onset cardiovascular disease at age 48. Her current medications and metrics can be found in Table C27.2.

References

1. Joy T, Kennedy BA, Al-Attar S, et al. Predicting abdominal adipose tissue among women with familial partial lipodystrophy. *Metabolism* 2009;58:828–834

2. Chan JL, Oral EA. Clinical classification and treatment of congenital and acquired lipodystrophy. *Endocr Pract* 2010;2010;310–323

3. Huang-Doran I, Sleigh A, Rochford JJ, et al. Lipodystrophy: metabolic insights from a rare disorder. *J Endocrinol* 2010;207:245–255

4. Fiorenza CG, Chou SH, Mantzoros CS. Lipodystrophy: pathophysiology and advances in treatment. *Nat Rev Endocrinol* 2011;7:137–150

5. Simha V, Subramanyam L, Szczepaniak L, et al. Comparison of efficacy and safety of leptin replacement therapy in moderately and severely hypoleptinemic patients with familial partial lipodystrophy of the Dunnigan variety. *J Clin Endocrinol Metab* 2001;97:785–792

Case 28:
Severe Insulin Resistance and Lipodystrophy

Kavya Mekala, MD;[1] and Joseph Aloi, MD[1]

Case

A 35-year-old African-American woman was referred to the Endocrine clinic for evaluation of severe insulin resistance and an abnormal body habitus. She had been on U500 insulin with total daily insulin requirements up to 1,000 units. Further details of the history revealed that she was diagnosed with diabetes at age 17 when she presented to the emergency department with glucose in the 400s mg/dL and HbA$_{1c}$ of 11.5%. She also was diagnosed with hypertension at that time. She had recurrent severe hypertriglyceridemia and developed pancreatitis complicated by pancreatic pseudocyst requiring resection during that admission. She also reported a history of bilateral ovarian cysts. She attained menarche in fourth grade and her periods were regular.

On evaluation, her physical characteristics were striking with appearance of fat redistribution (Figure C28.1). She had lipohypertrophy in the face, neck upper chest, axillary region, and anterior abdomen. She had relative absence of fat in the lower extremities with prominent veins and musculature. She exhibited severe acanthosis nigricans as well as hyperkeratosis.

Laboratory investigations revealed IGF-1 109 ng/mL, DHEAS 89 ng/mL, total testosterone 28 ng/dL, and free testosterone 3.2. Random

---

[1]Section on Endocrinology & Metabolism, Wake Forest School of Medicine, Winston-Salem, NC

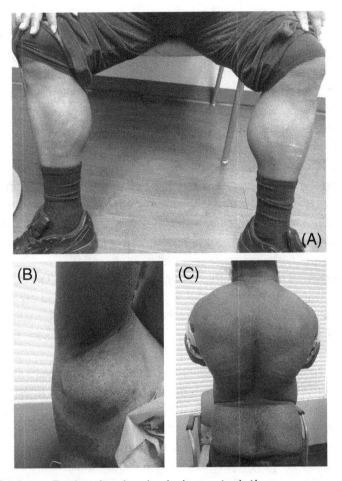

Figure C28.1—Patient's physical characteristics.

(A) prominent muscles and veins in lower extremities; (B) prominent axillary fat pad with severe acanthosis nigricans; (C) lipohypertrophy in upper back and neck

cortisol was 6.1 ug/dL with ACTH 25 pg/mL. 24-hour urine for free cortisol was 14.8 mcg/24 hrs. Her serum leptin level was low at 4 ng/mL (8–38.9).

Discussion

Lipodystrophy syndromes comprise a diverse group of disorders that are characterized by complete or partial loss of fat (lipoatrophy) or a combination of lipoatrophy and lipohypertrophy.[1] Lipodystrophy can be classified as partial, general, or localized based on the extent of fat loss.[1,2] The disease can be further categorized as congenital or acquired (Table C28.1). HIV-related lipodystrophy is the most commonly seen acquired lipodystrophy, associated with the use of highly active antiretroviral therapy (HAART).[1-3]

The pathophysiology of lipodystrophy involves the loss of functional, mature adipocytes owing to defects in adipogenesis, adipocyte apoptosis, or storage of excess triglycerides. Considerable progress has been made in discovery of the molecular basis of genetic lipodystrophies, although the molecular basis of some novel genetic syndromes remains unknown.

Most lipodystrophy syndromes predispose affected individuals to developing insulin resistance. Diabetes is typically diagnosed in adolescence and can be associated with ketoacidosis. Hypertriglyceridemia and pancreatitis, hepatic steatosis, and cirrhosis, polycystic ovary syndrome, and cardiovascular disease such as coronary artery disease and hypertrophic cardiomyopathy are other metabolic complications.

Diagnosis of lipodystrophy is primarily clinical but often challenging. Serial photographs may be useful to document the clinical course. Dual-energy X-ray absorptiometry and other imaging modalities can be used to measure fat mass and distribution but are typically used in research settings.

The mainstay of treatment involves addressing the individual metabolic derangements. Insulin sensitizers such as metformin and thiazolindiones can be used to treat insulin resistance (the efficacy of the latter agent is still being assessed in clinical trials). Insulin requirements may be significantly higher, as seen in our patient. Fibric acid derivatives and fish oil supplements help with hypertriglyceridemia, and clinical trials with therapies targeting APOC3 are currently underway. Low-fat diets can reduce chylomicronemia. Strenuous physical activity should be avoided in familial partial lipodystrophy with increased risk of cardiomyopathy. Cosmetic measures such as dermal fillers and liposuction may be used to improve appearance. Metreleptin therapy was approved by the FDA in 2014 for use in congenital or acquired generalized lipodystrophy. Concern over its use relates to development of neutralizing antibodies and risk of development of T-cell lymphoma. Tesamorelin, which is a growth hormone releasing factor, has been used in HIV-related lipodystrophy to decrease abdominal fat.

Our patient's phenotypic presentation appeared most consistent with familial partial lipodystrophy. She underwent gene testing that revealed an interesting LMNA mutation. She was switched to U500 insulin via pump, and this helped reduce her insulin requirement and slightly improve

Table 28.1—Classification of Lipodystrophy Syndromes

Type	Subtypes (gene mutation)	Clinical features
Congenital Generalized Lipodystrophy (CGL) OR Berardinelli-Seip Syndrome	CGL1 (AGPAT2) CGL2 (BSCL2) CGL3 (CAV1) CGL4 (PTRF)	• Autosomal recessive • Parental consanguinity • Total or near total loss of body fat in first 2 years of life • Muscular appearance, voracious appetite, and umbilical prominence • Postpubertal focal lytic lesions in long bones • Infertility and menstrual irregularities in women • Hypertrophic cardiomyopathy • Hepatic steatosis and cirrhosis • Hypertriglyceridemia and pancreatitis • Low serum adiponectin and leptin
Acquired Generalized Lipodystrophy (AGL)	Lawrence Syndrome	• Onset in childhood • Likely autoimmune mediated • May be associated with panniculitis (tender subcutaneous, inflammatory nodules)
Familial Partial Lipodystrophy (FPL)	FPLD1, Köbberling FPLD2, Dunnigan (LMNA) FLPD3 (PPARG) FLPD4 (AKT2) FLPD5 (PLIN1)	• Loss of fat in extremities (Köbberling) • Loss of fat in extremities and trunk sparing face and neck (Dunnigan) • Diagnosis challenging in men • Associated cardiomyopathy
Acquired Partial Lipodystrophy (APL)	Barraquer-Simons syndrome HIV-related lipodystrophy	• Hypocomplementinemia (low C3) • Renal disease (membranoproliferative glomerulonephritis) • Fat loss in upper body with sparing of lower abdomen and lower limbs • Typically following 2 years of HAART therapy (protease inhibitors and nucleoside reverse transcriptase inhibitors) • Loss of fat in face, arms and legs with fat deposition in neck and abdomen
Localized	Trauma, injections, pressure, autoimmune	• Typically not associated with other metabolic derangements

Sources: Garg A and Tsoukas MA, Mantzoros CS[1,2]

glycemic control. She is additionally being treated with metformin, fenofibrate, statin and fish oil. She is entering a clinical trial to explore other therapeutic options.

This case highlights the importance of delineating the reasons for high insulin requirements and severe insulin resistance in diabetes and investigating secondary causes of obesity.

References

1.   Garg A. Lipodystrophies: genetic and acquired body fat disorders. *J Clin Endocrinol Metab* 2011;96:3313–3325

2.   Tsoukas MA, Mantzoros CS. Lipodystrophy syndromes. *Endocrinology: Adult and Pediatric.* 7th ed. Jameson JL, DeGroot LJ, Eds. Philadelphia, Elsevier, 2016, p. 648–661

3.   Patni N, Garg A. Congenital generalized lipodystrophies—new insights into metabolic dysfunction. *Nat Rev Endocrinol* 2015;11:522–534

Case 29:
Lipodystrophy Due to PPAR-γ Gene Mutation

Aaron Hodes, MD;[1,2] Rebecca Brown, MD;[3] Elaine Cochran, CRNP;[3] and Mihail Zilbermint, MD[1,4,5]

Case report

A 51-year-old Caucasian female with long-standing diabetes and hypertriglyceridemia presented to the National Institutes of Health (NIH) for evaluation. She required multiple medications to control her diabetes of 30 years, and at the time of presentation, her noninsulin treatments included metformin, pioglitazone, and exenatide. After an episode of pancreatitis 25 years prior to presentation at NIH, insulin therapy was initiated with progressive escalation to using U-500 insulin, which has kept her HbA$_{1c}$ controlled around 6.5%. At the NIH, her total daily dose was 175 units of U-500 insulin via insulin pump. Complications from her diabetes included gastroparesis, toe amputation, progressive axonal sensory neuropathy, and bladder dysfunction.

[1]Eunice Kennedy Shriver National Institute of Child Health and Human Development, Bethesda, MD

[2]Albert Einstein College of Medicine, Department of Radiology, Jacobi Medical Center, Bronx, NY

[3]National Institute of Diabetes and Digestive and Kidney Diseases, Bethesda, MD

[4]Johns Hopkins University School of Medicine, Department of Endocrinology, Diabetes and Metabolism, Baltimore, MD

[5]Suburban Hospital, Department of Medicine, Bethesda, MD

DOI: 10.2337/9781580406666.04

Since age 11, she had hypertriglyceridemia, on many occasions higher than 5,000 mg/dL (normal <150 mg/dL), and only one episode of pancreatitis. At the time of the NIH evaluation, her triglycerides were normal on omega-3-fatty acids, fenofibrate, and a statin. She was also on lisinopril and spironolactone for hypertension.

She reported an unusually large appetite since her teenage years. Menarche occurred at 13 years, and she has always had irregular menses, controlled with oral progestin.

Family history was significant for extreme hypertriglyceridemia and diabetes. All five of her siblings are alive with diabetes and hypertriglyceridemia, and one sister has a similar body habitus, except with a more prominent abdomen and muscular limbs. Her mother had hypertriglyceridemia as high as 5,000–6,000 mg/dL and passed away at 73 years from myocardial infarction. Her father did not have diabetes and passed away at 82 years from congestive heart failure. No other known relatives had similar symptoms or conditions.

On initial assessment at the NIH, her vital signs were temperature 37.1°C, pulse 81 bpm, and blood pressure 118/74 mmHg. Weight was 83.1 kg, height 177.5 cm, and BMI 26.4 kg/m^2. Physical examination was significant for decreased fat in the upper extremities, absent fat with muscular appearance in the lower extremities and buttocks, abdominal obesity, and a normal amount of fat in the face and neck. She had mild acanthosis nigricans, clitoromegaly (clitoral index 135 mm^2), and mild hepatomegaly.

Given her diabetes with severe insulin resistance, hypertriglyceridemia, and unusual body habitus, a lipodystrophy syndrome was suspected. The patient was enrolled in the Natural History of Disorders of Insulin Resistance clinical research trial at the NIH (NCT00001987).

Laboratory tests revealed significant insulin resistance by fasting (Table C29.1) with optimized HbA$_{1c}$ and cholesterol levels and borderline high triglyceride levels, and evaluation of the pituitary and target organ axes was unremarkable (Table C29.2). Complement levels were within normal limits, and serum levels of CRP, anti-ENA screen, and anti-nuclear antibody were not elevated (Table C29.2). DEXA scanning revealed an overall adiposity of 27.6%, most in the arms (34.3–36.7%) and trunk (28.8%) and least in the legs (22.8–24.1%) and head (20.4%). Her leptin level was 10 ng/dL.

An outside provider had discontinued her pioglitazone shortly after presentation at the NIH, and her insulin requirements dramatically increased.

Table C29.1—Results of Oral Glucose Tolerance Test

Oral Glucose Tolerance Test	Serum Glucose (mg/dL)	Serum Insulin (mcU/mL)	Serum C-peptide (ng/mL)
–30 min	120	113.6	3.0
0 min	117	113.9	3.0
10 min	284	134.7	4.6
30 min	336	131.7	5.6
60 min	358	137.1	5.8
90 min	354	136.7	5.7
180 min	281	166.2	6.1

While the test requires the patient to be off insulin and fasting, this patient's insulin insensitivity required her to perform this test fasting while being infused with her basal insulin.

At a second visit 3 months later, pioglitazone was restarted with return to baseline insulin requirements and glucose levels.

Genetic investigation revealed a mutation in PPAR-γ. The patient was enrolled in additional NIH clinical research trials (NCT01778556 and NCT00025883), and subcutaneous 10 mg metreleptin daily therapy was initiated. Shortly thereafter, her insulin requirements and appetite significantly improved for 7 months, after which insulin requirements and hunger returned to pre-metreleptin levels. After 13 months of metreleptin, DEXA scanning revealed a global increase in adiposity, to a total of 32.0% with increases in her head (24.8%), legs (27.3–29.4%), trunk (32.6%), and arms (39.7–42.0%).

Discussion

Insulin resistance, hyperglycemia, and hypertriglyceridemia are usually associated with obesity and the metabolic syndrome. In cases where body habitus is atypical and relatively lean with high insulin requirements >2 units/kg/day, lipodystrophy should be considered. Lipodystrophy syndromes have the cardinal feature of deficient subcutaneous adipose tissue.[1] They are categorized as either acquired or congenital, and also as partial or complete, depending on extent of adipose deficiency. The reported prevalence of non–HIV-related forms of lipodystrophy syndromes is less than 0.001%, but this is likely an underestimate, especially for partial lipodystrophy (PL) syndromes.[2] Here we report a woman with diabetes,

Table C29.2—Initial laboratory Values

Laboratory Test	Value	Normal Range	Laboratory Test	Value	Normal Range
Luteinizing Hormone	9.3 units/L	Postmenopausal: 11–40 units/L	Creatine Kinase	92 units/L	38–252 units/L
Follicle Stimulating Hormone	15.5 units/L	Postmenopausal: 22–153 units/L	Total Cholesterol	118 mg/dL	Optimal: <200 mg/dL
Parathyroid Hormone	6.9 pg/mL	15.0–65.0 pg/mL	HDL	24 mg/dL	Low risk: >60; high risk: <40 mg/dL
Growth Hormone	0.12 ng/dL	0.00–8.00 ng/dL	LDL	60 mg/dL	Optimal: <100 mg/dL
Insulin-Like Growth Factor-1	151 ng/mL	Tanner V: 143–859 ng/mL	Triglycerides	172 mg/dL	Optimal: <150 mg/dL; Borderline 150–199 mg/dL
Thyroid Stimulating Hormone	1.32 mcIU/mL	0.27–4.20 mcIU/mL	HbA_{1c}	6.5%	4.8-6.4%
Thyroxine	12.2 mcg/dL	4.5–12.5 mcg/dL	Anti-Thyroglobulin Antibody	<20 IU/mL	0.0–40.0 IU/mL
Triiodothyronine	83 ng/dL	90–215 ng/dL	Anti-Thyroid Peroxidase Antibody	<10 IU/mL	0.0–34.9 IU/mL
Total Complement	124 CAE Units	55–145 CAE Units	C-Reactive Protein	0.31 mg/L	Low CV risk <1.0 mg/L
C3 Complement	124.0 mg/dL	90.0–180.0 mg/dL	Anti-ENA Screen*#	Negative	0-19 EU
C4 Complement	10.0 mg/dL	10.0–40.0 mg/dL	Anti-Nuclear Antibody*	Negative	0.0–0.9 EU

*These tests were done by ELISA method. #Anti-ENA Screen includes testing for anti-ribonuclear protein, anti-Smith, anti-SSA, anti-SSB, anti-Jo1, and anti-Scl70 antibodies.

hyperphagia, prominent muscularity, and abnormal fat distribution due to familial partial lipodystrophy (PL) with a peroxisome proliferating activator receptor-γ (PPAR-γ) gene mutation.

In this patient, the combination of severe insulin resistance, history of severe hypertriglyceridemia, unusual fat distribution, and strong family history led to the suspicion of familial PL. In patients requiring high doses of insulin (>2 units/kg/day) and persistently elevated triglyceride levels (>250 mg/dL) despite maximized therapy, physicians should perform careful physical examination for any unusual fat distribution.[1]

PL patients can present with a metabolic profile much worse than non-lipodystrophic patients with diabetes. Among a large cohort in Turkey of 2,022 type 2 diabetic patients, 16 patients had PL without identified genetic mutations. Distinctive characteristics of those 16 PL patients were being diagnosed with diabetes at a younger age (42 vs 50 years, $p = 0.005$) and had higher HbA_{1c} (8.9% vs 7.1%, $p = 0.001$), fasting glucose levels (10.55 vs 6.44 mmol/L, $p < 0.001$), triglycerides (2.09 vs 1.55 mmol/L, $p = 0.004$), LDL cholesterol (3.41 vs 2.92 mmol/L, $p = 0.025$), and total cholesterol levels (5.43 vs 4.89 mmol/L, $p = 0.007$), compared to non-lipodystrophic patients.[3]

PPAR-γ mutations have been shown to be important for adipocyte survival and differentiation. As of this report, thiazolidinediones, which are agonists of PPAR-γ, showed improved *in vitro* transcriptional activation of the mutated receptor from cell lines of patients with familial PL due to PPAR-γ mutations.[4] In our patient, pioglitazone was essential to optimize her glucose levels and insulin requirements. Metreleptin therapy for 12 months reduced insulin requirements and improved the metabolic profile in PL patients with baseline serum leptin <4 ng/mL, triglyceride levels >500 mg/dL, or $HbA_{1c} > 8\%$.[5] Despite the PPAR-γ mutation, our patient's HbA_{1c} and triglycerides were well controlled on conventional therapy, rendering improvement with metreleptin less likely.

In summary, we present a patient with familial PL due to PPAR-γ mutation that led to subcutaneous fat loss in her lower extremities, diabetes requiring high levels of insulin for glycemic control, and hypertriglyceridemia requiring fibrate and omega-3-fatty acid therapy. Clinicians encountering patients with difficult-to-control diabetes and unusual body habitus should consider further workup for lipodystrophy syndromes.

Acknowledgments

This research was supported in part by the Intramural Research Program of Eunice Kennedy Shriver National Institute of Child Health and Human Development, National Institutes of Health (NIH), National Institute of Diabetes and Digestive and Kidney Diseases. We thank Diane Cooper, MSLS, NIH Library, for providing assistance in writing this case.

References

1. Handelsman Y, Oral EA, Bloomgarden ZT, et al. The clinical approach to the detection of lipodystrophy - an AACE consensus statement. *Endocr Pract* 2013;19:107–116

2. Garg A. Lipodystrophies: genetic and acquired body fat disorders. *J Clin Endocrinol Metab* 2011;96:3313–3325

3. Demir T, Akinci B, Demir L, et al. Partial lipodystrophy of the limbs in a diabetes clinic setting. *Prim Care Diabetes* 2016;10:293–299

4. Ludtke A, Buettner J, Schmidt HH, Worman HJ. New PPARG mutation leads to lipodystrophy and loss of protein function that is partially restored by a synthetic ligand. *J Med Genet* 2007;44:e88

5. Diker-Cohen T, Cochran E, Gorden P, Brown RJ. Partial and generalized lipodystrophy: comparison of baseline characteristics and response to metreleptin. *J Clin Endocrinol Metab* 2015;100:1802–1810

Case 30:
Congenital Generalized Lipodystrophy

Henning Beck-Nielsen, MD, DMSc[1,2]

Case

A girl born to parents with normal subcutaneous fat deposition was diagnosed with congenital generalized lipodystrophy (CGL) at the age of 8 years old. She presented with almost no subcutaneous fat (fat content was less than 5% of her body weight), muscular hypertrophy (lipid deposition), hepatomegaly, and abdominal pain due to hepatomegaly. Biochemically, she presented with dyslipidemia, specifically increased plasma triglycerides, and reduced high-density lipoprotein (HDL) cholesterol. Initially, the patient was not treated pharmacologically, but with diet alone, and she was followed for some years before she was diagnosed with diabetes. She had delayed menarche and oligomenorrhea. An ultrasound showed polycystic ovary syndrome (PCOS), but normal androgen levels. The patient was 30 years of age when she developed frank diabetes, which was nonketotic (plasma C-peptide was 738 pmol/L with the reference value of 40–45 pmol/L) at the time of diagnosis, and glutamic acid decarboxylase (GAD) antibodies were negative. Clinically, her phenotype was similar to type 2 diabetes, even though she was lean, with hepatomegaly and an acromegalic facies. An insulin sensitivity test demonstrated severe insulin

[1]Department of Endocrinology, Odense University Hospital, Odense, Denmark
[2]Department of Clinical Research, University of Southern Denmark, Odense, Denmark

DOI: 10.2337/9781580406666.04

resistance in the presence of hyperinsulinemia. At the time of diagnosis of diabetes, her fasting plasma glucose was about 20 mmol/L (360 mg/dL), whereas HDL cholesterol was below 1 mmol/L, and plasma triglycerides were about 30 mmol/L. Low-density lipoprotein (LDL) cholesterol was normal. The patient did not have insulin receptor antibodies or acanthosis nigricans and was treated with insulin (basal-bolus regimen), and, as of today, she receives 75 units of NovoRapid and degludec together with simvastatin (40 mg), gemfibrozil (500 mg), and acipimox (250 mg) daily to normalize dyslipidemia. At present, her fasting plasma triglyceride level is 3.4 mmol/L, LDL cholesterol is 1.2 mmol/L, and HDL cholesterol is 1.2 mmol/L. She has mild retinopathy, which may be due to lipid deposition in the retina. There have been no macrovascular complications until now (the patient is 50 years old). She still requires pain medications for abdominal pain and muscle pain. Her muscle and liver enzymes as well as alanine transaminase and creatine phosphokinase (CPK) are slightly elevated. Physically, the patient is able to play golf with a low handicap.

Discussion

Congenital generalized lipodystrophy (CGL) is an uncommon, but severe disease where subcutaneous lipid deposition is severely reduced due to loss of adipose tissue. The disease is autosomal recessive inherited and cannot be cured, but it can be treated pharmacologically. When lipid intake cannot be deposed in fat cells in subcutaneous tissue, it is redirected for deposition ectopically, for example in liver and muscle cells, as well as sometimes in skin and β-cells. The consequences of ectopic lipid deposition are severe insulin resistance and eventually frank diabetes.[1]

The disease is due to a mutation in the lipogenic genes such as BSCL2 and AGPAT2.[2] It is important to diagnose the disease based on the loss of subcutaneous adipose tissue already at school age since early treatment seems to be important because fat deposition in the liver can result in non-alcoholic steatohepatitis (NASH) and finally liver cirrhosis.

Ectopic lipid deposition due to obesity or CGL seems to induce the same kind of insulin resistance in liver and skeletal muscle cells. The accumulation of lipids, specifically diacylglycerol (DAG) and ceramides, inhibits insulin signaling mainly via serine phosphorylation of the insulin receptor and the insulin receptor substrate (IRS) complex.[3] In the 1970s, we have described that the binding of insulin to the insulin receptor in a boy with Berardinelli-Seip syndrome was significantly reduced.[4] Later on, the reduced activity of the insulin receptor signaling was demonstrated to reduce glycogen synthase kinase (GSK) and phosphoinositide 3-kinase (PI3K) activity and thereby glucose uptake and utilization.[3]

Surgical treatment shunting lipids away from intestinal absorption has also been shown to be able to "cure" diabetes and dyslipidemia in patients with CGL, emphasizing the role of ectopic lipid deposition in the development of diabetes.[5]

Normally, insulin resistance is not sufficient to induce hyperglycemia, but β-cell function seems to be reduced in those patients where hyperglycemia develops. The cause may be exhaustion of β-cells due to insulin resistance or lipid accumulation in β-cells resulting in reduced glucose oxidation and thereby diminished insulin secretion.

The long-term prognosis is still difficult to predict since few patients have been treated for a longer period. However, treatment has improved in patients with CGL over the years, thanks to earlier diagnosis and more efficient drug therapy.

Conclusion

Early diagnosis based on the absence of subcutaneous fat and proper pharmacological treatment of diabetes and dyslipidemia seem to be able to improve dysmetabolism and thereby the quality of life and life expectancy in patients with CGL.

References

1.   Lima JG, Nobrega LHC, de Lima NN, Santos MGdN, Baracho MFP, Jeronimo SMB. Clinical and laboratory data of large series of patients with congenital generalized lipodystrophy. *Diabetol Metab Syndr* 2016;8:23

2.   Magre J, Delepine M, Khallouf E, Gedde-Dahl T Jr, Van Maldergem L, Sobel E, et al. Identification of the gene altered in Berardinelli-Seip congenital lipodystrophy on chromosome 11q13. *Nat Genet* 2011;28:365–370

3.   Softic S, Boucher J, Solheim MH, Fujisaka S, Haering MF, Homan EP, Winnay J, Perez-Atayde AR, Kahn CR. Lipodystrophy due to adipose tissue-specific insulin receptor knockout results in progressive NAFLD. *Diabetes* 2016; 65:2187–2200

4.   Oseid S, Beck-Nielsen H, Pedersen O, Sovik O. Decreased binding of insulin to its receptor in patients with congenital generalized lipodystrophy. *N Engl J Med* 1977;296:245–248

5. Mingrone G, Henriksen FL, Greco AV, Krogh LN, Capristo E, Gastaldelli A, Castagneto M, Ferrannini E, Gasbarrini G, Beck-Nielsen H. Triglyceride-induced diabetes associated with familial lipoprotein lipase deficiency. *Diabetes* 1999; 48:1258–1263

Case 31:
Pancreatogenic Diabetes

Nadezhda Zherdeva, MD;[1] and Boris Mankovsky, MD, PhD[1]

Case

Patient PI, 55-year-old white male, was admitted to the Department of Diabetology due to significant deterioration of metabolic control, which occurred over the last few months.

Past Medical History

The patient was diagnosed with diabetes in December 2007. The manifestation of diabetes occurred immediately after the onset of acute pancreatitis. However, despite the diagnosis, the patient required insulin for the correction of hyperglycemia at the onset of the disease. He was prescribed insulin glargine 20 units per day. He took insulin glargine for 3 consecutive years after diagnosis, but in 2010, insulin was discontinued and he was prescribed sulfonylurea—gliclazide 120 mg daily. From today's perspective, that change of antihyperglycemic treatment does not seem to be well justified.

After the switch to oral antihyperglycemic medication, the patient did not attend the diabetes clinic and just occasionally checked blood glucose levels at fasting at home. According to the patient, fasting glucose levels

[1]Diabetology Department, National Medical Academy for Postgraduate Education, Kiev, Ukraine

DOI: 10.2337/9781580406666.04

were always around 12 mmol/L (216 mg/dL). No postprandial blood glucose or HbA$_{1c}$ levels had been checked since 2010.

Medical history is remarkable for episodes of alcohol abuse. There is no history of any surgery or gallstones. Family history is unremarkable; there is no family history of diabetes.

At the current admission, the patient presented with complaints of dizziness, fatigue, impaired sleep, and impaired vision. He complained of episodes of blood glucose spikes to 20 mmol/L (360 mg/dL) and elevation of arterial blood pressure to 160/90 mmHg.

The physical exam was unremarkable: body weight was 82 kg, height was 178 cm, BMI was 25.9 kg/m². Heart rate was 100 beats per minute, and blood pressure was 146/90 mmHg. Laboratory tests confirmed poor metabolic control; HbA$_{1c}$ level was 11.2%. The blood glucose levels during the day ranged between 14.05 mmol/L (253 mg/dL) and 20.9 mmol/L (376 mg/dL).

The urine analysis showed increased levels of ketones, protein – 0.099 g/L, without signs of urinary infection (leukocytes 1–2 per field, no bacteria). Liver functional tests revealed significant elevation of alanine aminotransferase (ALT) – 158 units/L and less marked elevation of aspartate aminotransferase (AST) – 76 units/L (the upper limit for both tests is 40 units/L).

Creatinine was 128 mmol/L and glomerular filtration rate (GFR) was 51 mL/min/1.73 m² (by Modification of Diet in Renal Disease formula). Based on the history of alcohol abuse and acute pancreatitis, the levels of amylase in the blood and urine were tested and found to be within the normal range. C-peptide level was measured at 1.95 ng/mL (normal range – 0.9 – 7.10 ng/mL). Despite this seemingly normal level of C-peptide, we believe that this test reflects inappropriate insulin production by β-cells as the level of glycemia exactly at the time of blood drawing was rather high, 20.9 mmol/L (376 mg/dL).

The test for antibodies to glutamate amino decarboxylase (anti-GAD antibodies) was performed and no increased levels were found – 4.81 mU/mL (less than 10 mU/mL considered as negative test).

Based on the results of examination, lab tests, and history of disease, the patient was prescribed insulin while oral sulfonylurea was discontinued. Intensive insulin treatment was prescribed – insulin glargine 36 units at night time and insulin glulisine 3 times a day immediately before or just after the meal – 2 units of insulin per 15 g of carbohydrate. The appropriate rehydration was performed.

After the treatment was initiated, the levels of glycemia decreased significantly and fluctuated within 6–10 mm/L during the day. There was no ketonuria. There were slight positive changes of GFR – increased to 78 mL/min/1.73m^2, ALT 135 units/L, AST 61 units/L.

Discussion

Based on the medical history, the results of the examination, and lab tests we summarized that this patient seems to be a continued alcohol abuser. As no other risk factors for acute pancreatitis were revealed, we can assume that the case of acute pancreatitis in this patient could be attributed to his alcohol abuse. The revealed changes of liver functional tests can confirm the role of alcohol abuse.

Diabetes manifested immediately after the onset of acute pancreatitis. We believe that in this patient we can diagnose diabetes induced by acute pancreatitis. Of course, it does not seem to be possible to answer the question whether acute pancreatitis was the single causative factor for the development of diabetes or acted as a significant triggering factor for the manifestation of diabetes in an already predisposed subject.

Despite the original diagnosis of type 2 diabetes, this patient does not appear similar to typical patients with this type of disease. He is not over-weight. The oral antihyperglycemic medication did not seem to be effective in his case, and he presented to our clinic with severe deterioration of glycemic control and even ketonuria. It is important to note that his endogenous production of insulin was inappropriate with relative low level of C-peptide relative to the very high level of blood glucose.

Taken into consideration these clinical features and the course of diabetes, it is reasonable to exclude latent autoimmune diabetes of adults (LADA). In addition, the negative results of test on anti-GAD antibodies do not support the possibility of LADA.

The data regarding the incidence of pancreatogenic diabetic (also referred to as type 3c diabetes) are scarce and quite controversial. Cui and Andersen[1] reviewed the available literature and found that pancreatogenic diabetes occurs in 5–10% of all cases of diabetes in the Western world, and is associated with mild to severe acute pancreatitis. In the more recent study, which followed 100 patients with acute pancreatitis for 2.7 years, diabetes developed in 14% of patients studied.[2] Recently, in a large study, which enrolled 2,966 patients after an episode of acute pancreatitis and 11,864 age-matched control subjects, the hazard ratio for diabetes in the first 3 months after acute pancreatitis was 5.90 (60.8 and 8.0 per 1,000 person-years in acute pancreatitis and control groups, respectively), and during the following time period, the risk of diabetes remained increased by 2.54 (22.5 and 6.7 per 1,000 person-years in acute pancreatitis and control groups, respectively).[3] The severity of acute pancreatitis did not seem to play a role in the increased risk of developing diabetes. The clinical course of pancreatogenic diabetes is characterized by an increased hepatic glucose production leading to the severe and persistent hyperglycemia and high sensitivity of the peripheral tissues to insulin, which taken together can lead to so called "brittle diabetes" with frequent episodes of hyper- and hypoglycemia.[4,5]

To summarize, the presented case of pancreatogenic diabetes highlights the following clinical and laboratory peculiarities of this form of disease. In this patient, the onset was linked directly to onset of acute pancreatitis, which in turn was probably caused by alcohol abuse. The patient is not overweight and resistant to oral antihyperglycemic treatment. While it was not type 1 diabetes, the course of the disease looked similar to these types of diabetes and required insulin treatment. We can conclude that patients with pancreatogenic diabetes should be followed more closely and intensively than other type 2 diabetic patients with appropriate, on-time prescription of insulin, and monitoring of blood glucose and urine ketones levels.

References

1. Cui Y, Andersen DK. Pancreatogenic diabetes: special considerations for management. *Pancreatology* 2011;11:279–294

2. Vujasinovic M, Tepes B, Makuc J, Rudolf S, et al. Pancreatic exocrine insufficiency, diabetes mellitus and serum nutritional markers after acute pancreatitis. *World J Gastroenterol* 2014;20:18432–18438

3. Shen HN, Yang CC, Chang YH, Lu CL, Li CY. Risk of diabetes mellitus after first-attack acute pancreatitis: a national population-based study. *Am J Gastroenterol* 2015;110:1698–1706

4. Andersen DK. The practical importance of recognizing pancreatogenic or type 3c diabetes. *Diabetes Metab Res Rev* 2012;28:326–328

5. Magruder JT, Elahi D, Andersen DK. Diabetes and pancreatic cancer: chicken or egg? *Pancreas* 2011;40:339–351

Case 32:
A Case of Pancreatogenic Diabetes Due to Alcohol Abuse

Bushra Z. Osmani, MD;[1] Janice L. Gilden, MS, MD;[1] and Alvia Moid, DO[1]

Case

A 66-year-old African-American male with a past history of heavy long-term alcohol use since age 11 and substance abuse presented to the emergency department with a three-day history of nausea, vomiting, and "feeling dazed." His blood glucose level was 467 mg/dL (225.9 mmol/L), blood pH 7.2 (normal = 7.38–7.46), positive for small serum ketones, serum bicarbonate was 11 mmol/L (normal = 21–32 mmol/L), and anion gap was 23 mmol/L (normal = 8–20 mmol/L). He was found to have a urinary tract infection (UTI). BMI = 23 kg/m². Glycosylated hemoglobin (HbA_{1c}) was 12.4% (normal = 4.0–6.0%). The patient denied a prior knowledge of diabetes. However, he did admit to many years duration of hyperglycemic symptoms (polyuria, polydipsia), as well as numbness and tingling of his fingers and toes.

The American Diabetes Association defines diabetes as the presence of HbA_{1c} ≥6.5%, fasting plasma glucose (FPG) ≥126 mg/dL (7.0 mmol/L), 2-hour plasma glucose ≥200 mg/dL (11.1 mmol/L) during an oral glucose tolerance test (OGTT), or a random plasma glucose (RPG) ≥200 mg/dL (11.1 mmol/L) in a patient with symptoms of hyperglycemia or hyperglycemic crisis.[1]

[1]Rosalind Franklin University of Medicine and Science/Chicago Medical School and Captain James A. Lovell Federal Health Care Center, North Chicago, IL

DOI: 10.2337/9781580406666.04

Our patient fulfilled the above criteria since HbA$_{1c}$ was 12.4% with an RPG > 400 mg/dL (>22.2 mmol/L) and the presence of symptoms of polyuria and polydipsia.

Medical history was significant for chronic pancreatitis with pancreatic pseudocyst removal (25 years ago), difficult-to-control paranoid schizoaffective disorder (treated with a variety of medications and multiple hospitalizations), and hypertension. He is a current cigarette smoker. Although he has had heavy alcohol usage for many years, he now states that he only consumes occasional beer. His family history was significant for diabetes in his mother (unknown age of onset and unknown therapy). A review of past medical records revealed that 3 years ago, the patient was noted to have laboratory blood glucose measurements of >300 mg/dL (>16.7 mmol/L), treated with insulin, while admitted for sepsis, although HbA$_{1c}$ at that time was normal (5.3%). Following this episode, a few sporadic laboratory blood glucose levels were done up to 4 months ago and were normal. However, subsequently he did not seek any type of medical care until the present time.

During the current hospitalization, an insulin infusion was administered until the ketoacidosis resolved. He was then transitioned to low-dose subcutaneous insulin therapy: insulin detemir 10 units daily with insulin aspart correction with meals. Laboratory testing revealed C-peptide 0.40 ng/mL (normal = 0.81–3.85 ng/mL) with concomitant blood glucose = 233 mg/dL (12.9 mmol/L), negative 65-glutamic acid decarboxylase (GAD) antibodies, and 25-hydroxy (25-OH) vitamin D level of 17.7 ng/mL (normal = 30–100 ng/mL).

While an inpatient, the blood glucose levels had been difficult to control with marked sensitivity to small changes in therapeutic insulin doses. By day 5 of admission, the insulin doses were: insulin detemir 18 units daily and insulin aspart 8 units with meals. At that time, the patient decided to leave the hospital against medical advice.

One week later, he returned to the emergency room due to continuing symptoms of hyperglycemia with a blood glucose level of 605 mg/dL (33.6 mmol/L) and recurrence of diabetic ketoacidosis. He had not taken any insulin at home. He was readmitted to the inpatient unit, where an insulin infusion was again started. He was transitioned to subcutaneous insulin doses and discharged home with recommendations to take insulin detemir 20 units/day and insulin aspart 8 units with meals.

The American Diabetes Association classifies diabetes into four major types, summarized in Table C32.1. We, therefore, considered the diagnosis

Table C32.1—Classification of Diabetes and Other Associated Conditions

	Characteristics
Type 1 diabetes	Autoimmune β-cell destruction, usually leading to absolute insulin deficiency
Type 2 diabetes	Progressive loss of β-cell insulin secretions frequently on the background of insulin resistance
Specific types of diabetes due to other causes	A. Monogenic diabetes syndromes (such as neonatal diabetes and maturity-onset diabetes of the young or MODY) B. Diseases of the exocrine pancreas (such as cystic fibrosis) C. Drug- or chemical-induced diabetes (such as glucocorticoid use, in the treatment of HIV/AIDS, or after organ transplantation) *Other conditions associated with diabetes* Drugs/chemicals (Vacor, pentamidine, nicotinic acid, diazoxide, beta-adrenergic agonists, thiazides, Dilantin, Υ-interferon) Uncommon forms of immune-mediation (stiff-man syndrome, anti-insulin receptor antibodies) Genetic syndromes (Down syndrome, Klinefelter syndrome, Turner Syndrome, Wolfram syndrome, Friedreich's ataxia, Huntington's chorea, Laurence-Moon-Biedl syndrome, myotonic dystrophy, porphyria, Prader-Willi syndrome) Genetic defects in insulin action (Type A insulin resistance, leprechaunism, Rabson-Mendenhall syndrome, lipoatrophic diabetes) Exocrine pancreatic disease (pancreatitis, trauma/pancreatectomy, neoplasia, hemochromatosis, fibrocalculous pancreatopathy) Endocrinopathies (acromegaly, Cushing's, glucagonoma, pheochromocytoma, hyperthyroidism, somatostatinoma, aldosteronomas)
Gestational diabetes	Diabetes diagnosed in the second or third trimester of pregnancy that was not clearly overt diabetes prior to gestation

Source: Adapted from the American Diabetes Association's 2017 Standards of Care[1]

of pancreatogenic diabetes (sometimes referred to as type 3c diabetes) in our patient, with a history of heavy alcohol abuse, chronic pancreatitis, and previous pancreatic pseudocyst removal.

Pancreatogenic diabetes has a prevalence of 5–10% among all patients with diabetes in the Western populations.[1] It is important to diagnose this condition accurately, due to specific implications for therapeutic management, as well as long-term care and complications.

Patients with chronic pancreatitis develop diabetes as a consequence of islet cell destruction by pancreatic inflammation. Additionally, there is decreased insulin release from remaining β-cells due to nutrient maldigestion leading to impaired secretion of incretins.[2]

Up to 25% of patients with pancreatogenic diabetes have rapid swings in blood glucose levels.[4] They commonly have hyperglycemia (due to unsuppressed glucose production by the liver), followed by severe hypoglycemia (due to administration of exogenous insulin, enhanced peripheral sensitivity of insulin, decreased secretion of glucagon in response to hypoglycemia, and inconsistent eating patterns due to pain, nausea, or chronic alcohol abuse).[3,4]

Patients with pancreatogenic diabetes often have other comorbidities, such as malabsorption and qualitative malnutrition, leading to fat-soluble vitamin deficiencies (especially vitamin D), impaired fat hydrolysis and impaired incretin secretion. Greater than 90% of patients with chronic pancreatitis have vitamin D deficiency, which can manifest as osteoporosis or alterations in bone metabolism. Therefore, it is important to measure serum 25-hydroxyvitamin D levels and supplement patients who are deficient.[2]

One proposed diagnostic criteria for pancreatogenic diabetes consists of major and minor criteria that must be present to make this diagnosis. The major criteria are as follows: 1) exocrine pancreatic insufficiency, 2) pathological pancreatic imaging, and 3) absent autoimmune markers associated with type 1 diabetes (T1D). Minor criteria consist of impaired incretin secretion, absent pancreatic polypeptide secretion, impaired β-cell function, low serum levels of lipid soluble vitamins, and the absence of excessive insulin resistance.[2]

Our patient had a low C-peptide level with a high blood glucose level, which implies low pancreatic reserve of insulin. With this in mind, the patient can be considered as having T1D. However, he did not demonstrate the presence of autoantibodies to pancreatic β-cells. Thus, he meets the criteria for the diagnosis of pancreatogenic diabetes. Our patient also had low levels of Vitamin D, a lipid-soluble vitamin, which further supports the diagnosis of pancreatogenic diabetes. However, he refused to have an evaluation to assess malabsorption.

Management of pancreatogenic diabetes consists of blood glucose control, counseling about lifestyle modifications (including diet, physical activity, smoking cessation, and abstinence from alcohol), as well as management of the exocrine pancreatic deficiency.[2] The pharmacologic treatment for pancreatogenic diabetes is the same as that for type 2 diabetes. Therefore, metformin is usually the drug of first choice. Oral agents like sulfonylureas and glinides may also be used, but thiazolidinediones should be avoided due to potential side effects of fluid retention, congestive heart failure, and bone fractures.[2] While incretin-based therapies like glucagon-like peptide-1 (GLP-1) analogues and dipeptidyl peptidase (DPP)-IV inhibitors enhance insulin secretion, use of these should be avoided in patients with pancreatogenic diabetes, due to a possible increase in risks for pancreatitis and pancreatic cancer, as well as the possibility of causing more gastrointestinal side effects.[5] Since chronic pancreatitis is a progressive condition, many patients will eventually require therapy with insulin.

Exocrine pancreatic insufficiency and malabsorption may not be clinically significant until over a 90% decrease in exocrine pancreatic function. Therefore, it is important to also look for qualitative malnutrition, demonstrated by deficiencies of fat-soluble vitamins (A, D, E, and K). Oral pancreatic enzyme replacement may be necessary to prevent steatorrhea, as well as to prevent other metabolic complications (such as impaired incretin release) and qualitative malnutrition.[2]

This case demonstrates the presentation of one type of pancreatogenic diabetes, due to complications from alcohol abuse. Other etiologies of endocrine pancreatic disease include other causes of pancreatitis (such as hypertriglyceridemia, hypercalcemia, idiopathic, and other), trauma, pancreatectomy, neoplasia, cystic fibrosis, hemochromatosis, and fibrocalculous pancreatopathy.

This research was supported in part by the Captain James A. Lovell Federal Health Care Center.

References

1. American Diabetes Association. Diagnosis and classification of diabetes mellitus. *Diabetes Care* 2014;37(Suppl. 1):S81–S90

2. Ebert R, Creutzfeldt W. Reversal of impaired GIP and insulin secretion in patients with pancreatogenic steatorrhea following enzyme substitution. *Diabetologia.* 1980;19:198–204

3. Ewald N, Hardt PD. Diagnosis and treatment of diabetes mellitus in chronic pancreatitis. *World J Gastroenterol* 2013;19(42):7276–7281

4. Duggan SN, Ewald N, Kelleher L, Griffin O, Gibney J, Conlon KC. The nutritional management of type 3c (pancreatogenic) diabetes in chronic pancreatitis. *Eur J Clin Nutr* 2017;71:3–8

5. Alves C, Batel-Marques F, Macedo AF. A meta-analysis of serious adverse events reported with exenatide and liraglutide: acute pancreatitis and cancer. *Diabetes Res Clin Pract* 2012;98:271–284

Case 33:
Post-Pancreatectomy Diabetes

Eric Dale Buras, MD, PhD;[1] Roma Y. Gianchandani, MD;[1] and Jennifer Wyckoff, MD[1]

Case

A 44-year-old woman presented with post-pancreatectomy diabetes (PPD). She was diagnosed with hereditary pancreatitis at age 18 in the setting of persistent abdominal pain, and pancreatic duct (PD) stricture. At age 19, she underwent a pancreaticojejeunostomy, with transient resolution of symptoms. Due to continued disease flares and a history of pancreatic adenocarcinoma in her father, she underwent genetic testing that revealed a mutation in the cationic trypsinogen gene. Surveillance imaging alternating magnetic resonance imaging with endoscopic ultrasound was performed every 6 months. She continued to have severe abdominal pain and required bile duct stenting; however, stricture progressed until an endoscopic retrograde cholangiopancreatogram probe could not traverse the PD. She underwent a total pancreatectomy and splenectomy with concurrent takedown of the pancreaticojejeunostomy.

At age 36, BMI was 30.9 kg/m² and HbA$_{1c}$ was <6.5% without use of anti-hyperglycemic medications. Following surgery at age 39, she required a basal-bolus insulin regimen of 20–25 units daily. Her long-acting insulin was down-titrated to prevent fasting hypoglycemia, and mealtime insulin

[1]Division of Endocrinology, Department of Medicine, University of Michigan, Ann Arbor, MI

DOI: 10.2337/9781580406666.04

increased to cover postprandial hyperglycemia. One year postoperatively, she maintained HbA_{1c} values ranging from 6.5–7.0% on a regimen of glargine 7 units, mealtime insulin/carbohydrate ratio of 1:15, and sensitivity of 1:50. Sensitivity was ultimately reduced to 1:150 to preclude hypoglycemic events. Due to continued hypoglycemia, she was started on a continuous glucose monitoring system at age 42, and shortly thereafter transitioned to an insulin pump. At no point did she develop ketoacidosis.

Discussion

Definition

"Pancreatogenic diabetes" was initially defined by Minkowski in 1889 based on the observation of hyperglycemia in pancreatectomized dogs. In humans, the first case of pancreatic diabetes was described in 1942 in a patient who underwent total pancreatectomy for an "islet cell adenoma." With increasing postoperative survival times due to advanced surgical techniques and improved chemotherapy regimens for pancreatic cancer, PPD has gained increasing clinical relevance.[1] At present, PPD is classified a subset of type 3, or secondary, diabetes. Although it constitutes an insulin-deficient state, like type 1 diabetes (T1D), unique aspects of PPD pathophysiology must be appropriately managed to limit long-term morbidity and mortality.

Epidemiology

Total pancreatectomy is relatively rare (4,000 performed in the United States between 1998 and 2006).[1] While this procedure uniformly causes insulin-requiring diabetes, more commonly performed partial resection procedures may also be complicated by PPD. PPD prevalence in these cases depends on the underlying disease and specific operative procedure. In the setting of tumor resection, retrospective case series demonstrate 9% diabetes risk 21 months after distal pancreatectomy, and 20% risk during a 3–10-year follow-up period. Rates are higher following proximal pancreatectomy, reaching 44% in a single-center series with average follow-up of 5–7 years. Central pancreatectomy is comparatively benign with no demonstrated PPD risk in a 50-patient series.[2] Chronic pancreatitis itself carries a high risk of secondary diabetes—up to 83% in one large single-center retrospective analysis; although, even in this population, distal pancreatectomy represented an independent risk factor for disease development.[3] While total pancreatectomy represents the prototype for PPD pathophysiology, the phenomena outlined below occur to varying extents even in the setting of these subtotal procedures.[4]

Pathogenesis

PPD pathogenesis is driven by absence of all islet components and, to some extent, exocrine hormone deficiency. While PPD patients lack endogenous insulin production, the condition differs from T1D based on a concurrent absence of glucagon. Unable to mount appropriate counter-regulatory responses to falling blood glucose, PPD patients are subject to frequent and severe hypoglycemia. Conversely, glucagon deficiency largely spares PPD patients from diabetic ketoacidosis.[2] Pancreatic exocrine hormone deficiency may contribute to rapid intestinal transit states making glucose absorption unpredictable and further complicating management.[4] PPD patients have increased peripheral insulin sensitivity due to an unexplained upregulation of insulin binding sites. Paradoxically, hepatic insulin receptor number and insulin sensitivity are reduced in PPD (as in chronic pancreatitis), owing to pancreatic polypeptide deficiency.[5]

Glycemic Control and Complications

While no large-scale trials have compared glycemic parameters in PPD versus T1D, PPD is generally considered difficult to manage, with up to 25% of patients classified as "brittle."[1] Hepatic insulin resistance yields significant hyperglycemia, while enhanced peripheral insulin sensitivity and glucagon deficiency risk severe hypoglycemia with exogenous insulin. Rates of microvascular and macrovascular complications are difficult to estimate given the diversity of prepancreatectomy diseases and limited follow-up duration in most studies. Based on available analyses, retinopathy frequency and severity are similar to T1D, and neuropathy is common. While microalbuminuria is frequently seen in PPD, end-stage renal disease is rare. Although rates of macrovascular complications are difficult to estimate, they are believed to be lower in PPD, due in part to compromised lipid absorption post-pancreatectomy.[1]

Management

Treatment of PPD is generally similar to that of T1D; however specific perioperative and long-term management issues deserve consideration. As with other major surgeries, postoperative hyperglycemia after pancreatectomy is an independent risk factor for morbidity and mortality, especially with blood glucose >140 mg/dL.[6] These findings have led some to recommend a blood glucose target <140 mg/dL, which is lower than the American Diabetes Association target of 140–180 mg/dL (7.7–10 mmol/L).

PPD patients generally have lower basal and higher postprandial insulin requirements. On basal-bolus regimens, long-acting insulin may be dosed in the morning to mitigate risk of overnight hypoglycemia. Patients should be encouraged to eat frequent small meals, avoid alcohol, and rigorously monitor blood glucose (particularly during exercise) to prevent hypoglycemia.[1] As in this case, continuous glucose monitoring and insulin pump therapy (allowing for variation of basal insulin delivery) can be helpful. Islet autotransplantaton has been evaluated after pancreatectomy for benign disease, and >50% rates of insulin independence have been achieved during the initial hospitalization. Nonetheless, insulin independence rates are considerably lower on long-term follow-up.[1] Given the essential component of glucagon deficiency in PPD pathophysiology, closed-loop dual-chamber insulin pump therapy represents an attractive future option for these patients.[2]

References

1.   Scavini M, Dugnani E, Pasquale V, Liberati D, Aleotti F, Di Terlizzi G, Petrella G, Balzano G, Piemonti L. Diabetes after pancreatic surgery: novel issues. *Curr Diab Rep* 2015;15:16

2.   Maeda H, Hanazaki K. Pancreatogenic diabetes after pancreatic resection. *Pancreatology* 2011;11:268–276

3.   Malka D, Hammel P, Sauvanet A, Rufat P, O'Toole D, Bardet P, Belghiti J, Bernades P, Ruszniewski P, Lévy P. Risk factors for diabetes mellitus in chronic pancreatitis. *Gastroenterology* 2000;119:1324–1332

4.   Cui Y, Andersen DK. Pancreatogenic diabetes: special considerations for management. *Pancreatology* 2011;11:279–294

5.   Andersen DK, Ruiz CL, Burant CF. Insulin regulation of hepatic glucose transporter protein is impaired in chronic pancreatitis. *Ann Surg* 1994;219:679–686

6.   Eshuis WJ, Hermanides J, van Dalen JW, van Samkar G, Busch OR, van Gulik TM, DeVries JH, Hoekstra JB, Gouma DJ. Early postoperative hyperglycemia is associated with postoperative complications after pancreatoduodenectomy. *Ann Surg* 2011;253:739–744

Case 34:
Diabetes and Hemochromatosis

Davide Maggi, MD, PhD;[1] Anna Aleo, MD;[1] Lucia Briatore, MD;[1] Chiara Mazzucchelli, MD;[1] Luigi Fontana, MD;[1] and Renzo Cordera, MD[1]

Case 1

A 72-year-old Caucasian male came to our observation for evaluation and classification for the possibility of type 2 diabetes (T2D). Hyperglycemia was discovered a few months before after a small hemorrhagic stroke, and he was treated from then with basal insulin 0.3 unit/kg. He did not report systemic symptoms; at physical examination, his BMI was 21 kg/m², and he presented hepathomegaly. Lab test results were: HbA$_{1c}$ was 7.9% during insulin therapy 0.3 unit/kg, LDL 105 mg/dL, HDL 65 mg/dL, and triglycerides 128 mg/dL. A T2D diagnosis was unlikely because of the apparent absence of insulin resistance, the low BMI, and the responsiveness to exogenous insulin. Next, a negative GAD antibodies test did not support a diagnosis of latent autoimmune diabetes of adults, and diabetes secondary to other diseases was hypothesized. The patient reported a 5 kg unintentional weight loss during the last year. Among other tests, ferritin was 1,325 ug/L, s-transferrin 96%, and transferrin 1.88 g/L. A diagnosis of hemochromatosis was suspected and a genetic analysis was carried out. The HFE gene C282Y recessive mutation was present in a homozygous state. Severe iron accumulation was detected by nuclear magnetic resonance (NMR), in the liver and

[1]Diabetes Unit, Department of Internal Medicine, IRCCS San Martino and University of Genova, Genova, Italy

DOI: 10.2337/9781580406666.04

pancreas. Pituitary function was normal; testosterone was low/normal 2.9 ng/mL, while fasting C-peptide was 0.89 ng/mL.

The diagnosis was made of diabetes secondary to iron overload due to genetic C282Y Type 1 hemochromatosis.

C282Y homozygous mutation of HFE gene can cause hemochromatosis independently from environment. It is now recognized that iron absorption from intestinal cells, as well as iron exit from macrophage is regulated by ferroportin. In the case of C282Y mutation, hepcidin deficiency increases expression of ferroportin, which increases iron transport from intestinal cells and iron exit from macrophages, resulting in increased iron not bound to transferrin, and thus available for parenchymal cell capitation. Intracellular iron overload activates the generation of reactive oxygen species and lipid peroxidation. Cells with lower antioxidant activity are more sensitive to oxygen damage, thus explaining the iron damage to hepatocytes, endocrine, and cardiac cells. In this case, NMR spectroscopy confirmed iron overload in pancreatic cells making insulin deficiency the mechanism underlying hyperglycemia.

Case 2

A 51-year-old Caucasian male came to our observation with a diagnosis of T2D. Family history for diabetes was negative. He was treated for hypertension in the last decade with a fixed combination of renin-angiotensin-aldosterone inhibitors, diuretics, and metformin (2 g/day). On physical examination, visceral obesity (BMI 32 kg/m^2; waist circumference 111 cm) was present, lasting from his early twenties. HbA$_{1c}$ was 7.8%, HDL cholesterol was 72 mg/dL, and triglycerides (TG) level was 85 mg/dL. The patient's skin appeared reddish in color and blood analysis revealed erythrocytosis (Hgb 18.5 mg/mL, Hct 53%). Increased plasma ferritin (up to 935 ng/mL), saturated-transferrin fraction (>53%), and transferrin (253 ug/mL) were consistent with a provisional diagnosis of hemochromatosis. Genetic analysis was carried out and showed the homozygous mutation H63D in the HFE gene. Penetrance of H63D mutation is extremely low and this mutation does not cause hemochromatosis, but it can facilitate iron overload when associated with other risk factors such as heavy alcohol intake, visceral obesity, and inflammation.[1] The patient reported a moderate alcohol intake on social occasions.

At initial evalution, polyglobulia was unexplained and not justified by HFE mutation. Since the patient's ancestors originated from central Italy, we searched for thalassemia with hemoglobin variant, in particular lepore

Hb. Genetic analysis was negative. Next, we searched for a secondary polyglobulia; erythropoietin was elevated, suggesting a reactive secondary polyglobulia. The patient was again questioned on possible cause of hypoxemia: he smoked two cigars weekly and suffered from chronic sinusitis and morning headaches. Sleep apnea was previously diagnosed and this finding was enough to cause desaturation and to explain elevated erythropoietin and secondary polyglobulia. Finally, testosterone was measured and found to be in the high normal range. In summary, this patient presented with iron overload due to complementary action of genetic H63D mutation and environmentally increased erythropoietin secondary to hypoxemia due to sleep apnea, visceral obesity, and elevated testosterone. HFE mutations, testosterone, and erythropoietin act on a common substrate that represents a final common pathway regulating iron availability. All three decrease hepcidin activity, which in turn activates ferroportin. This latter facilitates iron transport and deposition inside parenchymal cells. Iron overload initiates cellular damage by generation of reactive oxygen species and lipid peroxidation. Cells, like pancreatic β-cells and the endocrine cells in general, with higher mitochondrial activity are less resistant to oxygen toxicity. In this case, a diagnosis of T2D does not fit the complete clinical presentation, suggesting instead a diagnosis of diabetes secondary to hemochromatosis.

Discussion

The relationship between body iron overload and diabetes is complex and bidirectional; primary genetic iron overload (hemochromatosis) might cause diabetes by β-cell dysfunction. Conversely diabetes, obesity, metabolic syndrome, and low-grade inflammation increase iron body deposition. In the latter circumstances, hyperglycemia and diabetes are mostly secondary to insulin resistance.[2] In both conditions a common pathway resulting in iron cellular overload is activated.[3] Excess intracellular iron causes cell damage while iron depletion by phlebotomy results in a better diabetes control.

Here we report two cases of diabetes illustrative of this relationship: high ferritin plasma concentration and a saturated transferrin fraction >50%, suggesting a diagnosis of hemochromatosis. Genetic analysis showed two different homozygous mutations in the HFE gene but only one with significant penetrance. These two patients carry a genetic profile associated with iron overload and support a diagnostic challenge: diabetes secondary to hemochromatosis or is it T2D? These cases illustrate that even a straightforward diagnosis of T2D might be misleading and can potentially delay the most appropriate therapy.

These two cases are representative of the wide spectrum of genes/environment mutual relationships.

Case 1 represents typical hemochromatosis: mutation of C282Y leads to deregulation of hepcidin which in turn up-regulates ferroportin, resulting in increased intestinal iron absorption and macrophage depletion with iron deposition in parenchymal liver cells and endocrine cells. Case 2 is more complex since three different abnormalities (each one subclinical) contributed to a definite clinical picture. In this case, neither mutation H63D alone nor increased erythropoietin or testosterone can explain the complete clinical presentation, in particular iron overload and polyglobulia.[4,5]

In both cases, phlebotomy was started and soon after both metabolic and vascular abnormalities improved.

References

1. Kelley M, Joshi N, Xie Y, Borgaonkar M. Iron overload is rare in patients homozygous for the H63D mutation. *Can J Gastroenterol Hepatol* 2014;28:198–202

2. Simcox JA, McClain DA. Iron and diabetes risk. *Cell Metab* 2013;17:329–341

3. Powell LW, Seckington RC, Deugnier Y. Haemochromatosis. *Lancet* 2016; 388:706–716

4. Shah YM, Xie L. Hypoxia-inducible factors link iron homeostasis and erythropoiesis. *Gastroenterology* 2014;146:630–642

5. Dhinsha S, Ghanim H, Batra M, Kuhadiya ND, Abuaysheh S, Green K, Makdissi A, Chauduri A, Dandona P. Effect of testosterone on hepcidin, ferroportin, ferritin and iron binding capacity in patients with hypogonadotropic hypogonadism and T2DM. *Clin Endocrinol (Oxf)* 2016;85:772–780

Case 35:
Bronze Diabetes

Erin K.P. Meyerhoff, RN, FNP-C, CDE[1]

Case

SM is a very fair-skinned white male of German heritage, born in 1975. He presented to the clinic in March 2007 at age 32. He was diagnosed with diabetes in 2006. He reported increased thirst and urination at diagnosis. His primary concern was blurry vision. He reported inability to see further than 3 feet. He was unable to recall his presenting blood glucose but stated it was around 500 mg/dL without ketosis and HbA$_{1c}$ was around 9%. He had been feeling poorly for 3–6 months.

His primary care provider placed him on metformin and glipizide for 3–6 months. SM reported he had repeated and sudden hypoglycemia. SM then requested switching to insulin so he could achieve better control and prevent hypoglycemia.

On his first visit to our clinic, his HbA$_{1c}$ was 6.0% and he reported no symptomatic hypoglycemia (Table C35.1). He was on insulin 75/25 – 10 units in the morning and 20 units in the afternoon. His weight was 159 pounds (72.3 kg) and BMI was 22.8 kg/m^2. Past medical history was unremarkable. Family history revealed two paternal uncles with type two diabetes and a mother with hypothyroidism. A negative screening of hepatitis A, B, and C followed.

---

[1]Division of Endocrinology, Diabetes and Metabolism, Department of Medicine, University of Colorado Anschutz Medical Campus, Aurora, CO

DOI: 10.2337/9781580406666.04

Table C35.1 — Baseline Laboratory Testing (Only Pertinent Results Provided)

Component Latest Reference Range	3/26/2007
Glucose Random Serum/Plasma 60–199 milligrams per deciliter	197
Alk. Phos. 39 - 117 units per liter	158 (H)
Aspartate Aminotransferase 0–47 units per liter	62 (H)
Alanine Aminotransferase 0–47 units per liter	82 (H)
Bilirubin Total 0.0 - 1.0 milligrams per deciliter	1.1 (H)
Glutamic Acid Decarboxylase AB 0.0–1.45 units per milliliter	< 1
C-Peptide, Serum or Plasma 0.8–3.5 ng/ml	2.5
A1C Glycohemoglobin 4.3–6.5 percent	6.0

Table C35.2 — Patient Iron Studies

Component Latest Reference Range	4/12/2007
Iron 45–160 ug/dL	187 (H)
Unsat. Iron Binding Capacity 110–370 ug/dL	<17
Total Iron Binding Capacity 210–390 ug/dL	<204
Transferrin Saturation % 20–70 percent	>92%
Ferritin, Serum/Plasma 10–388 ng/ml	3,778 (H)

In May of 2007 DNA testing for hemochromatosis detected two copies of the C282Y mutation in his HFE genes, homozygous for hemochromatosis (Table C35.2). He was referred to hepatology for a complete workup and started phlebotomies. Liver biopsy was positive for stage 3–4 fibrosis. Computed tomography of chest showed no cardiomegaly.

He was lost to follow-up from 2007 to 2011 due to changing careers, going back to school, and being uninsured. He was getting phlebotomies through blood donation at this time. He quit smoking.

In January 2011, he complained of reduced sexual desire and function. He stated that he did not need to shave his beard anymore due to reduced facial hair. He was diagnosed with central hypogonadism (Table C35.3). Pituitary magnetic resonance imaging was unremarkable. All other pituitary labs were normal. He was started on testosterone with return of secondary hair, sexual desire, and function.

Table C35.3—Patient Hormone Studies

Component *Latest Reference Range*	9/13/2011
Free Testosterone *9.0–30.0 ng/dL*	0.4 (L)
Total Testosterone 348–1197 *ng/dL*	27
Follicle Stimulating Hormone *1–18 mIU/mL*	1
Luteinizing Hormone 1.5–9.3 *mIU/mL*	1.0

On September 13, 2011, his HbA_{1c} was 5.2%. Between January 2012 and April 2014, he was in excellent glycemic control: HbA_{1c} 5.6% to 5.8% with highest home BG postmeal value of 152 mg/dL.

In March of 2016 his HbA_{1c} was 5.9% and blood glucose ranged between 90 and 130 mg/dL through the day with no hypoglycemia. He continued with Humalog 75/25 14-15 units in A.M. on weekends and 12 units on workdays with 29 units in the evening. Total daily insulin dose was 44 units at 0.5 unit/kg.

Discussion

Hereditary hemochromatosis (HH) is an autosomal recessive disorder associated with increased intestinal absorption of iron and deposition of iron in the organs. It is most commonly found in those with northern European heritage. Upon diagnosis, most people will have elevated levels of iron. Transferrin saturation percentage will be high. A level greater than 60% in men and 50% in women is accurate in detecting over 90% of patients with HH.[1] They may have elevated ferritin especially later in the disease process when iron stores are full. It often takes up to 40 years for iron storage to be excessive and cause secondary disease. Many are not diagnosed with HH until their fourth decade of life.[2]

Mutations of the HFE (hereditary Fe) gene are involved. Two-point mutations have been designated C282Y and H63D. Homozygous C282Y mutation is the most commonly associated mutation and found in 60 to 93% of individuals with HH. Compound heterozygotes, with one copy of C282Y and one of H63D, have minimal risk for HH and it is usually of lesser severity.[2] A significant percent of subjects found to have homozygous HH at the time of screening have no evidence of iron overload at the time of screening[3] or after 12 or more years of follow-up.[4]

The most common sequelae from HH are bronzing of the skin, cirrhosis, liver cancer, cardiomegaly, arrhythmias, heart failure, joint pains, infections, secondary hypogonadism, primary hypothyroidism, and "bronzed diabetes."[2] According to Simcox and McClain,[5] iron overload is associated with β-cell failure and insulin resistance.

SM has been counseled on basal/bolus therapy but prefers his current premixed insulin regimen. Testosterone levels are well controlled on topical therapy. Thyroid function remains normal. Liver function remains stable.

His disease and frequent phlebotomies likely affect the accuracy of his HbA_{1c}. He does check his BG fasting and random times through the day (after large meals, pre and post exercise) with great results. He may need more consistent fasting and mealtime BG monitoring.

References

1.   Edwards CQ, Kushner JP. Screening for hemochromatosis. *N Engl J Med* 1993;328:1616–1620

2.   Brandhagen DJ, Fairbanks VF, Baldus W. Recognition and management of hereditary hemochromatosis. *Am Fam Physician* 2002;65:853–860

3.   Beutler E, Felitti VJ, Koziol JA, Ho NJ, Gelbart T. Penetrance of 845G->A (C282Y) HFE hereditary hemochromatosis mutation in the USA. *Lancet* 2002;359:211–218

4.   Whitlock EP, Garlitz BA, Harris EL, Beil TL, Smith PR. Screening for hereditary hemochromatosis: a systematic review for the U.S. Preventive Services Task Force. *Ann Intern Med* 2006;145:209–223

5.   Simcox JA, McClain DA. Iron and diabetes risk. *Cell Metab* 2013;17:329–341

Case 36:
Type 2 Diabetes in Liver Cirrhosis and Hepatocellular Carcinoma

Sarena Ravi, MD, MPH;[1] Alvia Moid, DO;[1] Janice L. Gilden, MS, MD;[1] and Dhauna Karam, MD[1]

Case

A 64-year-old Caucasian male with uncontrolled type 2 diabetes of 13 years' duration and liver cirrhosis secondary to hepatitis C and alcohol abuse, taking 90–100 units total insulin per day (per records), presented to the emergency department with one-week duration of worsening abdominal pain, swelling, pedal edema, nausea, and nonbloody emesis. He had multiple hospitalizations over the past year for hepatic encephalopathy and was readmitted for decompensated liver cirrhosis and hepatic encephalopathy.

On Day 1 of hospitalization, his blood glucose decreased to 46 mg/dL (2.6 mmol/L) 4 hours after being given a dose of basal insulin detemir 40 units (Table C36.1) (home dose = 60 units). Blood glucose (BG) then increased to 84 mg/dL (4.7 mmol/L) 1 hour later following an ampule of D50 and a meal. Three hours later, the BG dropped to 54 mg/dL (3.0 mmol/L), and the patient received another ampule of D50. By day 2, 28 hours after receiving the one-time dose of basal insulin, BG again dropped to 42 mg/dL (2.3 mmol/L), despite consuming three full meals daily. During the remainder of the hospitalization, point-of-care BG done premeals and bedtime

[1]Rosalind Franklin University of Medicine and Science/Chicago Medical School and Captain James A. Lovell Federal Health Center, North Chicago, IL

DOI: 10.2337/9781580406666.04

Table C36.1 — Table of Blood Glucose Values Below 70 mg/dL (3.9 mmol/L)

	Glucose Value/Time	Insulin Given/Time	Dextrose Given/Time
Day 1	46 mg/dL at 6:00 A.M. 54 mg/dL at 9:40 A.M.	Detemir 40 units-2:00 P.M.	1 ampule D50 6:00 1 ampule D50 9:40
Day 2	42 mg/dL at 5:20 A.M.	None	1 ampule D50 5:20
Day 3 to day 7 (discharge)	69 mg/dL at 12:00 A.M. on day 6	None	None

were maintained between 60 and 100 mg/dL (3.3 and 5.5 mmol/L), despite eating three meals with three snacks. Glucagon was never administered.

After standard treatment for hepatic encephalopathy, with subsequent improvement of mental status, the patient admitted that he had not been taking insulin for several weeks prior to the current hospitalization. This was verified by his family and also confirmed by outpatient pharmacy. The patient and family recalled that at home, fingerstick BG was either normal or low, despite not taking insulin for "several weeks," and possibly months.

Laboratory data confirmed that HbA_{1c} was 4.7% (4–6%). Patient had HbA_{1c} of 7.9% three months previously and 11.6% six months prior to this hospitalization. Hemoglobin during hospitalization ranged from 8–9 g/dL (normal 13–17 g/dL). Fasting C-peptide was 2.15 ng/mL (normal 0.81–3.85 ng/mL) with a concurrent glucose of 196 mg/dL (11.0 mmol/L). Alpha-fetoprotein levels were somewhat elevated (46.9 ng/mL; normal range is 0–8.0), and computed tomography (CT) scan was negative 8 months ago. However, the alpha fetoprotein increased to 20,000 ng/mL and CT scan of abdomen and pelvis now revealed a large $11 \times 10.6 \times 17.6$ cm heterogeneous liver mass occupying most of the right lobe, suggestive of hepatocellular carcinoma.

Before comprehensive evaluation of hypoglycemia could be undertaken, the patient chose hospice care. Posthospitalization, three weeks after diagnosis, while in the nursing home, the patient experienced 10 hypoglycemic episodes in one week with point-of-care BG values less than 60 mg/dL (<3.3 mmol/L) per nursing records, with the lowest being 27 mg/dl (1.5 mmol/L). It is to be noted that he was able to consume regular meals and snacks, had experienced no hyperglycemic glucose values, and no longer required insulin since day 1 of hospitalization.

Discussion

Gluconeogenesis is the process by which the liver produces glucose from noncarbohydrate precursors. In hepatic failure the destruction of hepatocytes, hyperinsulinemia, and inadequate storage of glucose in other organs may all contribute to hypoglycemia. Cirrhotic patients have been found to have elevated insulin levels, indicating either insulin resistance or reduced metabolism of the insulin by the diseased liver. Hypoglycemia may develop in these patients from insulin autoantibodies.[1]

Various neoplasms of epithelial and mesenchymal origin are associated with hypoglycemia and are classified as nonislet cell tumor hypoglycemia (NICTH), insulin-secreting tumors, myeloma, lymphoma, leukemia, and metastatic neoplasia.[2,3] These are about 25% as common as an insulinoma.

Hepatocellular carcinoma accounts for about 23% of total cases in patients with NICTH. The NICTH is thought to be due to an overproduction of an aberrant form of IGF-2 (insulin-like growth factor-II).[2–4] At the cellular level, IGF-1, IGF-2, and insulin can bind to 4 or more types of IGF-1 receptors. Each receptor-ligand binding then leads to different, as well as overlapping actions.[3] Overproduction of aberrant IGF-2 or "big IGF-2" then suppresses growth hormone (GH) biosynthesis and thus decreases GH-dependent production of IGF and IGF-binding protein-3 (IGFBP-3), causing hypoglycemia.

This condition presents with severe fasting hypoglycemia, as well as low plasma nonesterified fatty acid, beta-hydroxybutyrate, undetectable plasma insulin, C-peptide, proinsulin levels, and low GH levels. There is a high ratio of IGF-2: IGF-1 of 10:1 (normal = 3:1).

Other rare causes of NICTH include: autoantibodies to the insulin receptor, destruction of the liver, production of tumor necrosis factor, and other hypoglycemic cytokines, adrenocortical carcinoma, fibrosarcoma, and mesotheliomas (Table C36.2).

This case demonstrates a rare cause of hypoglycemia in a patient with type 2 diabetes who presented with decompensated liver cirrhosis from hepatitis C and developed a suspected IGF-2 secreting hepatocellular carcinoma. As mentioned earlier, diagnostic workup was not able to be completed due to hospice. Laboratory values of insulin, proinsulin, and C-peptide were not drawn during hypoglycemia, as glucose was corrected quickly by nursing staff before venous draw. Iatrogenic cause was not suspected because he continued to have hypoglycemia 24 hours after the

Table C36.2—Laboratory Test Results for Various Etiologies of Hypoglycemia

Diagnosis:	Insulin	Proinsulin	C-peptide	IGF-1	IGF-2	IGF2:1GF1 ratio	Pro-1GF2	OHA Screen	Insulin Antibody
OHA	High	High	High	N	N	N	N	+	–
Exogenous insulin	High	Low	Low	N	N	N	N	–	–
Insulinoma, post-GP	High	High	High	N	N	N	N	–	–
IAS	High	High	High	N	N	N	N	–	+
IGF-mediated	Low or low-normal	Low or low-normal	Low or low-normal	Low	High or N	High	High	–	–
NICTH	<3	<5	<.2	<100	>275	>3:1			
Noninsulin or IGF-mediated	<3	<5	<.2	N	N	N	N	–	–

N, normal; IAS, Insulin autoimmune syndrome
OHA, Oral hypoglycemic agent; post-GP, postgastric bypass
Source: Adapted from Bodnar T, Acevedo MJ, Pietropaolo M[5]

last dose of insulin was given. Insulin requirements dropped from 90 units daily to zero units without hyperglycemia, which prompted other etiologies to be entertained (e.g., IGF secretion).

Although advanced cirrhosis and liver failure, insulin autoantibodies, and poor glycogen stores can all present as an etiology for hypoglycemia, this case highlights the importance of considering hepatic malignancy as a possible cause. In addition, insulin dose requirements may decrease in severe liver disease and should not be based upon body weight.

Our case also demonstrates the potential for rapidly changing insulin requirements in a patient with type 2 diabetes and liver cirrhosis, since his insulin requirements decreased from 90–100 total daily insulin units to 0 units over the suspected course of three months. Therefore, close monitoring of glucose levels and adjustment and readjustment of pharmacologic treatment are essential in patients with diabetes and liver cirrhosis.

In addition to iatrogenic hypoglycemia, and/or impaired hepatic function, sudden development of normo- or hypoglycemia in a patient with diabetes prompts rapid investigation for an underlying malignancy.

This research was supported, in part, by the Captain James A. Lovell Federal Health Care Center.

References

1. Levinthal G, Tavill A. Liver disease and diabetes. *Clin Diabetes* 1999;17

2. Marks V, Teale JD. Tumours producing hypoglycaemia. *Endocr Relat Cancer* 1998;5:111–129

3. Bourcigaux N, Arnault-Ouary G, Christol R, Perin L, Charbonnel B, Le Bouc Y. Treatment of hypoglycemia using combined glucocorticoidand recombinant human growth hormone in a patient with a metastatic non-islet cell tumor hypoglycemia. *Clin Ther* 2005;27:246–251

4. Dynkevich Y, Rother KI, Whitford I, et al. Tumors, IGF-2, and hypoglycemia: insights from the clinic, the laboratory, and the historical archive. *Endocr Rev* 2013;34:798–826

5. Bodnar TW, Acevedo MJ, Pietropaolo M. Management of non-islet cell tumor hypoglycemia: a clinical review. *J Clin Endocrinol Metab* 2014;99:713–722

Case 37:
Poor Glycemic Control in Insulin-Treated Diabetes Due to Anti-Insulin Antibodies

David S. Church, MRCP;[1,2] and Robert K. Semple, MB, PhD[1,2]

Case History

An 83-year-old white European man with a 60-year history of type 1 diabetes was referred by his primary care physician. Over the long course of his diabetes, his glycemic control had been stable, with the mean HbA$_{1c}$ over the 5 years prior to referral being 7.5% (range 4.8–5.7). In the nine months prior to referral, new instability in glycemia had emerged, however, characterized by a predictable and recurring pattern of severe hypoglycemia on waking before breakfast, with hyperglycemia during the rest of the day. He had a history of moderate, painless diabetic peripheral neuropathy without other documented diabetes-related complications, as well as seropositive rheumatoid arthritis, hypertension, hyperlipidemia, and carcinoma of the prostate. There was no recent weight loss.

Insulin therapy before this period of glycemic instability was with a basal-bolus regimen of insulin detemir (10 units morning and evening) and preprandial insulin lispro (7 units with each breakfast, lunch, and evening meal). In response to the morning hypoglycemia and daytime hyperglycemia, this regimen was altered iteratively in primary care over several

[1]The University of Cambridge Metabolic Research Laboratories, Wellcome Trust-MRC Institute of Metabolic Science, Cambridge, U.K.

[2]The National Institute for Health Research Cambridge Biochemical Research Centre, Cambridge, U.K.

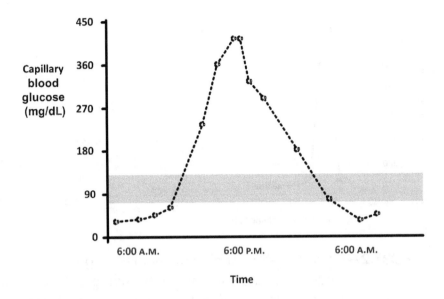

Figure C37.1—Daytime glycemic profile. Capillary blood glucose monitoring at presentation (mean of four weeks' home recording) demonstrating fasting hypoglycemia overnight with postprandial hyperglycemia during the day.

months, so that at referral insulin detemir was used once daily (4 units with breakfast), with an altered profile of insulin lispro preprandially (24, 20, and 3 units with breakfast, lunch, and evening meal, respectively). Despite this substantial reprofiling of daily insulin delivery, capillary blood glucose values on referral of ≤36 mg/dL (2 mmol/L) were regularly documented in the morning with few or no hypoglycemic symptoms, contrasting with significant hyperglycemia over the rest of the day (Figure C37.1).

On examination, the patient's body mass index was 27.2 kg/m², and there was no clinical evidence of lipohypertrophy or lipoatrophy at insulin injection sites, or acanthosis nigricans. Blood pressure was 132/63 mmHg lying and 129/62 mmHg on standing. Serum renal, hepatic, and thyroid functions were normal. Serum rheumatoid factor was raised at 194 (0–30) units/mL. HbA$_{1c}$ was 9.9%, and opportunistically measured plasma insulin in a sample taken 2 hours after breakfast and morning insulin dosing was <0.3 (0–86) µIU/mL, while plasma C-peptide concentration was undetectable (both assayed by PerkinElmer® AutoDELFIA®

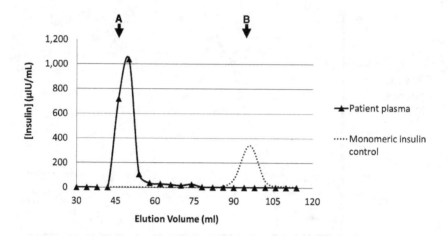

Figure C37.2—Demonstration of high molecular weight "macro-insulin" using gel filtration chromatography of plasma. Results of insulin immunoassay (Mercodia Iso-Insulin ELISA) of different elution volumes after gel filtration chromatography of (A) patient plasma and a monomeric ("free") insulin control sample are shown.

assay). The insulin assay used has been shown not to detect either insulin detemir or insulin lispro, and so these findings were consistent with bona fide type 1 diabetes, as demonstrated by absent endogenous insulin secretion.[1]

In view of the relatively acute onset of deranged glycemic control without any prior change in insulin regimen or other circumstances, the plasma sample initially obtained was examined in more detail. Insulin concentration was redetermined, this time using an enzyme-linked immunoassay with a broader specificity (Mercodia Iso-Insulin) that was able to detect most currently used insulin analogs. This revealed an extremely high plasma insulin concentration of 5,343 µIU/mL, one to two orders of magnitude higher than expected at the time sampled on the basal-bolus insulin regimen used. Insulin immunosubtraction studies using polyethylene glycol; protein G and anti-IgM precipitation suggested the presence of anti-insulin IgG with a high capacity to bind insulin, while plasma gel filtration chromatography studies (Figure C37.2) demonstrated that essentially all immunodetectable insulin was present in high molecular complexes co-eluting with immunoglobulins, consistent with the presence of large amounts of antibody-bound "macroinsulin."[2]

Following confirmation of insulin-binding antibodies, the importance of a long-acting carbohydrate-containing snack before bed was emphasized. Although a variety of antibody-depleting therapies were considered, in view of the patient's frailty and comorbidities, he was prescribed only prednisolone 30 mg once daily. This abrogated morning hypoglycemia, but worsened later hyperglycemia, with daytime capillary blood glucose readings ranging from 180–270 mg/dL (10–15 mmol/L). The introduction of glucocorticoids had the additional benefit of improving the patient's symptoms from inflammatory arthritis. Subsequently, the prednisolone was titrated downward, guided by symptoms, to 10 mg daily. At this level, daytime glucose readings ranged from 108–216 mg/dL (6–12 mmol/L) without morning hypoglycemia, and HbA_{1c} improved slightly to 9.3%. The morning insulin detemir dose was increased to 6 units with insulin lispro increasing to 20, 12, and 6 units before meals. Fourteen months later the patient died from acute left ventricular failure.

Discussion

Anti-insulin antibodies are common in patients with type 1 diabetes, but only rarely do they have insulin-binding characteristics sufficient to alter insulin kinetics to a clinically significant degree.[3] Insulin sequestration by antibody can buffer acute insulin delivery and thus attenuate insulin action, leading to postprandial hyperglycemia, while also effectively acting as an extremely slow–release insulin, with bound insulin leaching from antibody complexes to generate free bioactive insulin at physiologically inappropriate times such as overnight.[4] This phenomenon was demonstrated in this patient who showed daytime hyperglycemia and nocturnal (fasting) hypoglycemia despite concerted insulin dose titration to combat this. This was the key clinical clue to the presence of insulin binding by antibodies.

While the presence of immunodetectable anti-insulin autoantibodies alone is consistent with the diagnosis, precipitation and immunosubtraction techniques to remove insulin-antibody complexes, coupled to insulin immunoassays with the ability to detect analog insulin species, are required to prove derangement of the proportion of "bound" and "free" insulin in plasma. Analytic challenges to identifying clinically significant anti-insulin antibodies include variable detection of different insulin analog by most insulin assays,[1] interference in insulin measurement by antibodies,[2] and limited routine access to specialist assays in many diagnostic laboratories.

Insulin autoantibodies are commonly identified at the onset of type 1 diabetes even before insulin treatment but only very rarely perturb insulin kinetics to a clinically significant extent. The immunogenicity of exogenous insulin was first reported in 1936 by Banting who observed an insulin neutralizing factor in plasma following a course of "insulin shock" treatment. Insulin antibodies were heavily studied from the 1940s to the 1980s, when immune reactions to exogenous insulins were commonly described in an era of animal-derived insulins. In the modern era, synthetic insulin analogs pose a new immunogenic challenge, and severe insulin antibody-mediated dysglycemia can occur even after many years of insulin therapy in patients treated with insulin analogs, as this case demonstrates.

The therapeutic approach to pathogenic anti-insulin antibodies includes close glucose monitoring, usually coupled to empirical alterations of the insulin analog used; however, in severe cases some form of antibody-depleting therapy is likely to be required. Plasmapheresis may provide short-term relief of dysglycemia and provide proof of principle for antibody depletion, but definitive therapy may be required using glucocorticoids, rituximab, mycophenolate mofetil, or other immunosuppressive therapies, often in combination. A small case literature has emerged supporting these agents in individual cases, but there is currently no clarity on the optimal approach to antibody depletion.[4–6] In the case described, hypoglycemic episodes were pragmatically mitigated by steroid therapy alone; however, this had no discernible effect on the underlying macroinsulin on repeat biochemical evaluation.

Acknowledgments

Dr. David Halsall, The Pathology Partnership, Department of Clinical Biochemistry and Immunology, Addenbrooke's Hospital, Cambridge, U.K. Mr. Peter Barker, Core Biochemical Assay Laboratory, Addenbrooke's Hospital, Cambridge, U.K.

References

1.   Parfitt C, Church D, Armston A, Couchman L, Evans C, et al. Commercial insulin immunoassays fail to detect commonly prescribed insulin analogues. *Clin Biochem* 2015;48:1354–1357

2.   Church D, Cardoso L, Bradbury S, Clarke C, Stears A, Dover A, et al. Diagnosis of insulin autoimmune syndrome using polyethylene glycol precipitation and gel filtration chromatography with *ex vivo* insulin exchange. *Clin Endocrinol (Oxf)* 2016;86:347–353

3.   Lampasona V, Liberati D. Islet autoantibodies. *Curr Diab Rep* 2016;16:53

4.   Dozio N, Scavini M, Beretta A, Sarugeri E, Sartori S, Belloni C, et al. Imaging of the buffering effect of insulin antibodies in the autoimmune hypoglycemic syndrome. *J Clin Endocrinol Metab* 1998;83:643–648

5.   Philippon M, Sejil S, Mugnier M, Rocher L, Guibergia C, Vialettes B, et al. Use of the continuous glucose monitoring system to treat insulin autoimmune syndrome: quantification of glucose excursions and evaluation of treatment efficacy. *Diabet Med* 2014;31:e20–e24

6.   Saxon DR, McDermott MT, Michels AW. Novel management of insulin autoimmune syndrome with rituximab and continuous glucose monitoring. *J Clin Endocrinol Metab* 2016;101:1831–1834

Case 38:
Cystic Fibrosis–Related Diabetes

Ravi Iyengar, MD;[1] Roma Y. Gianchandani, MD;[1] and Jennifer Wyckoff, MD[1]

Case

A 31-year-old woman with cystic fibrosis (CF) presented for management of cystic fibrosis–related diabetes (CFRD). Her initial manifestation of CF at 6 months old was pancreatic insufficiency. She later developed pulmonary complications, including chronic sinusitis and bronchopulmonary aspergillosis. She maintained an appropriate growth curve through childhood but suffered recurrent respiratory disease treated with chronic low-dose prednisone (5–10 mg). Her fasting glucose values remained normal until age 21 when a routine oral glucose tolerance test (OGTT) revealed a 2-hour blood glucose of 327 mg/dL (18.2 mmol/L) with a concurrent HbA$_{1c}$ of 7.4%. Prandial insulin was started but discontinued at age 24 due to noncompliance. A C-peptide level was then checked to distinguish insulin deficiency from resistance and found to be elevated at 5.6 ng/mL. She started repaglinide 0.5 mg with meals and increased to 1.0 mg, which she continued for three years. However, her HbA$_{1c}$ continued to rise and was up to 9.9% by age 26 with the development of fasting hyperglycemia. She was restarted on insulin aspart with a carbohydrate ratio of 1:45, with

[1]Department of Metabolism, Endocrinology, & Diabetes, University of Michigan, Ann Arbor, MI

eventual titration to 1:15. NPH insulin 4 units at bedtime was added to address fasting hyperglycemia. Her HbA_{1c} improved on insulin, reaching the goal of <7%. At age 28, she was transitioned to an insulin pump. Her glycemic control has remained in the target range, with no complications of diabetes.

Discussion

CF is an autosomal recessive disorder with over 1,500 identified mutations in the cystic fibrosis transmembrane regulator (CFTR) gene and a higher prevalence in the Caucasian population.[1] Manifestations may include recurrent sinopulmonary infections, pancreatic insufficiency, chronic pancreatitis, distal intestinal obstruction, focal biliary cirrhosis, nephrolithiasis, male infertility, and severe fat-soluble vitamin deficiencies, leading to bone disease. Disease manifestations vary widely in individuals depending on specific mutations.

Due to improved treatment, the median survival age is increased to 47 years, requiring a new focus on CF complications in adults.[2] CFRD occurs in up to 40–50% of persons with CF over the age of 30.[3] Median survival age was thought to be lower in women with CFRD, though this gender disparity is no longer noted in the recent literature due to improved treatment and detection.[2-4]

CFRD is multifaceted in etiology, presentation, and prognosis with progressive β-cell dysfunction resulting in insulin deficiency and variable insulin resistance due to infections and treatments. Mechanisms for this include variable pancreatic dysfunction related to genotypic variation in CF genes, chronic CF-related pancreatitis, and pancreatic amyloid deposition as seen in type 2 diabetes.[5] Additionally, CF patients often have acute and chronic infections resulting in a chronic inflammatory state, glucocorticoid treatment, and, in some, lung transplants with corresponding insulin resistance–inducing medications. Thus, CFRD shares features of both type 1 and type 2 diabetes.

Diagnosis of CFRD remains a topic of debate but it is clear that early diagnosis is a key in preventing worsening outcomes. Current guidelines from the American Diabetes Association (ADA) and Cystic Fibrosis Foundation (CFF) recommend two separate oral glucose tolerance tests (OGTT) using 75 g glucose solution with a 2-hour cutoff of 200 mg/dL annually in patients over the age of 10.[6] An HbA_{1c} ≥6.5% or fasting plasma glucose ≥126 mg/dL (7 mmol/L) can be used for confirmatory testing in a stable state of health but is not recommended alone to make the diagnosis. Early use of impaired fasting glucose to determine need for a subsequent OGTT can promptly identify patients with CFRD. HbA$_{1c}$ can underestimate mean glucose values in CF patients; however, recent data suggest its use as a marker of CFRD progression in place of OGTT, which is time-consuming. Patients often have repetitive illness requiring frequent hospitalizations or nutritional deficiencies warranting enteral feeding; CFRD can still be confirmed in the acute setting by an OGTT ≥200 mg/dL (11.1 mmol/L) or fasting plasma glucose ≥126 mg/dL (7 mmol/L) that persists for 48 hours.

Insulin remains the mainstay of drug therapy in CFRD. A multidisciplinary team with expertise in CF and CFRD nutrition is essential, given the complexity of these patients. Early identification and treatment with insulin can slow the decline in pulmonary function, with the added benefit of weight gain. Oral agents including sulfonylureas evaluated in CFRD have shown minimal benefit and increased risk for adverse effects.[2] Our patient had a detectable C-peptide level, which helped determine whether diabetes was secondary to pancreatic insufficiency or chronic steroid use. Repaglinide has a mild effect in reducing postprandial hyperglycemia. When our patient's HbA$_{1c}$ and fasting glucose started rising, insulin therapy was restarted. Current guidelines no longer differentiate between fasting hyperglycemia and postprandial hyperglycemia in CFRD.[5] For monitoring glucose, CFRD patients are recommended to check capillary glucose four times daily. The ADA and CFF currently recommend quarterly HbA$_{1c}$ measurements in CFRD.[6] Transition to continuous subcutaneous insulin therapy, as occurred with our patient, has been demonstrated to be safe and beneficial in reducing future complications. Ratios of basal to bolus insulin doses are lower than in patients with type 1 diabetes.

CFRD patients have significantly fewer macrovascular complications versus patients with type 1 or type 2 diabetes, and essentially no reported cases of death from cardiovascular events.[7] The risk of microvascular complications in CFRD is similar to that for patients with other forms of diabetes. Given the number of risk factors for chronic kidney disease, careful attention to preserving kidney health is important. A direct correlation between insulin insufficiency and decline in pulmonary function has been established, though this disparity continues to decrease due to early detection and treatment.[3] There is an increased risk of complications with impaired fasting glucose and CFRD duration greater than 10 years. Annual screening for complications is recommended using ADA guidelines starting five years after diagnosis of CFRD.

Medical innovations continue to enhance diagnosis and therapies for CF with increasing emphasis on CF-related complications including CFRD. Early treatment remains crucial to preventing microvascular complications, slowing the decline in pulmonary function, and improving overall survival.

References

1. Adler AI, Shine BSF, Chamnan P, Haworth C, Bilton D. Genetic determinants and epidemiology of cystic fibrosis-related diabetes. *Diabetes Care* 2008;31:1789–1794

2. Zirbes J, Milla CE. Cystic fibrosis related diabetes. *Paediatr Respir Rev* 2009;10:118–123

3. Moran A, Saeed A, Dunitz J, Holme B, Nathan B, Thomas W. Cystic fibrosis-related diabetes: current trends in prevalence, incidence, and mortality. *Diabetes Care* 2009;32:1626–1631

4. Milla CE, Billings J, Moran A. Diabetes is associated with dramatically decreased survival in female but not male subjects with cystic fibrosis. *Diabetes Care* 2005;28:2141–2144

5. Kelly A, Moran A. Update on cystic fibrosis-related diabetes. *J Cyst Fibros* 2013;12:318–331

6. Moran A, Brunzell C, Cohen RC, et al. Clinical care guidelines for cystic fibrosis-related diabetes. *Diabetes Care* 2010;33:2697–2708

7. Konrad K, Scheuing N, Badenhoop K, Borkenstein MH, Gohlke B, Schofl C, Seufert J, Thon A, Holl RW. Cystic fibrosis-related diabetes compared with type 1 and type 2 diabetes in adults. *Diabetes Metab Res Rev* 2013;29:568–575

Case 39:
Pembrolizumab and Diabetic Ketoacidosis

Francesca Cottini, MD;[1] and Kathleen Dungan, MD, MPH[1]

Case

A 48-year-old male with metastatic adenocarcinoma of the colon presented to our emergency department with nausea, vomiting, and generalized malaise. He denied chills, fevers, diarrhea, or abdominal pain. He had a previous history of seminoma and underwent left radical orchiectomy and radiation seventeen years before the current presentation. The patient had no known allergies. He lived with his wife, denied sick contacts, did not smoke tobacco or use illicit drugs, and drank alcohol socially. He had a positive family history of type 2 diabetes on his maternal side.

Two months before the current presentation he was diagnosed with adenocarcinoma of the colon with intraabdominal and hepatic metastases, after reporting several episodes of hematochezia. Six weeks later, he started a clinical trial and received three doses of FOLFOX (folinic acid, fluorouracil, oxaliplatin), and pembrolizumab. The last infusion of FOLFOX-pembrolizumab was five days before the current presentation. At that time, he was in his usual state of health, though with mild nausea and a macular-papular rash on his arms. Laboratory tests were unremarkable, except for a nonfasting blood glucose of 215 mg/dL, and carcinoembryonic antigen (CEA) of 188 ng/mL improved from one month prior. One day before the

[1]Department of Internal Medicine, Division of Endocrinology, Diabetes & Metabolism, The Ohio State University, Columbus, OH

current presentation, he was feeling well and played golf outdoors. That night, he developed worsening nausea, vomiting, polydipsia, and hiccups and was seen in the emergency department.

On examination, the patient was alert and oriented to person, place, and time. The pulse was 108 beats per minute, the blood pressure 131/79 mm Hg, the respiratory rate 24 breaths per minute, and the oxygen saturation 96% while breathing ambient air. His weight was 178 pounds and his height was 5' 8" with a BMI of 26.1. The abdomen was soft, nontender, and nonguarded, and the remainder of the examination was normal.

Blood counts and lipase were normal. Blood glucose was 732 mg/dL, beta-hydroxybutyrate was >24 mmol/L, calculated anion gap was 30, and serum creatinine was 1.84 mg/dL (Table C39.1). Urinalysis was positive for glucose and large ketones. He was started on intravenous insulin, fluids, and potassium supplementation with resolution of symptoms. HbA$_{1c}$ was 6.9%. Anti-GAD (glutamic acid decarboxylase) and antipancreatic islet antibodies were positive, while IA-2, anti-insulin and zinc transporter 8 antibodies were negative. C-peptide was 0.5 ng/mL with a concomitant glucose of 215 mg/dl. C-peptide levels were then repeated with glucose normalization together with insulin, proinsulin and glucose levels, showing the following values: C-peptide 0.1 ng/mL, 17.7 mIU/mL, 8.1 pmol/L and 96 mg/dL, respectively. He was then discharged home on both short- and long-acting insulin with plans to continue treatment with pembrolizumab.

Discussion

Medications promoting an immune response against tumoral cells are novel and promising approaches for cancer therapeutics. Specifically, anti–programmed cell death-1 (PD-1) antibodies (pembrolizumab and nivolumab) have been approved for the treatment of advanced melanoma and non–small cell carcinoma and are currently under evaluation in clinical trials of other types of cancers. However, endocrine autoimmune syndromes have been described as a result of anti–PD-1 therapy, including thyroid dysfunction, autoimmune hypophysitis, and adrenalitis, as early as 2–8 weeks after beginning treatment. Diabetic ketoacidosis (DKA) has been reported in only a few cases.[1,2] Our case describes a patient with rapid-onset type 1 diabetes presenting in DKA in the setting of pembrolizumab therapy.

Our patient received three doses of pembrolizumab, a PD-1 receptor inhibitor, before being admitted to the hospital with DKA. Less than ten

Table C39.1—Laboratory Data

Variable	Normal Lab Ranges (Units of Measure)	Forty Days before Admission	Five Days before Admission	On Admission
Sodium	133–143 (mmol/L)	136	139	128
Potassium	3.5–5.0 (mmol/L)	3.9	4.0	5.5
Chloride	98–108 (mmol/L)	103	105	92
Carbon dioxide	22–30 (mmol/L)	26	26	7
BUN	7–22 (mg/dL)	14	15	34
Serum creatinine	0.7–1.3 (mg/dL)	0.92	1.05	1.84
Glucose	70–99 (mg/dL)	75	215	732
Calculated anion gap	7–17 (mmol/L)	7	8	29
beta-Hydroxybutyrate	<0.4 (mmol/L)			>24
Amylase	20–103 (units/L)			27
Lipase	11–82 (units/L)			17
Arterial blood gases pH pCO$_2$ (mm Hg) pO$_2$ (mm Hg) Bicarbonate	7.35–7.45 32–48 (mmHg) 83–108 (mmHg) 22–26 (mmol/L)			7.244 20.1 99.3 9.8
C-peptide	0.2–2.7 (ng/mL)			0.5
Insulin	0–29.1 (uIU/mL)			17.7
Proinsulin	≤18.8 (pmol/L)			8.1
Antibodies anti-: • GAD65 • Islet cell • IA-2 • Insulin • Zinc transporter 8	<5 (IU/mL) <1.25 (JDF) <0.8 (units/mL) <0.4 (units/mL) <15 (units/mL)			>250 (Positive) 2,560 (Positive) <0.8 (Negative) <0.4 (Negative) <10 (Negative)

cases of rapid-onset diabetes have been reported in the literature. As with other reported cases, our patient did not have an established diagnosis of diabetes.[1,2] He had risk factors for type 2 diabetes, such as a positive family history and being overweight. However, the rapid progression to DKA after the first indication of hyperglycemia five days earlier and positive autoantibodies were more consistent with type 1 diabetes (T1D).

PD-1 functions as an inhibitory costimulatory molecule and is expressed on activated T cells (CD4+ and CD8+), T regulatory cells, B cells, and dendritic cells. PD-1 is crucial for inducing peripheral immune tolerance, by weakening the magnitude of the antigen-specific immune response to infection or self-antigens[3] and by triggering the numerical expansion and function of T regulatory cells[4] binding to the PD-L1/PD-L2 molecule. Blocking PD-1 has been proven beneficial as a cancer therapy by reactivating the natural antitumoral immunity.

Even though the pathogenesis of T1D is not fully understood, it has been associated with an abnormal immune response. In T1D, CD8+ T lymphocytes are the main mediators of β-cell destruction by both direct cytotoxic effects and by the release of cytokines such as TNF-α, INF-α, and IL-1 α, β, while autoantibodies are involved in autoantigen processing and presentation to dendritic cells, magnifying the action of autoreactive T cells. Studies in prediabetic female nonobese diabetic (NOD) mice have shown that blockade of PD-1 or PD-L1 can cause rapid onset of diabetes, inducing autoantibodies and IFN-producing GAD-reactive T cells.[1,5] Since PD-1 inhibition potentiates T cell and B cell immune responses and promotes the release of cytokines, it is not surprising that it can induce a rapid-onset diabetes that is more similar to T1D in terms of presentation and pathogenesis. However, despite a high penetrance in the NOD mouse models, rapid-onset diabetes is uncommon after pembrolizumab treatment in humans. Polymorphisms in the HLA complex, such as HLA DR3 and/or DR4 haplotype (DRB1*03:01-DQA1*05:01-DQB1*02, -DR3 and DRB1*04:01/02/04/05/08-DQA1*03:01-DQB1*02-DR4) and in the insulin (INS), the CTLA-4, and PTPN22 genes have been reported in patients with T1D. Our patient was HLA DRB103 positive, but we did not test for other polymorphisms.

Hence, we propose that PD-1 inhibition might have been the trigger necessary to unveil an underlying smoldering autoimmune process that otherwise was silent (Figure C39.1).

In conclusion, rapid-onset diabetes with DKA is a rare complication of novel immunomodulatory agents. Serial glucose monitoring and urinalysis potentially with autoantibody testing and genotyping of patients should be considered in patients receiving PD-1/PDL-1 inhibitors. Furthermore, clinicians should immediately initiate insulin therapy in any patient who develops hyperglycemia while receiving these therapies in order to prevent DKA.

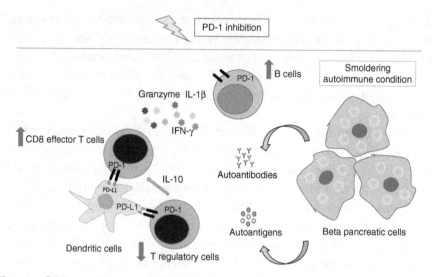

Figure C39.1—Proposed model for rapid-onset of diabetes upon PD-1 inhibition.

PD-1 inhibition counteracts the inhibitory response on activated T cells and B cells and blocks T regulatory function. In the presence of a smoldering autoimmune process with autoantibodies and autoantigen release, pancreatic beta cells can be targeted by direct cytotoxic effects or by cytokine release.

References

1. Hughes J, Vudattu N, Sznol M, Gettinger S, Kluger H, Lupsa B, Herold KC. Precipitation of autoimmune diabetes with anti-PD-1 immunotherapy. *Diabetes Care* 2015;38:e55–e57

2. Mellati M, Eaton KD, Brooks-Worrell BM, Hagopian WA, Martins R, Palmer JP, Hirsch IB. Anti-PD-1 and Anti-PDL-1 monoclonal antibodies causing type 1 diabetes. *Diabetes Care* 2015;38:e137–138

3. Keir ME, Liang SC, Guleria I, Latchman YE, Qipo A, Albacker LA, Koulmanda M, Freeman GJ, Sayegh MH, Sharpe AH. Tissue expression of PD-L1 mediates peripheral T cell tolerance. *J Exp Med* 2006;203:883–895

4. Francisco LM, Sage PT, Sharpe AH. The PD-1 pathway in tolerance and autoimmunity. *Immunol Rev* 2010;236:219–242

5. Ansari MJ, Salama AD, Chitnis T, Smith RN, Yagita H, Akiba H, Yamazaki T, Azuma M, Iwai H, Khoury SJ, et al. The programmed death-1 (PD-1) pathway regulates autoimmune diabetes in nonobese diabetic (NOD) mice. *J Exp Med* 2003;198:63–69

Case 40:
Glycemic Control in Patient with Multiple Chronic Complications

Amena Iqbal, MD;[1] Janice L. Gilden, MS, MD;[1] Boby G. Theckedath, MD;[1] Alvia Moid, DO;[1] Srikar Rapaka;[1] and Degaulle Dai[1]

Case

A 57-year-old African-American male who had been using an insulin pump to manage his blood sugars for the last 10–15 years, presented to the Endocrinology Clinic for further evaluation and management of uncontrolled type 1 diabetes with chronic complications of peripheral and autonomic neuropathy (including gastroparesis), retinopathy, nephropathy, left below-knee amputation, hypertension, coronary artery disease, and hyperlipidemia despite many prior years of good glycemic control. He reported that his blood glucose had recently improved over the past month and that he was no longer having frequent hypoglycemic episodes. He was concerned that he was strongly advised by his primary care provider about the fact that his HbA$_{1c}$ was elevated, indicating poor glycemic control, and that he should immediately improve his glycemic control to achieve an HbA$_{1c}$ of 7%.

After physical examination, his BMI was 29.62 kg/m^2. Laboratory evaluation results are as follows: creatinine was .080 mg/dL (0.67–1.17), e-GFR was 40, hemoglobin was 10.6 g/dL (13–17), HbA$_{1c}$ was 8.3% (4–6), random

[1]Diabetes/Endocrinology Division, Rosalind Franklin University of Medicine and Science/Chicago Medical School and Captain James A. Lovell Federal Health Care Center, North Chicago, IL

DOI: 10.2337/9781580406666.04

blood glucose was 133 mg/dL (7.3 mmol/L), and urine microalbumin/creatinine ratio was 100.3 mg/g (0–30).

Due to renal insufficiency and patient reporting improvement in blood glucose control, fructosamine was ordered: 355 umol/L (190–270).

The importance of tight glycemic control has been recognized to reduce the development and progression of diabetes-related complications. HbA_{1c} has been regarded as the gold standard for measurement of glycemic control.

HbA_{1c} is formed in a nonenzymatic glycation pathway by exposure of hemoglobin to plasma glucose and has been shown to reflect the average glycemic control over 2–3 months.[1] Thus, the use of HbA_{1c} as a standard laboratory test has been the gold standard for assessing glycemic control. Studies evaluating pharmacological therapy and glycemic control, as well as chronic complications of diabetes, have used this measurement as a predictor of the development, as well as prevention of diabetic complications.

However, the HbA_{1c} does not measure glucose variability, now thought to possibly be a better predictor of diabetic complications. In addition, the measurement is an integrated average of glucose levels and does not adequately reflect episodes of hypoglycemia. Thus, the same HbA_{1c} could either represent similar levels of blood glucose or several higher levels averaging with many hypoglycemic episodes over the same time period. Thus, a lack of knowledge regarding the actual glucose levels and variability could adversely affect clinical decision making.

In addition, discordances between HbA_{1c} and other measures of glycemic control are commonly encountered. While correlations exist between plasma glucose concentrations and HbA_{1c} measurements in populations with type 1 and 2 diabetes and normal kidney function, the reliability of standard measures for assessing long-term glycemic control can be affected by chronic kidney disease (CKD), and these values may be falsely low or high.[2]

In addition, HbA_{1c} is influenced by other factors, such as changes in the life span of the red blood cell (RBC), recombinant human erythropoietin, the uremic environment, and blood transfusions in patients with CKD, especially those on hemodialysis. The RBC life span is significantly reduced by 20–50%. This increased hemoglobin turnover leads to decreased exposure time to ambient glucose, and lowers nonenzymatic binding of glucose to hemoglobin, thus decreasing the value obtained for HbA_{1c}.

Therefore, the interfering and confounding factors observed in patients with renal disease can lead to erroneous HbA_{1c} values. Other measures of glycemic control, such as glycated proteins and fructosamine, have been

Table C40.1—Comparison of Measures of Glycemic Control

Glucose (mg/dL)	Glucose mmol/L	Fructosamine	HbA$_{1c}$ (%)
97	5.3	212.5	5.0
126	7	250	6.0
154	8.5	287.5	7.0
183	10.1	325	8.0
212	11.7	362.5	9.0
240	13.3	400	10.0
269	14.9	437.5	11.0
326	18.1	475	12.0
355	19.7	512.5	13.0
360	20	550	14.0
390	21.6	587.5	15.0

Source: Adapted from Radin MS.[4]

suggested to better reflect glycemic control in these situations. These nonenzymatic levels measure the reactions of proteins with glucose in a similar manner to HbA$_{1c}$. Since the turnover of plasma proteins is much shorter than hemoglobin (half-life about 2–3 weeks), glycated plasma proteins can provide an index of glycemia over a shorter period of time. Table C40.1 shows different markers of glycemic control with mean and median glucose in patients with diabetes.[3]

Fructosamine originates from nonenzymatic glycation of mainly albumin (~90%) and various proteins and therefore reflects the concentration of each protein and measures short-term control of blood glucose levels over the past 1–3 weeks.

As in Table C40.1, for each fructosamine change of 75 mmol/L there is approximately an increase or decrease of 60 mg/dL blood sugar or 2% HbA$_{1c}$.[4]

Further studies observed an underestimation of glycemic control by HbA$_{1c}$ in a number of studies that led to uncertainty regarding the usefulness of HbA$_{1c}$ as an indicator of glycemic control in CKD.[5]

Therefore, measurement of fructosamine may be a more accurate measurement for the current degree of glycemic control in patients with chronic renal failure, iron deficiency anemia, pregnancy, chronic liver disease, and variant hemoglobins. As in Table C40.2, hypoproteinemia and hypothyroidism can cause a false lower value of fructosamine.

Table C40.2 — Conditions Resulting in High and Low Levels of Fructosamine

High Level	Low Level
Persistent hyperglycemia	Hypoproteinemia
	Hypothyroidism

In addition to the confounding factors of measurement, recent recommendations are for individualized glycemic control goals with higher levels acceptable for patients with multiple chronic diabetic complications and long-standing disease duration, as well as for patients with high risks for hypoglycemia, as in this patient. This case also highlights the fact that some patients with type 1 diabetes develop long-term chronic complications, despite tight glycemic control.

References

1. American Diabetes Association. Standards of medical care in diabetes—2017. *Diabetes Care* 2012;35(Suppl. 1):S11–S24

2. Vos FE, Schollum JB, Coulter CV, Manning PJ, Duffull SB, Walker RJ. Assessment of markers of glycemic control in diabetic patients with chronic kidney disease using continuous glucose monitoring. *Nephrology (Carlton)* 2012;17:182–188

3. Cohen RM, Holmes YR, Chenier TC, Joiner CH. Discordance between HbA_{1c} and fructosamine. *Diabetes Care* 2003;26:163–167

4. Radin MS. Pitfalls in hemoglobin A1c measurement: when results may be misleading. *J Gen Intern Med* 2014;29:388–394

5. Youssef D, El Abbassi A, Jordan RM, Peiris AN. Fructosamine—an underutilized tool in diabetes management: case report and literature review. *Tenn Med* 2008;101:31–33

Case 41:
Diabetes and Exposure to Agent Orange

Bushra Z. Osmani, MD;[1] Janice L. Gilden, MS, MD;[1] and Charles Harris, BS[1]

Case 1

A 68-year-old African-American male veteran presented to the Diabetes Clinic with a 40 year history of type 2 diabetes (T2D), diagnosed from routine blood tests, done when he was being discharged from the Armed Forces. During the Vietnam War, the patient had been exposed to Agent Orange (AO).

At the time of presentation to our clinic, BMI = 35 kg/m². He also had peripheral neuropathy, hypertension, hyperlipidemia, and degenerative joint disease. He had a gastric bypass surgery done at an unknown time, many years ago. There is no family history of diabetes. HbA_{1c} was 7.1% (normal = 4–6).

Case 2

A 60-year-old Caucasian male (British and Irish ancestry) presented to the Diabetes Clinic with a 22-year history of T2D. The patient was initially diagnosed with diabetes at age 38, 4–5 years after being discharged following service in the Vietnam War. While he was not part of Operation Ranch Hand, he did run through fields in Vietnam where AO was sprayed

[1]Rosalind Franklin University of Medicine and Science/Chicago Medical School and Captain James A. Lovell Federal Health Care Center, North Chicago, IL

and was therefore exposed to it. He was initially treated with diet and gly-buride. Eighteen years later, metformin was added to this regimen (doses unknown). He is currently taking 40 units of basal insulin (glargine) and 5 units of short-acting insulin (aspart) for meals, in addition to 1,000 mg of metformin daily.

Upon presentation, BMI was 26.67 kg/m^2, his HbA$_{1c}$ was 8.2% with neuropathy, nephropathy, and retinopathy. He also had hypertension, hyperlipidemia, and gout. There was no family history of diabetes.

Discussion

Between 1965 and 1971, 17.6 million gallons of AO and other herbicides were sprayed by the U.S. Air Force on millions of acres of Vietnam.[1] AO was the most potent, deadly, and widely used of the tactical herbicides. AO was a mixture of 2,4-dichlorophenoxyacetic acid and 2,4,5-trichlorophenoxy-acetic acid in a 1:1 ratio. 2,3,7,8-tetrachlorodibenzo-p-diaxin (TCDD) was a contaminant of the defoliant and is from a class of chemicals called dioxins, classified by the United States Environmental Protection Agency as carcino-gens and teratogens.[1] TCDD has very low bioavailability in the environment, with low absorption, even if ground troops came into sprayed areas. Further-more, nearly 90% of the dioxin released would be destroyed by photodegra-dation before it reached the ground, making it less likely for ground troops to come into contact with it. Unfortunately, many people came into direct con-tact with AO, the highest exposure being by members of Operation Ranch Hand, which was the Air Force unit that was responsible for spraying herbi-cides from aircraft in Vietnam.[1]

The following conditions have been associated with AO exposure: acute and subacute peripheral neuropathy, chloracne, AL amyloidosis, Hodgkin's disease, chronic lymphocytic leukemia, B-cell leukemias, mul-tiple myeloma, non-Hodgkin's lymphoma, ischemic heart disease, T2D, Parkinson's disease, porphyria cutanea tarda, prostate cancer, respiratory cancers, and soft tissue sarcomas.[2]

A significant increase in the prevalence of diabetes and a decreased age at which diabetes was diagnosed has been observed in those veterans from Operation Ranch Hand who had high levels of TCDD in their blood.[1]

TCDD produces its biological effects by upregulating expression of TNF-α in different cell types.[1] The toxic effects of TCDD are thought to be a direct result of increased TNF-α expression. Studies have shown that TNF-α in adipose tissue is related to the insulin resistance of obesity. Since

TCDD stimulates expression of TNF-α, this may then promote insulin resistance. TCDD exposure also contributes to the adipose tissue–mediated proinflammatory condition that is associated with the metabolic syndrome, since TCDD is concentrated in adipose tissue.[1]

One hypothesis for the association between T2D and TCDD is that those individuals who have a slow elimination rate of TCDD retain it longer than those with high elimination rates of TCDD. Elimination rate is dependent on body fat, with heavier individuals having a decreased rate of elimination and leaner individuals having an increased rate of elimination. Therefore, the risk of T2D in veterans of Operation Ranch Hand may be higher from increased body fat.[3]

Case 1 describes an obese veteran with no family history of diabetes, who was diagnosed with T2D at a young age. Morbid obesity alone is a risk factor for insulin resistance and T2D. However, obesity can also be a risk factor for increased adipose tissue TNF-α, causing increased insulin resistance. Increased adipose tissue can also decrease the rate of elimination of TCDD, causing longer exposure to the chemical and increased susceptibility to toxic effects of TCDD.

In Case 2, this patient was exposed to AO and was diagnosed with T2D at the age of 38, with no family history of diabetes. Although the evidence linking AO to the development of diabetes is controversial, we cannot rule out exposure to TCDD as a cause of T2D.

Thus, evidence regarding the correlation between T2D and AO is quite controversial. Effects of metabolic dysfunction could be TCDD level dependent. There is no direct relationship between exposure to TCDD and diabetes, but when adjusted for service date and length of time spent in Operation Ranch Hand, there may be a correlation between high levels of TCDD exposure and T2D. It is suggested that high levels of TCDD can cause insulin dysfunction, and it is hypothesized that Ranch Hand veterans develop T2D over time due to the hyperinsulinemia caused by TCDD. Although some veterans with lower levels of TCDD (higher than control, lower than highest exposure) were found to have some of these metabolic abnormalities, the limited sample size of Operation Ranch Hand veterans does not allow us to completely rule out confounders (education level, rank, etc.). Therefore, the possibility exists that these two cases might have developed T2D secondary to exposure to AO.

Type 1 diabetes (T1D) has also been linked to toxins in food and water. Toxins are thought to activate autoimmune mechanisms resulting in pancreatic islet cell death in genetically susceptible individuals.[4] Some studies have shown that a high intake of nitrates and nitrites can increase the risk of T1D. Arsenic also has a possible link to development of diabetes.[5]

Certain medications can impair β-cells or disrupt insulin action and, therefore, cause diabetes, such as glucocorticoids, nicotinic acid and certain diuretics, antiseizure drugs, drugs used to treat human immunodeficiency virus, and psychiatric drugs. Pentamidine can increase the risk of diabetes by causing pancreatitis and β-cell damage.[5]

This research was supported in part by the Captain James A. Lovell Federal Health Care Center.

References

1.   Kern PA, Said S, Jackson WG Jr, Michalek JE. Insulin sensitivity following Agent Orange exposure in Vietnam veterans with high blood levels of 2,3,7,8-tetrachlorodibenzo-p-dioxin. *J Clin Endocrinol Metab* 2004;89:4665–4672

2.   Young AL, Cecil PF Sr. Agent Orange exposure and attributed health effects in Vietnam veterans. *Mil Med* 2011;176(Suppl. 7):29–34

3.   Michalek JE, Ketchum NS, Tripathi RC. Diabetes mellitus and 2,3,7,8-tetrachlorodibenzo-p-dioxin elimination in veterans of Operation Ranch Hand. *J Toxicol Environ Health A* 2003;66:211–221

4.   Rewers M, Ludvigsson J. Environmental risk factors for type 1 diabetes. *Lancet* 2016; 387:2340–2348

5.   Kuo CC, Moon K, Thayer KA, Navas-Acien A. Environmental chemicals and type 2 diabetes: an updated systematic review of the epidemiologic evidence. *Curr Diab Rep* 2013;13:831–849

Case 42: Pasireotide-Induced Hyperglycemia

Kaitlin Brau, MD[1] and Andjela Drincic, MD[1]

Case

A 40-year-old Caucasian male was diagnosed with Cushing's disease in 2008 when he presented with left-sided visual field loss, weight gain, low libido, and erectile dysfunction. He was found to have a pituitary macroadenoma (2.0 × 2.2 × 2.7 cm) with intrasellar and suprasellar extension, as well as right cavernous sinus invasion. That same year, he underwent resection of this macroadenoma, but residual disease in the cavernous sinus remained. He did not develop adrenal insufficiency postsurgery.

On routine outpatient follow-up over the next five years, this patient continued to have persistently elevated salivary cortisol and 24-hour urinary free cortisol levels, followed by signs and symptoms of progressive Cushing's disease, including weight gain, facial rounding with minor flushing of the skin, development of supraclavicular fat pads, as well as pre-diabetes with HbA$_{1c}$ of 6.2%. Therapeutic options were discussed and the patient chose to start therapy. At the start of therapy, urinary free cortisol was 79.1 mcg/d (<60 mcg/d) and salivary cortisol 0.206 mcg/dL, 0.320 mcg/dL, 0.223 mcg/dL (ULN 0.112 mcg/dL). He was instructed to monitor blood glucose four times per day. His urinary free and salivary cortisol levels decreased during the therapy; urinary free cortisol decreased to 65.4

[1]Division of Diabetes, Endocrinology, and Metabolism, University of Nebraska Medical Center, Omaha, NE

DOI: 10.2337/9781580406666.04

Table C42.1—Patient's Blood Glucose Log, Days 14–20 of Pasireotide Use

Days Post First Injection	Fasting A.M. Blood Glucose (mg/dL)	Blood Glucose before Lunch (mg/dL)	Blood Glucose before Dinner (mg/dL)	Blood Glucose before Bedtime (mg/dL)
14	132	79	107	156
15	114	89	122	106
16	120	66	104	124
17	119	91	104	145
18	112	72	125	103
19	121	67	108	184
20	121	81	99	198

mcg/d (<60 mcg/d) and salivary cortisol to 0.117 mcg/dL, 0.151 mcg/dL, 0.092 mcg/dL (ULN 0.112 mcg/dL). Seven days after starting pasireotide 0.6 mg bid, the patient began noticing elevated fasting blood glucose levels. See Table C42.1 for the blood glucose log of days 14–20 of pasireotide therapy. He chose to stop the medication 1 month into therapy. His HbA$_{1c}$, a year after stopping pasireotide therapy, remained <5.7%.

Discussion

Patients with chronically elevated cortisol levels, similar to the above patient, are at greater risk of mortality and of comorbidities such as cardiovascular disease, dyslipidemia, insulin resistance, impaired glucose tolerance, diabetes, osteoporosis, and related fractures.[1] Hypercortisolism causes disorders of glucose metabolism due to 1) increased insulin resistance and 2) pancreatic β-cell dysfunction, inhibiting insulin release. The reduced insulin sensitivity affects the liver, skeletal muscle, and adipose tissue, either directly or indirectly. The inhibitory effect of cortisol on insulin secretion at the level of the pancreatic β-cell can further worsen impaired glucose tolerance.[2] Glucose metabolism disorders occur in about half of patients with Cushing's syndrome; diabetes has the potential to develop in two-thirds of these cases.[2]

Pasireotide is a novel medication used for treatment of Cushing's disease that results in improvement of hypercortisolemia as well as other manifestations of Cushing's disease such as hypertension, obesity, and dyslipidemia.[1] However, despite improvement in hypercortisolemia, pasireotide can also cause hyperglycemia but does so in a different manner, separate from that of Cushing's disease. Pasireotide is a somatostatin analog that exerts its therapeutic effect by binding to somatostatin receptors, subtypes 2 and 5, blocking the release of ACTH from corticotropes. Because these somatostatin receptor subtypes are expressed not only by pituitary cells but by other cell types, including pancreatic islet cells, the binding of pasireotide can lead to reduction of insulin secretion by β-cells as well as reduction of intestinal secretion of glucagon-like peptide and glucose-dependent insulinotropic peptide. These effects can be seen in as little as eight days. Pasireotide does not affect hepatic or peripheral insulin sensitivity.[2,3]

In a study published in 2014 by Colao et al., pasireotide was associated with hyperglycemia-related adverse events in 118 of 162 (72.8%) patients. Despite declines in cortisol levels, blood glucose and glycated hemoglobin levels increased soon after treatment initiation and then stabilized. Forty-six percent of these patients required treatment with a glucose-lowering medication.[2]

A separate study was extended to evaluate the efficacy and safety of extended treatment with pasireotide therapy. Hyperglycemia-related adverse events were reported in 68% of patients (13 out of 19). Seven of these patients completed therapy on treatment for hyperglycemia. Five patients continued therapy with no medication treatment for hyperglycemia. One patient discontinued pasireotide therapy.[4]

When starting pasireotide therapy, patients with normal glucose metabolism should be advised to self-monitor their fasting and postprandial glucose levels, twice weekly in the first week and once weekly thereafter. Patients with impaired fasting glucose or impaired glucose tolerance and patients with preexisting diabetes should be monitored on a daily basis at the start of pasireotide therapy. Treatment should then be adjusted to control further hyperglycemia.[1]

Based on the above-described pathophysiologic mechanisms, specific recommendations for treatment of pasireotide-induced hyperglycemia have been proposed by Colao et al. It is recommended that treatment for pasireotide-induced hyperglycemia be initiated with metformin. If that patient has failed to achieve glycemic control with metformin, it is suggested that a DPP-4 inhibitor will be added. If hemoglobin A1C remains greater than 7.0%, then a GLP-1 receptor agonist is recommended to

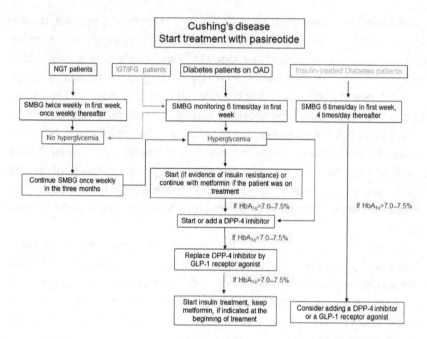

Figure C42.1—Recommendations on monitoring frequency and treatment of patients with Cushing's disease treated with pasireotide therapy. DDP-4, dipeptidyl peptidase-4; GLP-1, glucagon-like peptide-1; HbA$_{1c}$, glycated hemoglobin; IFG, impaired fasting glycemia; IGT, impaired glucose tolerance; NGT, normal glucose tolerance; OAD, oral antidiabetic drugs; SMBG, self-monitoring of blood glucose.

Source: Reprinted with permission from Colao A et al.[2]

replace the DPP-4 inhibitor, given their superior glucose-lowering effect. If neither the DPP-4 inhibitor nor the GLP-1 receptor agonist provides glucose control, then it is suggested that insulin treatment be initiated in addition to metformin treatment.[1] Figure C42.1 illustrates recommendations for pasireotide monitoring frequency and treatment.

As a result of his Cushing's disease, the above patient had prediabetes prior to starting pasireotide therapy. The unequal balance of reduced insulin sensitivity, in the case of Cushing's disease, and reduced insulin secretion seen during pasireotide therapy led to worsening of his hyperglycemia. This patient illustrates, uniquely, both mechanisms of hyperglycemia.

References

1. Nieman LK, Biller BM, Findling JW, Murad MH, Newell-Price J, Savage MO, et al. Treatment of Cushing's syndrome: an Endocrine Society clinical practice guideline. *J Clin Endocrinol Metab* 2015;100:2807–2831

2. Colao A, De Block C, Gaztambide MS, Kumar S, Seufert J, Casanueva FF. Managing hyperglycemia in patients with Cushing's disease treated with pasireotide: medical expert recommendations. *Pituitary* 2014;17:180–186

3. Silverstein JM. Hyperglycemia induced by pasireotide in patients with Cushing's disease or acromegaly. *Pituitary* 2016;19:536–543

4. Boscaro M, Bertherat J, Findling J, Fleseriu M, Atkinson AB, Petersenn S, et al. Extended treatment of Cushing's disease with pasireotide: results from a 2-year, phase II study. *Pituitary* 2014;17:320–326

Case 43:
Hemoglobin A1C vs. Fructosamine

Amena Iqbal, MD;[1] Janice L. Gilden, MS, MD;[1] Boby G. Theckedath, MD; [1] Srikar Rapaka;[1] and Degaulle Dai[1]

Case

A 64-year-old African-American male was referred to Endocrinology Clinic for management of uncontrolled type 2 diabetes, incidentally diagnosed in 2004, when he was admitted for pneumonia. He was started on oral anti-hyperglycemic therapy, metformin, for one month, and then stopped taking this medication on his own accord, due to improvement of blood glucose levels. Since that time, he stated that he followed a calorie-controlled, low-carbohydrate, and low-fat diet.

However, 12 years later, he experienced a 12-pound weight loss (over two months) with frequent urination and increased thirst for 3 weeks. Laboratory testing revealed blood glucose of 405 mg/dL (22.5 mmol/L).

Physical examination showed his BMI was 31.13 kg/m², but he was otherwise normal without acanthosis nigricans, skin tags, xanthoma, abdominal striae, muscle wasting, or peripheral neuropathy.

Laboratory evaluation results were as follows: random blood glucose was 198 mg/dL (10.9 mmol/L), creatinine was 1.79 mg/dL (0.64–1.17), e-GFR was 46.5, hemoglobin was 12.2 g/dL (13–17), Hemoglobin A1C

[1]Diabetes/Endocrinology Division, Rosalind Franklin University of Medicine and Science/Chicago Medical School and Captain James A. Lovell Federal Health Care Center, North Chicago, IL

(HbA$_{1c}$) was 2.3% (4–6), and microalbumin/ creatinine was 329.3 mg/g (0–30).

The concern was that this patient had significant hypoglycemia. Further laboratory testing showed hemoglobin electrophoresis: hemoglobin sickle cell (SC) disease. Subsequent fructosamine confirmed poor glycemic control (347 umol/L; 190–270).

Glycosylated hemoglobin, as commonly measured by HbA$_{1c}$ is regarded as the gold standard for measurement of glycemic control. It has been used as a predictor of diabetic complications, and for interventions that reduce HbA$_{1c}$, and, correspondingly reduce the risk of complications. However, discordances between HbA$_{1c}$ and other measures of glycemic control are commonly encountered.[1] The difference between plasma glucose and HbA$_{1c}$ is that the former reflects the physiology of glucose in the extracellular space and that HbA$_{1c}$ reflects the physiology of glucose in the extracellular space and is the nonenzymatic glycosylation product of hemoglobin in the intra-erythrocyte compartment. This nonenzymatic glycosylation of hemoglobin is glucose dependent.

Fructosamine differs from HbA$_{1c}$ because of the difference in turnover times of the underlying glycation targets: hemoglobin versus serum proteins.[2] In addition, fructosamine reflects plasma glucose, whereas HbA$_{1c}$ reflects intracellular glucose. We therefore selected the fructosamine measurement for comparison.

Hemoglobin S and E are prevalent variants in people of African, Mediterranean, or Southeast Asian descent. These variants interfere with the HbA$_{1c}$ test—both laboratory and point-of-care tests. Table C43.1 lists common medical conditions in which HbA$_{1c}$ may be falsely increased or decreased.[3]

Health-care providers should suspect the presence of a hemoglobinopathy when the HbA$_{1c}$ result is different from what is expected and includes the following conditions: 1) HbA$_{1c}$ result is above 15%, 2) results of self-monitoring of blood glucose have a low correlation with HbA$_{1c}$ results, 3) the HbA$_{1c}$ result is radically different from the previous result, when there is a change in laboratory methodology for this test and the glucose levels have not significantly changed. With certain assay methods, HbA$_{1c}$ values in patients with hemoglobinopathies result in falsely higher numbers, overestimating actual average blood glucose levels for the previous 3 months. Health-care providers may then falsely diagnose patients or prescribe more aggressive treatments, resulting in increased episodes of hypoglycemia.

Table C43.1 — Conditions with Falsely High and Low Glycosylated Hemoglobin Measurements

Falsely Elevated HbA$_{1c}$	Falsely Lower HbA$_{1c}$
Kidney failure (uremia), liver disease	Acute or chronic blood loss,
Chronic excessive alcohol intake	Sickle cell disease, Hb C and Hb S, thalassemia
Hypertriglyceridemia, lead poisoning	Blood transfusions, erythropoietin use
Drugs: corticosteroids, such as prednisone, and the antiseizure medication phenytoin (Dilantin). Some antiviral medications used to treat human immunodeficiency virus can also elevate blood sugar, including fosamprenavir (Lexiva) and saquinavir (Invirase)	Pregnancy

In situations of suspected unreliable HbA$_{1c}$ results when the patient has a hemoglobinopathy, the fructosamine test, which measures glycated serum protein or glycated albumin, may be more useful in assessing glycemic control.

Thus, fructosamine, while not routinely ordered, can also be useful in confirming the current level of glycemic control in other diabetic patients with iron deficiency anemia, pregnancy, chronic liver disease, chronic renal failure, and variant hemoglobins.[4] In such patients, HbA$_{1c}$ values are unreliable for diagnosing or monitoring diabetes and prediabetes in patients with hemoglobinopathies. This test of glycemic control may also be used in addition to HbA$_{1c}$.[5]

Since it is uncommon to observe a low HbA$_{1c}$ value, our case demonstrates the importance of suspecting that an unusual condition exists, when there is lack of correlation with the clinical situation. In these types of patients, alternative markers such as fructosamine levels may be useful, not only to confirm the presence of an unusual condition, but can also assist in a more accurate evaluation of glycemic control, thus avoiding errors in clinical decision-making that can result in either over or under treatment recommendations.

This research was supported, in part, by the Captain James A. Lovell Federal Health Care Center.

References

1. American Diabetes Association. Standards of medical care in diabetes—2017. *Diabetes Care* 2017;40(Suppl. 1):S11–S24

2. Cohen RM, Holmes YR, Chenier TC, Joiner CH. Discordance between HbA$_{1c}$ and fructosamine. *Diabetes Care* 2003;26:163–167

3. Ribeiro RT, Macedo MP, Raposo JF. HbA$_{1c}$, fructosamine, and glycated albumin in the detection of dysglycaemic conditions. *Curr Diabetes Rev* 2016;12:14–19

4. Bhat VS, Dewan KK, Krishnaswamym PR. Diagnostic dilemma of HbA$_{1c}$ detection in presence of a hemoglobinopathy: a case report. *Indian J Clin Biochem* 2011;26:91–95

5. Smart LM, Howie AF, Young RJ, Walker SW, Clarke BF, Smith AF. Comparison of fructosamine with glycosylated hemoglobin and plasma proteins as measures of glycemic control. *Diabetes Care* 1988;11:433–436

Part III:
Endocrinopathies, Immune-Mediated Diabetes, Diabetes of Unknown Cause, and Other Genetic Syndromes Sometimes Associated with Diabetes

5
Diabetes Secondary to Endocrinopathies

Julie M. Silverstein, MD;[1] Karin Sterl, MD;[1] Jacqueline L. Cartier, MD;[1] Paulina Cruz-Bravo, MD;[1] Cecilia A. Davis, MD;[1] Sobia Sadiq, MD;[1] and Janet B. McGill, MD, MA[1]

Introduction

D iabetes is a common complication of many endocrine diseases, acromegaly and Cushing's syndrome (CS) being the most prominent. The etiology of glucose intolerance varies among endocrine disorders, but physiologic studies generally identify either insulin resistance or insulin deficiency as the primary causative factor.[1] Diabetes risk is impacted by patient age, obesity, and family history in patients with endocrinopathies, but as most of the hormone excess syndromes occur in middle age, diabetes becomes an important comorbidity.[1]

Insulin resistance is found in patients with excess growth hormone (GH), glucocorticoid, catecholamine, or thyroid hormone levels.[2–5] Patients with acromegaly and cortisol excess often have metabolic syndrome characteristics, including hypertension, hyperlipidemia, vascular damage, a prothrombotic state (especially CS), and atherosclerosis.[2,3] Obesity is a concomitant condition that presents management difficulties in CS and to a lesser degree in acromegaly.[3]

---

[1]Division of Endocrinology, Metabolism and Lipid Research, Washington University School of Medicine, St. Louis, MO

DOI: 10.2337/9781580406666.05

325

Accelerated metabolism from excess catecholamine or thyroid hormone secretion typically causes weight loss, but increased demand for insulin and insulin resistance through hormone-specific mechanisms.[4,5] Diabetes or glucose intolerance associated with any of these endocrine disorders increases the risk of morbidity and mortality.

Insulin secretion is subject to dysregulation from a number of influences, including electrolyte disturbances and inhibition or reduced secretion from hormone excess or imbalance. The pancreatic neuroendocrine tumors and the catecholamine-producing tumors cause glucose intolerance or frank diabetes in susceptible individuals by these mechanisms.[6] Somatostatin, which is produced in excess by stomatostatinomas, and catecholamines from pheochromocytomas and ganglioneuromas inhibit insulin secretion through receptor-mediated mechanisms. Glucagon, the product of glucagonomas, impairs insulin secretion indirectly, but its major target is to increase glycogenolysis and gluconeogenesis from the liver.[7] The treatment of pancreatic and duodenal tumors often includes partial pancreatectomy, which further reduces insulin secretory capacity. Treatment of acromegaly, adrenocorticotrophic secreting tumors, and some of the neuroendocrine tumors (NETs) such as glucagonoma with somatostatin further inhibits insulin secretion and may cause or worsen glucose intolerance.

Diabetic ketoacidosis (DKA) is a life-threatening condition marking extreme metabolic decompensation. Patients with hyperthyroidism, pheochromocytoma, and somatostatinoma have presented with DKA as the initial manifestation of their illness.[8,9] Hyperthyroid patients presenting in DKA may have undiagnosed type 1 diabetes (T1D) or may have mild type 2 diabetes (T2D) after hyperthyroidism is corrected. Extreme insulin resistance has been blamed for DKA that occurs in untreated acromegaly and pheochromocytoma. This chapter will review the endocrinopathies that have been associated with diabetes as a concomitant condition, including treatment of the disorders and the impact of current treatments on glucose intolerance.

Acromegaly

Acromegaly is a rare condition that is caused by excessive production of GH, almost always from a somatotroph pituitary adenoma. Acromegaly has an annual incidence of 6 per 1 million people; the mean age at diagnosis is 40 to 45 years and the distribution between men and women is equal.[10] Due to the insidious nature of acromegaly and slow progression of the signs and symptoms of the disease, there is often a delay of up to 10 years before the diagnosis is made.[11]

Symptoms of acromegaly are related to compression of the surrounding structures by the pituitary mass and the effects of GH and insulin-like growth factor 1 (IGF-1) excess. The tumor mass can result in headaches, visual field defects, and other neurologic symptoms. Compression of the normal pituitary gland can cause decreased secretion of other pituitary hormones, leading to either partial or complete pituitary insufficiency. The most common hormone deficiencies are the gonadotrophins. Women may present with menstrual irregularities and men with decreased libido, erectile dysfunction, and decreased facial hair growth.[11] Other pituitary hormone deficiencies, such as thyroid-stimulating hormone (TSH) and adrenocorticotropic hormone (ACTH) deficiency occur less commonly. Approximately 30% of patients with acromegaly have GH and prolactin cosecreting adenomas. Most of the clinical manifestations of acromegaly result from excess GH that stimulates hepatic IGF-1 secretion. Common findings are acral and soft tissue overgrowth, skin thickening, bone and joint enlargement, visceromegaly, cardiovascular disease, and sleep apnea.[12,13]

The prevalence of diabetes in acromegaly ranges from 19 to 56% and is a predictive factor for increased mortality among acromegalic patients.[10,11,13] The risk of developing glucose intolerance is increased in those with older age, longer disease duration, higher GH levels, and family history of diabetes.[14,15] The mechanism of glucose intolerance in acromegaly is multifactorial; however, the direct diabetogenic effects of GH have been well described. Excess or sustained levels of GH cause increased lipolysis and lipid oxidation, which leads to inhibition of glycolytic enzymes, reduced muscle glucose uptake and oxidation, and increased hepatic glucose output, the hallmarks of insulin resistance.[16,17] Insulin levels may be normal or increased in patients with acromegaly, despite glucose intolerance. Increased secretion and clearance of insulin have been described with GH excess; however, the increases in visceral adiposity and insulin resistance commonly lead to glucose intolerance or diabetes.[18] IGF-1 also has metabolic effects such as nitrogen retention, lipolysis, and insulin antagonism.

Cases of diabetes presenting with DKA in patients with acromegaly have been reported, suggesting that accelerated lipolysis and insulin deficiency can also occur.[19] These cases have not had an autoimmune component, but appear to be due to extreme insulin resistance and functional insulin secretory deficits. The insulin resistance, impaired glucose tolerance, and diabetes related to acromegaly generally improve with treatment of the underlying disease, though various pharmacological agents used to treat acromegaly have different effects on glucose homeostasis.[13,14,20]

The mainstay of treatment in acromegaly is surgical resection of the GH-producing pituitary adenoma. Insulin resistance and fasting insulin levels have been found to improve significantly by three months after surgery.[20] Pharmacological therapy is used when surgery alone has not resulted in biochemical remission of acromegaly (normalization of GH and IGF-1 levels). Somatostatin analogs, such as octreotide, lanreotide, and pasireotide work by inhibiting GH production from somatotrophs and suppressing tumor growth. Octreotide and lanreotide transiently inhibit insulin secretion, but have minimal clinical impact on glucose homeostasis.[21] Conversely, pasireotide, due to its unique somatostatin receptor ligand–binding profile, has been associated with a greater degree of hyperglycemia and diabetes as a result of decreased insulin and incretin secretion.[22] Pegvisomant is a GH receptor antagonist that works by blocking GH from binding to its receptors. Therapy with pegvisomant has been shown to improve fasting glucose, insulin, and HbA_{1c} levels in patients with acromegaly.[23] In fact, in patients treated with pegvisomant, GH no longer stimulates lipolysis due to the blockade of its receptor, while insulin action is unabated. Independent of pharmacological therapies, gain in body weight could also be an important predictor of deterioration of glucose tolerance after surgery for acromegaly.[23] Moreover, in rare cases, patients who did not have hyperglycemia associated with acromegaly can develop diabetes following surgical removal of their pituitary adenoma.[24]

Management of diabetes in patients with acromegaly is similar to management of T2D and treatment goals are similar. However, there are currently no published guidelines addressing the management of pasireotide-induced hyperglycemia in patients with acromegaly. Established recommendations for pasireotide-induced hyperglycemia in Cushing's disease (CD) patients include treatment with metformin and either a DPP-4 inhibitor, GLP-1 agonist, or insulin, and it is likely that these agents would have similar efficacy in patients with acromegaly.[25] Lifestyle management is also important in these patients, but comorbidities may be limiting.

Diabetes complications occur in patients with acromegaly, but vary in both risk and natural history compared to persons with diabetes without acromegaly. For example, retinopathy is not common unless diabetes has had a prolonged duration, but cases of severe nonproliferative and proliferative retinopathy have been reported.[26,27] In one such case, severe nonproliferative retinopathy was accompanied by optic disc swelling, and both regressed after partially successful surgery to remove the pituitary adenoma.[27] Several cases have been described in which severe proliferative retinopathy was found despite modest hyperglycemia, including one in which elevated intravitreal IGF-1 and vascular endothelial growth factor levels were documented at vitrectomy.[28] Elevated GH or the effects of GH have been implicated in the development and progression of diabetic retinopathy for years, and even prompted hypophysectomy in patients with normal pituitary function many years ago. The relationship between acromegaly and retinopathy is less clear, since retinopathy is generally not present or mild at the time of diagnosis of acromegaly.[26]

GH excess may also play a role in the pathogenesis of diabetic nephropathy.[29] Renal growth and function are partially mediated by the actions of GH and IGF-1, and chronic exposure to excessive GH and IGF-1 has been associated with changes in kidney function and morphology. Although the relationship between acromegaly and diabetic nephropathy has not been clearly elucidated, patients with acromegaly have higher rates of microalbuminuria when compared to controls.[30]

The relationship between GH and IGF-1 excess and diabetic macroangiopathy is controversial, with some studies showing that acromegaly may protect against atherosclerosis despite the fact that patients with acromegaly and diabetes are more likely to have hypertension and proatherogenic lipid profiles as compared to patients with acromegaly who do not have diabetes.[10,13,14] Furthermore, the coexistence of hypertension and diabetes in acromegalic patients has been associated with more severe damage to cardiac function and higher risk of cardiovascular death.[11,13]

A potential link between cancer and increased mortality has been widely studied in patients with acromegaly. Although it is well known that acromegaly is associated with an increased risk of malignancies, specifically thyroid cancer, colon cancer, and urinary tract carcinomas, studies have not shown an increase in cancer mortality in patients with acromegaly.[13] Additionally, diabetes and obesity have been found to increase the risk of different cancers, and acromegalic patients with diabetes develop extrapituitary tumors more frequently than patients with acromegaly or diabetes alone.[31] Moreover, in patients with GH-producing tumors, survival rates of patients with diabetes are lower than those of nondiabetic patients.[32] In conclusion, acromegaly is rarely a disease associated with increased morbidity and mortality. The presence of diabetes and malignancy may influence the survival of patients with acromegaly, necessitating the need for vigilant monitoring and appropriate treatment of patients with acromegaly and coexistent diabetes.

Cushing's Syndrome

CS is a disorder characterized by excess exposure to glucocorticoids (GC) and is most commonly caused by ingestion of exogenous steroids. Endogenous CS, which is the topic of this chapter section, has multiple etiologies and an incidence of two to three cases per one million inhabitants per year.[33,34] Approximately 60–80% of CS is ACTH-dependent due to either a pituitary tumor (60%) or ectopic production of ACTH (10–15%) from non-pituitary tumors such as carcinoid tumors or small-cell carcinomas of the lung. The remaining 25% of cases are due to ACTH-independent production of cortisol from the adrenal gland, most commonly from an adrenal adenoma.[34]

The most common features of CS include truncal obesity, moon face, hypertension, easy bruising, diabetes or glucose intolerance, gonadal dysfunction, muscle weakness, hirsutism, mood disorders, dyslipidemia, and osteoporosis.[33] The prevalence of diabetes associated with CS ranges from 20–50%, and up to 70% of patients with CS are estimated to have impaired glucose tolerance.[35,36] These percentages may vary by population and background rates of obesity, glucose intolerance, and diabetes. Epidemiological data shows a higher prevalence of diabetes in overt CS compared to adrenal incidentalomas associated with subclinical CS.[35] Risk factors for the development of diabetes in patients with CS are similar to those for T2D and include older age, obesity, family history of diabetes, and biochemical evidence of glucose intolerance.

Under physiologic circumstances, GC are important for glucose metabolism and contribute to energy homeostasis, especially during the postprandial period. GC stimulate lipolysis and proteolysis, leading to production of fatty acids and amino acids. Glucose is produced through GC activation of gluconeogenesis and inhibition of glycogen synthesis in the liver, as depicted in Figure 5.1.[37] Diabetes develops in patients with CS from the combination of a decrease in insulin sensitivity at the muscle and liver and impairment in insulin secretion induced by GC excess.[37] Decreased insulin sensitivity stems from reduced insulin-stimulated glucose uptake in skeletal muscle and adipose tissue, increased proteolysis and lipolysis, and increased gluconeogenesis in the liver through direct and indirect effects on key enzymes involved in metabolic pathways, as shown in Figure 5.1.[37] Decreased insulin secretion occurs from glucocorticoid-mediated impairment in insulin exocytosis by modulation of gene expression leading to β cell dysfunction and apoptosis.[38] Other metabolic alterations in CS include increased leptin and decreased adiponectin levels, and the redistribution of adipose tissue from the subcutaneous to the visceral region in response to excess glucocorticoids.[37]

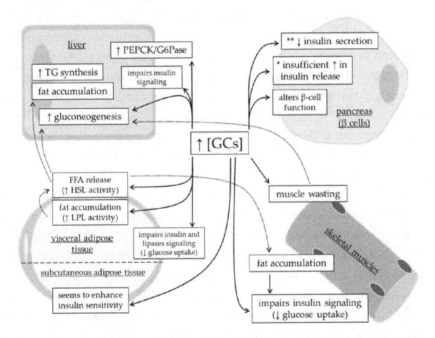

Figure 5.1—Adverse actions of glucocorticoids (GCs) on peripheral tissues involved in glucose homeostasis. Continuous lines mean direct effect, while dotted lines mean indirect action. FFA, free fatty acids; G6Pas, glucose-6-phosphatase; HSL, hormone-sensitive lipase; LPL, lipoprotein lipase; PEPCK, phosphoenolpyruvate carboxykinase; TG, triacylglycerol.

Source: Reprinted with permission from Pasieka AM, Rafacho A.[37]

Due to the pathophysiologic mechanisms outlined above, patients with CS are more likely to have hyperglycemia in the postprandial period rather than impaired fasting glucose. In fact, up to 50% of patients with diabetes and CS have normal fasting glucose levels.[36] In contrast to the general population in which the diagnosis of diabetes is often made on the basis of a fasting blood glucose level ≥126 mg/dL, the preferred test to diagnose diabetes or prediabetes in patients with CS is a 75-g oral glucose tolerance test (OGTT). No studies have validated using HbA_{1c} for diagnosis of glucose intolerance or diabetes in CS.

In order to prevent and decrease morbidity related to the complications of endogenous CS, the first priority in treatment is normalization of cortisol levels, keeping in mind that treatment modalities may have variable effects on glucose control. For patients with an ACTH-producing pituitary tumor (CD), surgery is considered the mainstay of treatment.[39] Surgical resection results in remission in approximately 82% of patients at ten years postsurgery with relapse occurring in 9–13% of cases.[40] In patients where surgical intervention is not feasible, or in whom persistent or recurrent CD occurs, additional treatments are required.[39] Conventional external beam radiation therapy, traditionally used in patients with residual or recurrent functioning pituitary adenomas, results in biochemical control in up to 78% of patients with CD.[41] Stereotactic radiosurgery, a technique that delivers a high dose of radiation to a more precise well-defined target, results in biochemical remission in 25–80% of patients with a mean follow-up of 2–17 years and a median time to normalization of cortisol levels ranging from 12–15 months. Hypopituitarism is the most commonly reported late complication of radiotherapy.[41] Bilateral adrenalectomy, an additional option for recurrent or persistent CD, results in rapid reduction of cortisol levels, but requires lifelong treatment with glucocorticoids and mineralocorticoids. Overtreatment of adrenal insufficiency may worsen persistent metabolic complications of CS such as diabetes.[42] Lastly, medical therapy to control cortisol secretion or action is frequently used as adjuvant therapy in patients not cured or who are not candidates for pituitary surgery, as a bridge until radiation therapy has had its full effect, and sometimes for presurgical treatment.[39] When decisions pertaining to therapeutic agents are considered, health-care providers must consider the degree of hyperglycemia in addition to hypercortisolism.[39]

Pasireotide, a new-generation multireceptor-targeted somatostatin receptor ligand, has been approved for the treatment of CD in patients when surgical resection has failed or is not a viable option.[43,44] Pasireotide works by decreasing production of ACTH from corticotroph adenomas and leads to reductions in tumor size. Response to pasireotide is monitored through measurements of cortisol in serum, urine, or late-night salivary secretions.[43,44] In clinical studies of pasireotide, hyperglycemia was frequently observed and was felt to be secondary to reduced incretin secretion.[45] Hyperglycemia-related adverse advents associated with pasireotide in clinical studies ranged from 68–73% and led to discontinuation in 5–6% of patients with CD.[45] Patients with risk factors for diabetes are at greater risk for pasireotide-induced hyperglycemia. Medical expert recommendations have been developed to treat hyperglycemia induced by pasireotide.[46] In patients with a fasting plasma glucose ≥ 126 g/dL or $HbA_{1c} > 6.5$ %, metformin should be initiated.[46] If euglycemia is not achieved by metformin alone, it is suggested that a DPP-4 inhibitor be added to the antidiabetic regimen.[46] Uncontrolled hyperglycemia ($HbA_{1c} > 7.0$%) on metformin and DDP-4 inhibitor therapy should prompt replacement of the DPP-4 inhibitor with a GLP-1 receptor agonist. In patients who cannot achieve glucose targets with a DPP-4 inhibitor or GLP-1 receptor agonist, consideration should be made regarding initiation of insulin therapy while continuing metformin treatment.[46] Pasireotide does not affect glucagon secretion and peripheral insulin sensitivity; consequently, hyperglycemia associated with pasireotide is temporary and is not expected to cause long-term effects if pasireotide is discontinued.[45]

Mifepristone is the first and only available glucocorticoid receptor antagonist and is FDA approved to control hyperglycemia in patients with endogenous CS.[47] Indications for initiating mifepristone treatment in CD are failed treatment with surgical interventions or medical therapy, or side effects, such as hyperglycemia associated with pasireotide or lastly as part of a multimodal approach.[47,48] Mifepristone is clinically better suited in patients in whom effects of diabetes are of critical concern.[48] Mifepristone was shown to improve glucose control in patients with CS who had failed other therapies and also had concurrent T2D, impaired glucose tolerance, or hypertension in the SIESMIC trial.[49] Clinical trial data have shown that mifepristone improves glycemic control and blood pressure, causes weight loss and a decrease in waist circumference, lessens depression, and improves overall well-being.[47–49] The majority of patients experience rapid resolution of the clinical signs of hypercortisolism. Blockade of the glucocorticoid receptor raises serum cortisol levels and increases the risk for adrenal insufficiency.[48] Furthermore, through activation of mineralocorticoid receptors, elevated serum cortisol levels can also lead to severe hypokalemia.[47,48] In women, mifepristone can cause endometrial thickening and vaginal bleeding.[49] In contrast to pasireotide, response to mifepristone is measured by variations in clinical symptoms such as hypertension, weight, and glucose control.[39,50]

Several non–FDA-approved medications with different mechanisms of action are used to treat patients with CS. Cabergoline, a dopamine agonist more commonly used in the treatment of prolactinomas and mild acromegaly, was shown to control cortisol secretion in 40% and induce tumor shrinkage in 20% of a group of 20 patients with CD.[51] Interestingly, improvements were seen in hypertension and glucose intolerance in patients who were resistant or escaped from therapy, suggesting a direct effect of dopamine agonists on glucose homeostasis.[51] Other agents used to control cortisol secretion from the adrenal glands, including ketoconazole, metyrapone, and mitotane, are not known to have any direct adverse effects on glucose metabolism and may improve glucose tolerance by reducing cortisol secretion.[39]

Patients with CS have a mortality rate four times higher than age-matched controls due to an increased risk of cardiovascular disease (Figure 5.2).[34,35] Causative factors include impaired endothelial function, impaired glucose tolerance, hypertension, hypercoagulability, dyslipidemia, atherosclerosis, and direct effects of hypercortisolism on the vasculature.[35] Regardless of the treatment modality, evidence suggests that resolution of hypercortisolism does not necessarily result in normalization of cardiovascular and cerebrovascular risk factors as evidenced by a higher prevalence of metabolic syndrome and atherosclerosis in patients in remission as compared to controls.[35] A more recent study, however, showed that serum biomarkers of endothelial dysfunction, intima media thickness, and other markers of micro- and macrovascular health were similar between CS patients in remission with controlled or no comorbidities when compared to healthy controls, highlighting the importance of identification and management of diabetes and the other sequelae of CS.[52]

Glucagonoma

Glucagonomas are extremely rare pancreatic neuroendocrine tumors with an estimated incidence of 1 per 20 million people.[53] Glucagonomas develop

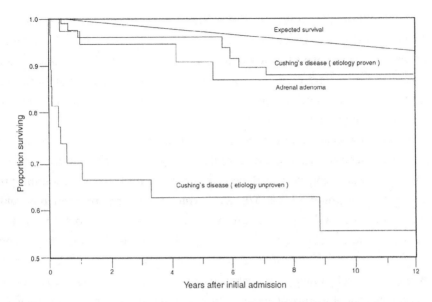

Figure 5.2—Survival of patients with Cushing's disease (proven and unproven) and with adrenocortical adenoma.

Source: Lindholm J et al.[34]

sporadically in 80–87% of cases while the remaining 13–20% of cases occur in patients with the multiple endocrine neoplasia (MEN) 1 syndrome.[54] Glucagonomas have an estimated male-to-female ratio of 0.8 and are most often diagnosed in middle-aged or older adults, mean age at onset 52.5 years, range 11–88 years.[54] Patients often present with the glucagonoma syndrome, which is characterized by necrolytic migratory erythema rash, cheilosis/stomatitis, diabetes, anemia, thrombosis, weight loss, and neuropsychiatric symptoms.[54-56] Although the syndrome can occur with or without tumor metastases, it is present in only 57% of patients with histologically proven glucagonomas.[54] Rash is more common than diabetes, possibly because of the weight loss and cachexia that occur with this unusual tumor.[54-57]

Glucagonomas develop within the pancreas in 97.3% of cases.[54] The majority are located in the pancreatic tail (53.7%) followed by the body (32.2%) and then the head of the pancreas (21.9%).[54,57] Extrapancreatic locations include the kidney, small intestine, lung, and liver. Glucagonomas are aggressive tumors and 75–90% have metastasized prior to diagnosis; typically to the liver, lymph nodes, adrenal glands, lung, and bone. There appears to be a close relationship between the size of the tumor and metastatic potential. Tumors below 2 cm were noted to have a low incidence of malignancy of 8.75% while tumors 2.1–5 cm had metastasized in 31.2% cases and finally metastatic risk in tumors greater than 5 cm was 66.7%. Tumors in patients with MEN 1 syndrome appear to have less malignant potential.[54]

Glucagon has many effects that impact glucose homeostasis. Glucagon's primary target is hepatocytes where it promotes glycogenolysis, gluconeogenesis, and ureagenesis.[7] Gluconeogenesis is dependent on other hormones to mobilize precursors, primarily amino acids and glycerol, which are severely reduced in patients with glucagonoma.[58] Glucagon has also been shown to increase proteolysis, amino acid oxidation, and urea production, which may be responsible for the net catabolism and weight loss that is common in patients with glucagonoma.[58,59] Interestingly, despite increased gluconeogenesis, severe hypoaminoacidemia that includes both gluconeogenic and nongluconeogenic amino acids is present in patients with glucagonoma.[58,60] Removal of the tumor, but not infusion of amino acids, restores blood and tissue amino acid levels to normal; however, infusion of amino acids and fatty acids helps with resolution of the rash.[60]

In T2D, glucagon secretion is stimulated in response to hyperglycemia, especially if insulin secretion is blunted. Furthermore, the ability of insulin to promote hepatic glucose uptake is attenuated by increased glucagon levels.[61] In subjects with impaired fasting glucose and impaired glucose tolerance, hyperglucagonemia heralds the onset of diabetes and loss of insulin secretion.[7] Findings from a randomized, double-blind, placebo-controlled phase two trial suggested that a glucagon receptor antagonist improved glucose control in patients with T2D, but this therapy has not been tested in patients with glucagonoma.[62] Glucagon levels are many times higher in patients with glucagon-producing tumors than they are in persons with diabetes, and are unregulated by other hormones or substrates. Despite this, and with likely insulin deficiency, glucose intolerance can be absent or mild, or severe enough to cause ketoacidosis in patients with glucagonomas.[54–57,58,63] Treatment with somatostatin analogs, while needed to manage symptoms from hyperglycagonemia, may worsen hyperglycemia and contribute to the risk of ketoacidosis.[63]

Patients with glucagonomas often experience symptoms for months to years before the diagnosis is made.[64] Surgical cure or prolonged survival without progression is possible with localized lesions, or those with limited local metastases.[54,64]

However, since many glucagonomas have metastasized by the time they are diagnosed, adjunctive therapy is required both to control tumor growth and to control symptoms from hyperglucagonemia.[64] Somatostatin analogs are the mainstay of adjuvant therapy, but their role is primarily to relieve symptoms of diarrhea, weight loss, and rash, since tumor response is generally negligible.[54,64] Glucose should be monitored in patients receiving a somatostatin analog, since hyperglycemia may worsen from suppression of insulin secretion. Amino acid infusion in the form of total parenteral nutrition is often needed to prevent cachexia. Hepatic embolization and chemotherapy are the preferred treatments for nonresectable metastases or recurrent disease, though response is variable.[64] Peptide receptor radionuclide therapy is a new therapy that has promise for patients who have not responded to chemotherapy (Table 5.1).[64]

Somatostatinoma

Somatostatin-producing tumors, known as somatostatinomas, arise from the D cells in the pancreas or spontaneously in other locations, and exhibit

Table 5.1 — Metabolic Effects of Drugs Used for Acromegaly, Cushing's Disease and Syndrome, and Glucagonoma

Drugs	Tumors, Syndromes			Metabolic Effects		
	Acromegaly	Cushing's Disease & Syndrome	Glucagonoma	Glucose Tolerance	Insulin Secretion	Insulin Resistance
Octreotide	X		X	↓	↓	
Lanreotide	X		X	↓	↓	
Pasireotide	X	X		↓↓	↓↓	
Bromocriptine				↑↔		?↓
Cabergoline	X	X		?↑	?↑	↓
Pegvisomant	X			↑↑		↓
Mifepristone		X		↑↑	↑	↓↓
Ketoconazole		X		↑	↑*	↓*
Metyrapone		X		↑	↑*	↓*
Mitotane		X		↑	↑*	↓*

*Indicates indirect effect.

more heterogeneity than the other gastrointestinal neuroendocrine tumors.[6,65] Only half of somatostatinomas are found in the pancreas, and comprise <4% of all pancreatic NETs.[65-69] The duodenum, specifically near the ampulla of Vater, is also a common site, and up to 26% of duodenal NETs stain for somatostatin.[68] Somatostatin staining tumors are also found in the bile ducts, the ovary, and in gangliocytic paragangliomas.[67] Somatostatinomas can occur sporadically but also occur in patients with MEN1, neurofibromastosis 1 (NF1), and von Hippel-Lindau (VHL) syndromes.[65,67] The sporadic tumors and those associated with NF1 and VHL syndromes are typically solitary, while the MEN1 associated tumors tend to be small and multiple.[65] Somatostatin-staining NETs have been found in conjunction with gastrointestinal stromal tumors or with other types of NETs, such as gastrinomas.[67,69] In a large series of somatostatinomas, only those arising from the duodenum were seen in patients with NF1.[67]

The somatostatinoma syndrome was described by Larsson et al. in 1977 and includes the following: 1) markedly elevated somatostatin levels in plasma or in the tumor, 2) diabetes of recent onset, 3) hypochlorhydria, 4) gallbladder disease, such as cholelithiasis, 5) diarrhea with or without steatorrhea, and 6) anemia and weight loss.[66] Within a few years, the likelihood of this defined clinical syndrome appearing with somatostatinomas was challenged by a number of authors; however, a few cases were subsequently reported of patients with the symptom complex.[67,70,71] In large case series, a small minority of patients with somatostatin-staining tumors expressed the key features of the somatostatinoma syndrome, largely because they presented with symptoms of localized disease, such as abdominal pain or jaundice.[67] Another reason for the lack of multiorgan symptoms is that most of the somatostatin staining tumors are well differentiated and metastasize locally to lymph nodes. Somatostatin staining may be found in nonfunctioning NETs of varying degrees of differentiation and in variable locations.[67,72] Tumors expressing somatostatin plus glucagon, pancreatic polypeptide, and other hormones are not uncommon. Lastly, somatostatinomas are sometimes found at autopsy, leaving the clinical correlations unclear.

The mechanism of somatostatin-induced diabetes is likely due to suppression of insulin secretion by somatostatin, but local effects from large pancreatic tumors may also play a role. Due to the rarity of somatostatinoma-associated diabetes, treatment recommendations are not established. It is likely that patients will require insulin, and management is no doubt complicated by symptoms such as abdominal pain and nausea due to biliary obstruction. Malabsorption due to pancreatic insufficiency or steatorrhea further complicates management. Since aggressive surgery is often curative, insulin replacement may be required after tumor resection due to pancreatic insufficiency.

Pheochromocytoma

Pheochromocytomas and paragangliomas are rare neuroendocrine tumors arising from adrenomedullary chromaffin cells and extra-adrenal ganglia respectively.[73] The incidence is 2 to 5 patients per million per year and is highest in those between 30 and 50 years of age.[74] The combined prevalence in patients with hypertension is 0.2 to 0.6%. Of patients with catecholamine hypersecretion, 80 to 85% will have a pheochromocytoma while 15 to 20% will have a paraganglioma. Pheochromocytoma is found in approximately 5% of adrenal incidentalomas.[75] Most of the cases are sporadic; however, up to 40% have germline mutations and these typically present at younger ages.[73,74] Between 10 and 17% of patients have malignant tumors; however, in those with mutations in the succinate dehydrogenase gene, the relative risk of metastases in nonchromaffin tissues is higher.[74,76] Pheochromocytoma or paraganglioma can occur in patients with the genetic syndromes MEN 2A, MEN 2B, neurofibromatosis 1 (NF1), and von Hippel-Lindau and the presence of an underlying genetic syndrome may alter the natural history of the disease.[73,74]

Symptoms are due to the hypersecretion of one or more catecholamines, including norepinephrine, epinephrine, and dopamine as well as metanephrine metabolites. Within chromaffin cells, catecholamines are metabolized to metanephrines: norepinephrine to normetanephrine and epinephrine to metanephrine.[75] Patients commonly present with the classic triad of episodic headaches, diaphoresis, and tachycardia and hypertension. Other symptoms include anxiety, tremor, and syncope. Weight loss can occur due to lipolysis and severe constipation due to the inhibition of peristalsis by catecholamines.[73,75]

Of note, patients with these tumors may present with new-onset hyperglycemia while those already diagnosed with diabetes can have worsening control.[77,78] Rare cases of DKA in patients with pheochromocytoma have been reported.[79] Glucose intolerance due to the effects of catecholamines is common.[80] Catecholamines have been shown to suppress β-cell insulin secretion by stimulation of alpha adrenergic receptors, decreased tissue utilization of glucose, and increased lipolysis.[81–83] Lipolysis stimulation is mediated by beta-1 and beta-3 adrenergic receptors.[84,85] Free fatty acids increase hepatic gluconeogenesis from lactate and alanine by stimulating gluconeogenic enzymes.[86] In the liver, an increase in epinephrine causes an initial activation of hepatic glycogenolysis, which is mediated by beta-2 receptors, and then a sustained increased rate of gluconeogenesis.[86,87] Furthermore, elevated catecholamine levels increase glycogenolysis in skeletal muscle and alter intrahepatic metabolism.[86,88] Gluconeogenic precursors from muscle and other extrasplanchnic tissues are diverted to glucose synthesis rather than oxidative pathways.[86] In addition, epinephrine causes decreased peristalsis and delayed absorption of glucose from the intestine. This causes insulin secretion from β-cells to be delayed, further contributing to glucose intolerance.[82]

While many patients with high plasma and urinary catecholamine levels have increased blood glucose levels, the development of diabetes is associated with age and longer known duration of hypertension.[89,90] Estimates vary; however, hyperglycemia is estimated to be present in about 40% of those with catecholamine-secreting tumors, while the prevalence of diabetes is approximately 35% and the incidence is 24%.[89-91] Treatment with α-adrenergic receptor blockade improves, but does not normalize, insulin sensitivity and blood glucose levels.[89-92] Even after adding a beta-blocking agent, euglycemia is not usually achieved, despite resolution of cardiovascular effects. Adrenoreceptors in various tissues may be activated by different levels of catecholamines, and the threshold at which adrenaline and related compounds elicit metabolic versus cardiovascular effects differs, precluding correction of the metabolic effects by using doses of blocking agents that are effective for cardiovascular purposes.[4]

Adrenalectomy is the recommended treatment for pheochromocytoma and resection for a paraganglioma.[75] Surgical removal of the tumor will correct the metabolic abnormalities caused by it but may not reverse hyperglycemia in all cases.[4,89-91] After surgery, close monitoring of blood sugar levels is necessary as hypoglycemia could be a complication. A sudden decrease in circulating catecholamines from interrupting blood flow to a tumor can prompt a rebound in insulin release and glucose uptake leading to interoperative and postoperative hypoglycemia.[93,94] Glucose monitoring in patients with catecholamine-secreting tumors should be part of the care of these patients, with special attention during the perioperative period for hypoglycemia. Persistent hyperglycemia after surgery should be investigated and treated appropriately.

Hyperthyroidism

Hyperthyroidism is caused by excess thyroid hormone synthesis and secretion from the thyroid gland or exogenous intake of thyroid hormone. Hyperthyroidism can range from a mild, asymptomatic problem detected on laboratory screening to a life-threatening emergency.[95,96] Overt hyperthyroidism is characterized by suppressed TSH concentration and raised levels of thyroxine (T4), triiodothyronine (T3), or both. Subclinical hyperthyroidism is defined as low TSH but normal T4 and T3, and is generally asymptomatic.[95] Overt hyperthyroidism, which is the topic of this chapter, affects 0.5–0.8% of the population in Europe and about 0.5% of the population in the U.S.[97,98] Women are more likely to develop hyperthyroidism than men; the female-to-male ratio was 4.2:1 in a population-based Swedish study.[99] Graves' disease is the most common etiology of hyperthyroidism in Europe and the U.S., but multinodular goiter is more common in iodine-deficient regions of the world.[97] Hyperthyroidism is diagnosed in every age group but shows a peak incidence in middle-aged adults in the fifth and sixth decades, while hyperthyroidism from multinodular goiter occurs most commonly in the elderly.[99]

The symptoms of hyperthyroidism stem from excess circulating thyroid hormones.[96] Patients are intolerant to heat, complain of sweating, lose weight, and note increased heart rate and tremor. Additional symptoms may include palpitations, irregular heartbeat, shortness of breath, and edema indicating possible cardiac arrhythmia or heart failure. People with Graves' disease may have symptoms related to ophthalmopathy or soft-tissue myxedema.[100]

Clinicians often note glucose intolerance in patients with previously normal glycemia, worsening hyperglycemia in patients with T2D, and increased insulin requirements in patients with T1D and insulin-requiring T2D despite weight loss in those with hyperthyroidism. While Graves' disease is known to occur more commonly in patients with T1D than in age-matched controls, similar prevalence data for T2D are limited.[101] Older studies of patients with thyrotoxicosis showed an increase in "nonphysiologic hyperglycemia" or diabetes ranging from 6.9% to 57%.[102,103] Follow-up of one of the cohorts found a reduction in diabetes prevalence from 57% to 30% at 8.8 months, but an increase in the same group to 43% at 11.6 years.[104] In a Chinese population, detection of prediabetes or diabetes by OGTT was 41.29% and 11.29% in patients with Graves' disease, compared to 19.45% and 10.03% in age-matched controls.[105]

HbA$_{1c}$ did not perform as well, diagnosing 33.23% with prediabetes and 4.52% with diabetes, compared to 22.8% and 8.51% respectively in controls.[105] The converse does not appear to be true, however. The HUNT2 population-based study looked for thyroid disease in patients with T2D in Norway and found a higher age-adjusted prevalence of hyperthyroidism (PR 1.75, 95% CI 1.12–2.73), also with undiagnosed hyperthyroidism (PR 2.16, 95% CI 1.30–3.60), in men, but not in women, but the relationship did not hold up in HUNT3.[106] Glucose intolerance is common and increased in patients with hyperthyroidism, but given the high background rates of prediabetes or diabetes in many populations worldwide, finding an excess of hyperthyroidism is unlikely.

Thyroid storm, which is a state of extreme hyperthyroidism with fever and multiorgan involvement or decompensation, occurs in up to 1% of patients hospitalized for thyrotoxicosis and is a life-threatening emergency with mortality of 10–75%.[107] Thyroid storm is often precipitated by other medical problems and has been described in numerous cases of patients presenting with concomitant DKA from regions around the world.[108–110] Patients not previously diagnosed with either T1D or T2D, or those with previously well-controlled diabetes, have experienced DKA when thyrotoxic, attesting to the severity of the metabolic derangement that can occur with excess circulating thyroid hormone.[8,108–110]

The cause of the disordered carbohydrate metabolism in hyperthyroidism has been extensively studied. In a sentinel report in 1985, Dimitriadis et al. showed that during thyrotoxicosis, insulin clearance was increased, insulin-induced suppression of hepatic glucose production was impaired, and that nonoxidative glucose uptake and disposal were reduced despite normal insulin receptor binding. In their otherwise normal (nondiabetic) study subjects, this was accompanied by an increase in insulin secretion and clearance.[111] These findings of hepatic and peripheral insulin resistance have been confirmed in later studies.[112,113] Interestingly, the level of T3 elevation correlated with the degree of peripheral insulin resistance as measured by homeostasis model assessments of insulin resistance (HOMA IR).[114] Maratou and colleagues[115] compared glucose and insulin parameters from OGTTs in subjects with hyperthyroidism and subclinical hyperthyroidism to euthyroid controls. Higher postprandial glucose levels were present in both hyperthyroid and subclinical groups compared to controls, and higher postprandial insulin levels were noted in the hyperthyroid group compared to controls. HOMA IR was increased in both hyperthyroid and subclinical hyperthyroid groups, while Matsuda and Belfiore indices were decreased in the postprandial period, confirming the presence of insulin resistance in both hyperthyroid and subclinical hyperthyroid patients.[115]

T3, the active thyroid hormone, has multiple direct and indirect effects on hepatocytes when studied in vitro. T3 has been shown to directly stimulate hepatic lipogenesis, but to decrease insulin-stimulated glycogen synthesis, insulin suppression of gluconeogenesis, and insulin-induced lipogenesis. The combined effects are increased lipogenesis, lipid oxidation, gluconeogenesis, and glucose oxidation.[116,117]

Hyperthyroidism has been shown to stimulate metabolism and thermogenesis. The underlying physiology is complex. While gluconeogenesis is stimulated in the liver, hyperthyroidism increases GLUT3 and GLUT4 expression in peripheral tissue, causing increased glucose flux and nonoxidative metabolism.[118] Since insulin cannot properly stimulate glycogen synthesis in hyperthyroid conditions, glycogen is depleted and glucose is converted to pyruvate, forming lactate via anaerobic metabolism. This metabolite promotes hepatic gluconeogenesis and increases the energy demand for glucose disposal.[118,119] Increased thermogenesis, reflecting increased energy demand, is a hallmark of hyperthyroidism. In a study using positron emission tomography, Lahesmaa and colleagues found that hyperthyroid patients had threefold higher glucose uptake in brown adipose tissue and markedly higher glucose uptake in skeletal muscle and lipid oxidation rates.[120] Energy expenditure (EE) was increased by 45% in hyperthyroid compared to healthy subjects, and they used more lipids as energy substrate. No difference was found in utilization of carbohydrates in this study. Interestingly, serum free T4 and free T3 levels correlated significantly with EE (R = 0.81 and R = 0.86, respectively, P<0.001).[120] The in vivo and in vitro metabolic effects of hyperthyroidism are comprehensively reviewed by Mitrou et al.[121]

How do these metabolic effects impact people? Importantly, individuals who develop hyperthyroidism have predisease metabolic signatures that interact with elevated thyroid hormone levels. Gonzalo et al.[122] studied a group of hyperthyroid women with intravenous, insulin-modified, glucose tolerance tests and confirmed lower insulin sensitivity by showing higher glucose levels with similar insulin secretion rates in the hyperthyroid patients compared to controls. Interestingly, women who were hyperthyroid showed a steeper decline in insulin sensitivity with increases in body weight than normal controls, suggesting that underlying insulin resistance from age or obesity may aggravate the glucose intolerance observed in hyperthyroidism.[122] In a study of 30 hyperthyroid patients, Al-Shoumer et al.[123] showed that elevated levels of fasting glucose, insulin, C-peptide, intact pro-insulin, and area under the curve of glucose during a 3-hour glucose tolerance test returned to normal after 1 month of antithyroid drug therapy and remained similar to controls at 6 months. Additionally, 3 patients who met OGTT criteria for diabetes, 9 of 10 patients with impaired glucose tolerance, and 4 of 5 patients with impaired fasting glucose had reversion to normal glucose tolerance at 1 and 6 months. One patient remained glucose intolerant at 1 month, but normalized at 6 months.[123] Patients with T1D and hyperthyroidism experience more episodes of DKA than euthyroid controls, indicating that the metabolic abnormalities can have serious consequences when insulin resistance occurs unexpectedly.[124]

There are no published guidelines addressing screening for glucose intolerance or diabetes in patients with hyperthyroidism. The American Thyroid Association did not address this problem in a recently published guideline on hyperthyroidism. Likewise, guidance for treatment of glucose intolerance in hyperthyroid patients is lacking. Since hyperthyroidism has many causes and affects persons across the entire age spectrum, consideration of predisease diabetes status including risk factors for glucose intolerance such as age and obesity are important factors in decisions to incorporate screening for diabetes. Clearly, diagnosis and treatment of hyperthyroidism should be undertaken urgently, and correction of the excess thyroid hormone milieu will have short-term and long-term metabolic benefits. Patients with diabetes should be monitored closely so that antidiabetic medications including insulin can be adjusted to meet the increased metabolic demands of hyperthyroidism, then readjusted when hyperthyroidism is treated and resolves. Prevention of DKA is critical for patients with T1D and susceptible individuals with T2D.

References

1. Resmini E, Minuto F, Colao A, Ferone D. Secondary diabetes associated with principal endocrinopathies: the impact of new treatment modalities. *Acta Diabetol* 2009;46:85–95

2. Olarescu NC, Bollerslev J. The impact of adipose tissue on insulin resistance in acromegaly. *Trends Endocrinol Metab* 2016;27:226–237.

3.   Valassi E, Crespo I, Santos A, Webb SM. Clinical consequences of Cushing's syndrome. *Pituitary* 2012;15:319–329

4.   Diamanti-Kandarakis E, Zapanti E, Peridis MH, Ntavos P, Mastorakos G. Insulin resistance in pheochromocytoma improves more by surgical rather than by medical treatment. *Hormones* 2003;2:61–66

5.   Kapadia KB, Bhatt PA, Shah JS. Association between altered thyroid state and insulin resistance. *J Pharmacol Pharmacother* 2012;3:156–160

6.   Grozinsky-Glasberg S, Mazeh H, Gross DJ. Clinical features of pancreatic neuroendocrine tumors. *J Hepatobiliary Pancreat Sci* 2015;22:578–585

7.   Wewer ANJ, Kuhre RE, Pedersen J, Knop FK, Holst JJ. The biology of glucagon and the consequences of hyperglycagonemia. *Biomark Med* 2016;10:1141–1151

8.   Mercer V, Burt V, Dhatariya KK. New onset type 1 diabetes presenting as ketoacidosis simultaneously presenting with autoimmune hyperthyroidism – a case report. *J Diab Complications* 2011;25:208–210

9.   Hirai H, Midorikawa S, Suzuki S, Sasano H, Watanabe T, Satoh H. Somatostatin-secreting pheochromocytoma mimicking insulin-dependent diabetes mellitus. *Intern Med* 2016;55:2985–2991

10. Fernandez A, Karavitaki N, Wass JAH. Prevalence of pituitary adenomas: a community-based, cross-sectional study in Banbury (Oxfordshire, UK). *Clin Endocrinol (Oxf)* 2010;72:377–382

11. Drange MR, Fram NR, Herman-Bonert V, Melmed S. Pituitary tumor registry: a novel clinical resource. *J Clin Endocrinol Metab* 2000;85:168–174

12. Lugo G, Pena L, Cordido F. Clinical manifestations and diagnosis of acromegaly. *Int J Endocrinol* 2012;2012

13. Colao A, Ferone D, Marzullo P, Lombardi G. Systemic complications of acromegaly: epidemiology, pathogenesis, and management. *Endocr Rev* 2004; 25:102–152

14. Nabarro JD. Acromegaly. *Clin Endocrinol (Oxf)* 1987;26:481–512

15. Kreze A, Kreze-Spirova E, Mikulecky M. Risk factors for glucose intolerance in active acromegaly. *Braz J Med Biol Res* 2001;34:1429–1433

16. Hansen I, Tsalikian E, Beaufrere B, Gerich J, Haymond M, Rizza R. Insulin resistance in acromegaly: defects in both hepatic and extrahepatic insulin action. *Am J Physiol* 1986;250:E269–273

17. Jap TS, Ho LT. Insulin secretion and sensitivity in acromegaly. *Clin Physiol Biochem* 1990;8:64–69

18. Foss MC, Saad MJ, Paccola GM, Paula FJ, Piccinato CE, Moreira AC. Peripheral glucose metabolism in acromegaly. *J Clin Endocrinol Metab* 1991;72:1048–1053

19. Kopff B, Mucha S, Wolffenbuttel BH, Drzewoski J. Diabetic ketoacidosis in a patient with acromegaly. *Med Sci Monit* 2001;7:142–147

20. Reyes-Vidal C, Fernandez JC, Bruce JN, et al. Prospective study of surgical treatment of acromegaly: effects on ghrelin, weight, adiposity, and markers of CV risk. *J Clin Endocrinol Metab* 2014;99:4124–4132

21. Colao A, Auriemma RS, Galdiero M, et al. Impact of somatostatin analogs versus surgery on glucose metabolism in acromegaly: results of a 5-year observational, open, prospective study. *J Clin Endocrinol Metab* 2009;94:528–537

22. Cuevas-Ramos D, Fleseriu M. Pasireotide: a novel treatment for patients with acromegaly. *Drug Des Devel Ther* 2016;10:227–239

23. Barkan AL, Burman P, Clemmons DR, et al. Glucose homeostasis and safety in patients with acromegaly converted from long-acting octreotide to pegvisomant. *J Clin Endocrinol Metab* 2005;90:5684–5691

24. Larijani B, Nakhjavani M, Baradar-Jalili R, Akrami SM, Bandarian F. Diabetes mellitus following pituitary adenomectomy in euglycemic patients with acromegaly. *J Coll Physicians Surg Pak* 2005;15:430–432

25. Frara S, Maffezzoni F, Mazziotti G, Giustina A. Current and emerging aspects of diabetes mellitus in acromegaly. *Trends Endocrinol Metab* 2016;27:470–483

26. Azzoug S, Chentli F. Diabetic retinopathy in acromegaly. *Indian J Endocrinol Metab* 2014;18:407–409

27. Tran HA, Petrovsky N, Field AJ. Severe diabetic retinopathy: a rare complication of acromegaly. *Int Med J* 2002;32:52–54

28. Inokuchi N, Ikeda T, Yasuda F, Shirai S, Uchihori Y. Severe proliferative diabetic retinopathy associated with acromegaly. *Br J Ophthalmol* 1999;83:628–633

29. Kamenicky P, Mazziotti G, Lombes M, Giustina A, Chanson P. Growth hormone, insulin-like growth factor-1, and the kidney: pathophysiological and clinical implications. *Endocr Rev* 2014;35:234–281

30. Baldelli R, De Marinis L, Bianchi A, Pivonello R, Gasco V, Auriemma R, Pasimeni G, Cimino V, Appetecchia M, Maccario M, Lombardi G, Pontecorvi A, Colao A,

Grottoli S. Microalbuminuria in insulin sensitivity in patients with growth hormone-secreting pituitary tumor. *J Clin Endocrinol Metab* 2008;93:710–714

31. Cheng S, Gomez K, Serri O, Chik C, Ezzat S. The role of diabetes in acromegaly associated neoplasia. *PLoS One* 2015;10:e0127276

32. Wen-Ko C, Szu-Tah C, Feng-Hsuan L, Chen-Nen C, Ming-Hsu W, Jen-Der L. The impact of diabetes mellitus on the survival of patients with acromegaly. *Endokrynol Pol* 2016;67:501–506

33. Nieman LK, Biller BM, Findling JW, Newell-Price J, Savage MO, Stewart PM, Montori VM. The diagnosis of Cushing's syndrome: an Endocrine Society clinical practice guideline. *J Clin Endocrinol Metab* 2008;93:1526–1540

34. Lindholm J, Juul S, Jorgensen JO, Astrup J, Bjerre P, Feldt-Rasmussen U, Hagen C, Jorgensen J, Kosteljanetz M, Kristensen L, Laurberg P, Schmidt K, Weeke J. Incidence and late prognosis of Cushing's syndrome: a population-based study. *J Clin Endocrinol Metab* 2001;86:117–123

35. Giordano R, Picu A, Marinazzo E, D'Angelo V, Berardelli R, Karamouzist I, Forno D, Zinna D, Maccariot M, Ghigo E, Arvatt E. Metabolic and cardiovascular outcomes in patients with Cushing's syndrome of different aetiologies during active disease and 1 year after remission. *Clin Endocrinol* 2011;75:354–360

36. Mancini T, Kola B, Mantero F, Boscaro M, Arnaldi G. High cardiovascular risk in patients with Cushing's syndrome according to 1999 WHO/ISH guidelines. *Clin Endocrinol* 2004; 61:768–777

37. Pasieka AM, Rafacho A. Impact of glucocorticoid excess on glucose tolerance: clinical and pre-clinical evidence. *Metabolites* 2016;6:E24

38. Tamez-Perez HE, Quintanilla-Flores DL, Rodriguez-Gutierrez R, Gerardo J, Gonzalez-Gonzalez JG, Tamez-Pena AL. Steroid hyperglycemia: prevalence, early detection and therapeutic recommendations: a narrative review. *World J Diabetes* 2015;6:1073–1081

39. Nieman LK, Biller BM, Findling JW, Murad MH, Newell-Price J, Savage MO, Tabarin A, Endocrine Society. Treatment of Cushing's syndrome: an Endocrine Society clinical practice guideline. *J Clin Endocrinol Metab* 2015;100:2807–2331

40. Hammer GD, Tyrrell JB, Lamborn KR, Applebury CB, Hannegan ET, Bell S, Rahl R, Lu A, Wilson CB. Transsphenoidal microsurgery for Cushing's disease: initial outcome and long-term results. *J Clin Endocrinol Metab* 2004;89: 6348–6357

41. Loeffler JS, Shih HA. Radiation therapy in the management of pituitary adenomas. *Clin Endocrinol Metab* 2011;96:1992–2003

42. Filipsson H. The impact of glucocorticoid replacement regimens on metabolic outcome and comorbidity in hypopituitary patients. *J Clin Endocrinol Metab* 2006;91:3954–3961

43. Colao A, De Block C, Gaztambide MS, Kumar S, Seufert J, Casanueva FF. Managing hyperglycemia in patients with Cushing's disease treated with pasireotide: medical expert recommendations. *Pituitary* 2014;17:180–186

44. Arnaldi G, Boscaro M. Pasireotide for the treatment of Cushing's disease. *Expert Opin Investig Drugs* 2010;19:889–898

45. Silverstein JM. Hyperglycemia induced by pasireotide in patients with Cushing's disease or acromegaly. *Pituitary* 2016;19:536–543

46. Reznik Y, Bertherat J, Borson-Chazot F, Brue T, Chanson P, Cortet-Rudelli C, Delemer B, Tabarin A, Bisot-Locard S, Verges B. Management of hyperglycaemia in Cushing's disease: experts' proposals on the use of pasireotide. *Diabetes Metab* 2013;39:34–41

47. Fleseriu M, Molitch ME, Gross C, Schteingart DE, Vaughan TB 3rd, Biller BM. A new therapeutic approach in the medical treatment of Cushing's syndrome: glucocorticoid receptor blockade with mifepristone. *Endocr Pract* 2013;19:313–326

48. Fleseriu M, Petersenn S. Medical therapy for Cushing's disease: adrenal steroidogenesis inhibitors and glucocorticoid receptor blockers. *Pituitary* 2015;18:245–252

49. Fleseriu M, Biller BM, Findling JW, Molitch ME, Schteingart DE, Gross C; SEISMIC Study Investigators. Mifepristone, a glucocorticoid receptor antagonist produces clinical and metabolic benefits in patients with Cushing's syndrome. *J Clin Endocrinol Metab* 2012;97:2039–2049

50. Fein HG, Vaughan TB 3rd, Kushner H, Cram D, Nguyen D. Sustained weight loss in patients treated with mifepristone for Cushing's syndrome: a follow-up analysis of the SEISMIC study and long-term extension. *BMC Endocr Disord* 2015;15:63

51. Pivonello R, De Martino MC, Cappabianca P, De Leo M, Faggiano A, Lombardi G, Hofland LJ, Lamberts SWJ, Colao A. The medical treatment of Cushing's disease: effectiveness of chronic treatment with the dopamine agonist cabergoline in patients unsuccessfully treated by surgery. *J Clin Endocrinol Metab* 2009;94:223–230

52. Wagenmakers MAEM, Roerink SHPP, Schreuder THA, Plantinga TS, Holewijn S, Thijssen DHJ, Smit JW, Rongen GA, Pereira AM, Wagenmakers AJM, Netea-Maier RT, Hermus ARMM. Vascular health in patients in remission of Cushing's syndrome is comparable with that in BMI-matched controls. *J Clin Endocrinol Metab* 2016;101:4142–4150

53. Boden G. Glucagonomas and insulinomas. *Gastroenterol Clin North Am* 1989;18:831–845

54. Soga J, Yakuwa Y. Glucagonomas/diabetico-dermatogenic syndrome (DDS): a statistical evaluation of 407 reported cases. *J Hepatobiliary Pancreat Surg* 1998;5:312–319

55. Mallison CN, Bloom SR, Warin AP, Salmon PR, Cox B. A glucagonoma syndrome. *Lancet* 1974;304:1–5

56. Wermers RA, Fatourechi V, Wynne AG, Kvols LK, Lloyd RV. The glucagonoma syndrome: clinical and pathologic features in 21 patients. *Medicine (Baltimore)* 1996;75:53–63

57. Kindmark H, Sundin A, Granberg D, Dunder K, Skogseid B, Janson ET, Welin S, Oberg K, Eriksson B. Endocrine pancreatic tumors with glucagon hypersecretion: a retrospective study of 23 cases during 20 years. *Med Oncol* 2007;24:330–337

58. Klein S, Jahoor F, Baba H, Townsend CM, Shepherd M, Wolfe RR. In vivo assessment of the metabolic alterations in glucagonoma syndrome. *Metabolism* 1992;41:1171–1175

59. Nair KS, Halliday D, Matthews DE, Welle SL. Hyperglucagonemia during insulin deficiency accelerates protein catabolism. *Am J Physiol* 1987;253:E208–E213

60. Roth E, Muhlbacher F, Karner J, Hamilton G, Funovics J. Free amino acid levels in muscle and liver of a patient with glucagonoma syndrome. *Metabolism* 1987;36:7–13

61. Unger RH, Cherrington AD. Glucagonocentric restructuring of diabetes: A pathophysiologic and therapeutic makeover. *J Clin Invest* 2012;122:4–12

62. Kazda CM, Ding Y, Kelly RP, Garhyan P, Shi C, Lim CN, Fu H, Watson DE, Lewin AJ, Landschulz WH, Deeg MA, Moller DE, Hardy TA. Evaluation of efficacy and safety of the glucagon receptor antagonist LY2409021 in patients with type 2 diabetes: 12- and 24-week phase 2 studies. *Diabetes Care* 2016;39:1241–1249

63. Fenkci SM, Yaylali GF, Sermez Y, Akdam H, Sabir N, Kirac S. Malign cystic gluca-gonoma presented with diabetic ketoacidosis: case report with an update. *Endocr Relat Cancer* 2005;12:449–454

64. Eldor R, Glaser B, Fraenkel M, Dovinert V, Salmon A, Gross DJ. Glucagonoma and the glucagonoma syndrome – cumulative experience with an elusive endo-crine tumor. *Clin Endocrinol* 2011;74:593–598

65. Garbrecht N, Anlauf M, Schmitt A, Henopp T, Sipos B, Raffel A, Eisenberger CF, Knoefel WT, Pavel M, Fottner C, Musholt TJ, Rinke A, Arnold R, Berndt U, Plockinger U, Wiedenmann B, Moch H, Heitz PU, Komminoth P, Perren A, Kloppel G. Somatostatin-producing neuroendocrine tumors of the duodenum and pancreas: incidence, types, biologic behavior, association with inherited syn-dromes, and functional activity. *Endocr Relat Cancer* 2008;15:229–241

66. Larsson LI, Hirsch MA, Holst JJ, Ingemansson S, Kuhl C, Jensen SL, Lundquist G, Rehfield JF, Schwartz TW. Pancreatic somatostatinoma. Clinical features and physiological implications. *Lancet* 1977;1:666–668

67. Soga J, Yakuwa Y. Somatostatinoma/inhibitory syndrome: a statistical evaluation of 173 reported cases as compared to other pancreatic endocrinomas. *J Exp Clin Cancer Res* 1999;18:13–22

68. House MG, Yeo CJ, Schulick RD. Periampullary pancreatic somatostatinoma. *Ann Surg Onc* 2002;9:869–874

69. Kumar T, Gupta B, Das P, Jain D, Jain HA, Madhusudhan KS, Dash NR, Gupta SD. Combined presence of multiple gastrointestinal stromal tumors along with duodenal submucosal somatostinoma in a patient with neurofibromatosis type 1. *Indian J Pathol Microbiol* 2016;59:359–361

70. Stacpoole PW, Kasselberg AG, Berelowitz M, Chey WY. Somatostatinoma syn-drome: does a clinical entity exist? *Acta Endocrinol (Copenh)* 1983;102:80–87

71. Green BT, Rockey DC. Duodenal somatostatinoma presenting with complete somatostatinoma syndrome. *J Clin Gastroenterol* 2001;33:415–417

72. Pipeleers D, Couturier E, Gepts W, Reynders J, Somers G. Five cases of somatostatinoma: clinical heterogeneity and diagnostic usefulness of basal and tolbutamide-induced hypersomatostatinemia. *J Clin Endocrinol Metab* 1983;56:1236–1242

73. Fishbein L. Pheochrochromocytoma and paraganglioma: genetics, diagnosis, and treatment. *Hematol Oncol Clin North Am* 2016;30:135–150

74. Pillai S, Gopalan V, Smith RA, Lam AK. Updates on the genetics and the clinical impacts on phaeochromocytoma and paraganglioma in the new era. *Crit Rev Oncol Hematol* 2016;100:190–208

75. Lenders JW, Duh QY, Eisenhofer G, Gimenez-Roqueplo AP, Grebe SKG, Murad MH, Naruse M, Pacak K, Young WF. Pheochromocytoma and paraganglioma: an Endocrine Society clinical practice guideline. *J Clin Endocrinol Metab* 2014;99:1915–1942

76. Amar L, Baudin E, Burnichon N, Peyrard S, Silvera S, Bertherat J, Bertagna X, Schlumberger M, Jeunemaitre X, Gimenez-Roqueplo AP, Plouin PF. Succinate dehydrogenase B gene mutations predict survival in patients with malignant pheochromocytomas or paragangliomas. *J Clin Endocrinol Metab* 2007; 92:3822–3828

77. Chen H, Sippel RS, O'Dorisio MS, et al. The North American Neuroendocrine Tumor Society consensus guideline for the diagnosis and management of neuro-endocrine tumors: pheochromocytoma, paraganglioma, and medullary thyroid cancer. *Pancreas* 2010;39:775–783

78. Manger WM, Gifford RW. Pheochromocytoma. *J Clin Hypertens (Greenwich)* 2002;4:62–72

79. Ishii C, Inoue K, Negishi K, Tane N, Awata T, Katayama S. Diabetic ketoacidosis in a case of pheochromocytoma. *Diabetes Res Clin Pract* 2001;54:137–142

80. Hamaji M. Pancreatic alpha- and beta-cell function in pheochromocytoma. *J Clin Endocrinol Metab* 1979;49:322–325

81. Khoury N, McGill JB. Reduction in insulin sensitivity following administration of the clinically used low-dose pressor, norepinephrine. *Diabetes Metab Res Rev* 2011;27:604–608

82. Vance JE, Buchanan KD, O'Hara D, Williams RH, Porte D. Insulin and glucagon responses in subjects with pheochromocytoma: effect of alpha adrenergic block-ade. *J Clin Endocrinol Metab* 1969;29:911–916

83. Lerner RL, Porte D. Epinephrine: selective inhibition of the acute insulin response to glucose. *J Clin Invest* 1971;50:2453–2457

84. Louis SN, Jackman GP, Nero TL, Iakovidis D, Louis WJ. Role of beta-adrenergic receptor subtypes in lipolysis. *Cardiovasc Drugs Ther* 2000;14:565–577

85. Germack R, Starzec AB, Vassy R, Perret GY. Beta-adrenoceptor subtype expres-sion and function in rat white adipocytes. *Br J Pharmacol* 1997;120:201–210

86. Saccà L, Vigorito C, Cicala M, Corso G, Sherwin RS. Role of gluconeogenesis in epinephrine-stimulated hepatic glucose production in humans. *Am J Physiol* 1983;245:E294–E302

87. Dufour S, Lebon V, Shulman GI, Petersen KF. Regulation of net hepatic glycogenolysis and gluconeogenesis by epinephrine in humans. *Am J Physiol Endocrinol Metab* 2009;297:E231–E235

88. Watt MJ, Howlett KF, Febbraio MA, Spriet LL, Hargreaves M. Adrenaline increases skeletal muscle glycogenolysis, pyruvate dehydrogenase activation and carbohydrate oxidation during moderate exercise in humans. *J Physiol* 2001;534:269–278

89. La Batide-Alanore A, Chatellier G, Plouin PF. Diabetes as a marker of pheochromocytoma in hypertensive patients. *J Hypertens* 2003;21:1703–1707

90. Stenström G, Sjöström L, Smith U. Diabetes mellitus in phaeochromocytoma. Fasting blood glucose levels before and after surgery in 60 patients with phaeochromocytoma. *Acta Endocrinol (Copenh)* 1984;106:511–515

91. Lenders JW, Eisenhofer G, Mannelli M, Pacak K. Phaeochromocytoma. *Lancet* 2005;366:665–675

92. Isles CG, Johnson JK. Phaeochromocytoma and diabetes mellitus: further evidence that alpha 2 receptors inhibit insulin release in man. *Clin Endocrinol (Oxf)* 1983;18:37–41

93. Akiba M, Kodama T, Ito Y, Obara T, Fujimoto Y. Hypoglycemia induced by excessive rebound secretion of insulin after removal of pheochromocytoma. *World J Surg* 1990;14:317–324

94. Chambers S, Espiner EA, Donald RA, Nicholls MG. Hypoglycaemia following removal of phaeochromocytoma: case report and review of the literature. *Postgrad Med J* 1982;58:503–506

95. Ross DS, Burch HB, Cooper DS, Greenlee MC, Laurberg P, Maia AL, Rivkees SA, Samuels M, Sosa JA, Stan MN, Walter MA. 2016 American Thyroid Association guidelines for diagnosis and management of hyperthyroidism and other causes of thyrotoxicosis. *Thyroid* 2016;26:1343–1421

96. De Leo S, Lee SY, Braverman LE. Hyperthyroidism. *Lancet* 2016;388:906–918

97. Garmendia MA, Santos Palacios S, Guillen-Grima F, Galofre JC. The incidence and prevalence of thyroid dysfunction in Europe: a meta-analysis. *J Clin Endocrinol Metab* 2014;99:923–931

98. Hollowell JC, Staehling NW, Flanders WD, Hannon HW, Spencer CA, Braverman LE. Serum TSH, T4 and thyroid antibodies in the United States population (1988 to 1994): National Health and Nutrition Examination Survey (NHANES III). *J Clin Endocrinol Metab* 2002;87:489–499

99. Abraham-Nordling M, Bystrom K, Torring O, Lantz M, Berg G, Calissendorff J, Nystrom HF, Jansson S, Jorneskog G, Karlsson FA, Hystrom E, Ohrling H, Orn T, Hallengran B, Wallin G. Incidence of hyperthyroidism in Sweden. *Eur J Endocrinol* 2011;165:899–905

100. Weetman AP. Graves' disease. *New Engl J Med* 2000;343:1236–1248

101. Nederstigt C, Corssmit EPM, Koning EJP, Dekkers OM. Incidence and prevalence of thyroid dysfunction in type 1 diabetes. *J Diabetes Complications* 2016;30:420–425

102. John HJ. Hyperthyroidism showing carbohydrate metabolism disturbances: ten years' study and follow-up of cases. *JAMA* 1932;99:620–627

103. Kreines K, Jett M, Knowles HC Jr. Observations in hyperthyroidism of abnormal glucose tolerance and other traits related to diabetes mellitus. *Diabetes* 1965;14:740–744

104. Maxon HR, Kreines KW, Goldsmith RE, Knowles HC Jr. Long-term observations of glucose tolerance in thyrotoxic patients. *Arch Intern Med* 1975;135:1477–1480

105. Yang L, Shen X, Yan S, Yuan X, Lu J, Wei W. HbA$_{1c}$ in the diagnosis and abnormal glucose tolerance in patients with Graves' hyperthyroidism. *Diabetes Res Clin Pract* 2013;101:28–34

106. Fleiner HF, Bjoro T, Midthjell K, Grill V, Asvold BO. Prevalence of thyroid dysfunction in autoimmune and type 2 diabetes: the population-based HUNT study in Norway. *J Clin Endocrinol Metab* 2016;101:669–677

107. Klubo-Gwiezdzinska J, Wartofsky L. Thyroid emergencies. *Med Clin North Am* 2012;96:385–403

108. Potenza M, Via MA, Yanagisawa RT. Excess thyroid hormone and carbohydrate metabolism. *Endocr Pract* 2009;15:254–262

109. Osada E, Hiroi N, Sue M, Nasai N, Iga R, Shigemitsu R, Oka R, Miyagi M, Iso K, Kuboki K, Yoshino G. Thyroid storm associated with Graves' disease covered by diabetic ketoacidosis: a case report. *Thyroid Res* 2011;4:8

110. Huang CY, Chen WL. Diabetic ketoacidosis as the initial presentation of hyperthyroidism. *Am J Emerg Med* 2015;33:1540.e1–1540.e2

111. Dimitriadis G, Baker B, Marsh H, Mandarino L, Rizza R, Bergman R, Haymond M, Gerich J. Effect of thyroid hormone excess on action, secretion, and metabolism of insulin in humans. *Am J Physiol* 1985;248:E593–601

112. Cavallo-Perin P, Bruno A, Boine L, Cassader M, Lenti G, Pagano G. Insulin resistance in Graves' disease: a quantitative in-vivo evaluation. *Eur J Clin Invest* 1988;18:607–613

113. Shen DC, Davidson MB, Kuo SW, Shew WH. Peripheral and hepatic insulin antagonism in hyperthyroidism. *J Clin Endocrinol Metab* 1988;66:565–569

114. Paul DT, Mollah FH, Alam MK, Fariduddin M, Azad K, Arslan MI. Glycemic status in hyperthyroid subjects. *Mymensing Med J* 2004;13:71–75

115. Maratou E, Hadjidakis DJ, Peppa M, Alevizaki M, Tsegka K, Lambadiari V, Mitrou P, Boutati E, Kollias A, Economopouloa T, Raptis S, Dimitriadis G. Studies of insulin resistance in patients with clinical and subclinical hyperthyroidism. *Eur J Endocrinol* 2010;163:625–630

116. Cachefo A, Boucher P, Vidon C, Dusserre E, Diraison F, Beylot M. Hepatic lipogenesis and cholesterol synthesis in hyperthyroid patients. *J Clin Endocrinol Metab* 2001;86:5353–5357

117. Betley S, Peak M, Agius L. Triiodo-L-thyronine stimulates glucogen synthesis in rat hepatocyte cultures. *Mol Cell Biochem* 1993;120:151–158

118. Weinstein SP, O'Boyle E, Haber RS. Thyroid hormone increases basal and insulin-stimulated glucose transport in skeletal muscle. The role of GLUT4 transporter expression. *Diabetes* 1994;43:1185–1189

119. Dimitriadis G, Pary-Billings M, Bevan S, Leighton B, Krause U, Piva T, Tegos K, Challiss RA, Wegener G, Newsholme EA. The effects of insulin on transport and metabolism of glucose in skeletal muscle from hyperthyroid and hypothyroid rats. *Eur J Clin Invest* 1997;27:475–483

120. Lahesmaa M, Orava J, Schalin-Jantti C, Soinio M, Hannukainen JC, Noponen T, Kirjavainen A, Iida H, Kudomi N, Enerback S, Virtanen KA, Nuutila P. Hyperthyroidism increases brown fat metabolism in humans. *J Clin Endocrinol* 2014;99:E28–E35

121. Mitrou P, Raptis SA, Dimitriadis G. Insulin action in hyperthyroidism: a focus on muscle and adipose tissue. *Endocr Rev* 2010;31:663–679

122. Gonzalo MA, Grant C, Moreno I, Garcia J, Suarez AI, Herrare-Pombo JL, Rovira A. Glucose tolerance, insulin secretion, insulin sensitivity and glucose effectiveness

in normal and overweight hyperthyroid women. *Clin Endocrinol* 1996;45: 689–697

123. Al-Shoumer KAS, Vasanthy BA, Al-Zaid MM. Effects of treatment of hyperthyroidism on glucose homeostasis, insulin secretion, and markers of bone turnover. *Endocr Pract* 2006;12:121–130

124. Dost A, Rohrer TR, Fröhlich-Reiterer E, Bollow E, Karges B, Bockmann A, Hamann J, Holl RW; for the DPV Initiative and the German Competence Network Diabetes Mellitus. Hyperthyroidism in 276 children and adolescents with type 1 diabetes from Germany and Austria. *Horm Res Paediatr* 2015;84:190–198

6
Immune-Mediated Diabetes

Maamoun F. Salam, MD;[1] Janet B. McGill, MD;[1] and
Jing W. Hughes, MD, PhD[1]

Latent Autoimmune Diabetes in Adults

Latent autoimmune diabetes in adults (LADA) is a common type of diabetes that has an autoimmune component but a different natural history than either type 1 diabetes (T1D) or type 2 diabetes (T2D). LADA shares genetic features and serologic markers with T1D, some genetic features with T2D, but patient phenotypic characteristics and management approaches are typically intermediary between T1D and T2D. While the World Health Organization considers LADA a slowly progressing subtype of T1D, individual patients may have a clinical picture that resembles T1D and progress to insulin dependency relatively rapidly, or patients can remain insulin independent for a long period of time, similar to patients with classic T2D. While LADA is considered as an admixture of the two major types of diabetes, it also represents incomplete destruction of β-cells by an autoimmune process that occurs in adults who present with variable body weight, insulin resistance, and other metabolic characteristics. In other words, T1D, LADA, and typical T2D form a continuum of varying severity of immune and metabolic dysfunction modified by genetic and nongenetic factors.[1-4]

[1]Washington University School of Medicine, St. Louis, MO

DOI: 10.2337/9781580406666.06

Definition and Diagnostic Criteria for LADA

Definitions and diagnostic criteria for LADA have varied over time and by different groups of investigators, but a consistent feature is the demonstration of autoimmunity or insulin deficiency. One definition of LADA proposed by the Immunology of Diabetes Society and Action LADA study includes: *1*) age 30–70 years at diagnosis, *2*) at least 6 months of non–insulin-requiring diabetes, and *3*) the presence of diabetes-associated autoantibodies like GAD 65, IA-2, or ZnT8.[1,5] Despite the global consensus on the autoimmune component of the definition, differences in the other two components are common, producing cohorts with different characteristics. The minimum age cutoff for LADA varies in studies from 25 to 40 years,[6–8] often without a clear rationale for the chosen criteria. Previously, the age cutoff for the diagnosis of T2D was established at 30 years,[9] but recognition of T2D in children and adolescents has markedly changed perception of this criterion, essentially invalidating age as a criterion for the diagnosis of T2D.[10] Likewise, patients of any age who present in diabetic ketoacidosis (DKA), or who develop it after being diagnosed with diabetes and are found to be insulin requiring after DKA, clearly merit a diagnosis of T1D, regardless of age. Patients with adult-onset T1D are generally excluded from studies of LADA patients and in general are an understudied population.

At least three factors influence the duration of the period between the diagnosis of diabetes and insulin initiation: *1*) the natural history of the disease, *2*) the timing of diagnosis in relation to natural history, and *3*) the therapeutic bias of the treating physician. These will vary from patient to patient.[5–8] For example, if diabetes is diagnosed on a mildly elevated glucose level in an asymptomatic person, this individual is likely to be diagnosed with T2D and may not require insulin for months to years. Conversely, if the same individual's presentation is delayed until he or she is symptomatic, the glucose is likely to be higher and insulin therapy may be started sooner. Patient characteristics and physician specialty and bias will determine whether testing of autoimmune markers or C-peptide is done, often resulting in delays making a correct diagnosis and starting insulin. Clearly, increased knowledge of the epidemiology, natural history, and pathogenesis of LADA is required to refine the diagnostic criteria across populations of age and ethnicity.[5]

LADA Epidemiology and Prevalence

Adult-onset autoimmune diabetes (including both T1D and LADA) is not rare. In the United Kingdom Prospective Diabetes Study (UKPDS), diabetes-related autoantibodies were found in ~10% of patients newly diagnosed with T2D.[1,6,11] Those with positive antibodies progressed to insulin therapy sooner than patients without antibodies. In a large cohort of adult-onset diabetes subjects diagnosed between 30 and 70 years of age attending primary and secondary care European centers, the prevalence of autoantibody positivity was 9.7%.[12] In this study, LADA was more prevalent than classic autoimmune T1D, odds ratio 3.3. Similar data from other ethnic groups are lacking, and the recent increases in rates of obesity and incidence of T2D have reduced the interest in screening all patients with T2D for islet autoimmunity.

LADA Pathogenesis

The natural history of preclinical LADA is unknown. The following two extreme possibilities are considered: patients with LADA could have either long-standing islet autoimmunity with slowly progressive β-cell damage over many years, or the onset of islet autoimmunity occurs in adulthood, corresponding with a shorter preclinical phase. The more logical notion, supported by leading investigators, is that autoimmune destruction of β-cells begins many years before diagnosis; however, this remains to be proven.[5]

An estimated 20–40% of LADA patients have at least one of the following antibodies: glutamic acid decarboxylase autoantibodies (GADA), tyrosine phosphatase autoantibodies (insulinoma-associated antigen-2 and 2B, designated IA-2 and IA-2beta), zinc-transporter 8 autoantibody (ZnT8A), or anti-insulin antibodies (valid if the patient has received insulin therapy for <2 weeks).[13-15] Figure 6.1 shows the percentage of the most common autoantibodies in autoimmune diabetes. Notably, a small percentage (4-5%) of nondiabetic populations may harbor GADA, suggesting that these disease markers require clinical correlation.[16,17]

All types of diabetes, including T1D, LADA, and T2D are polygenic in nature.

Genome-wide association studies showed that each major type of diabetes has a minimum of 50 associated genetic factors.[18,19] LADA shares genetic features with both T1D and T2D. Adult onset T1D and LADA have similar genetic features including human leukocyte antigen (HLA) types, insulin gene variable number of tandem repeats (INS VNTR), and protein tyrosine phosphatase nonreceptor type 22 (PTPN22).[2] The HLA locus confers most of the genetic susceptibility to T1D and LADA and is located on the short arm of chromosome 6.[20] Both T1D and LADA share HLA haplotypes including HLA

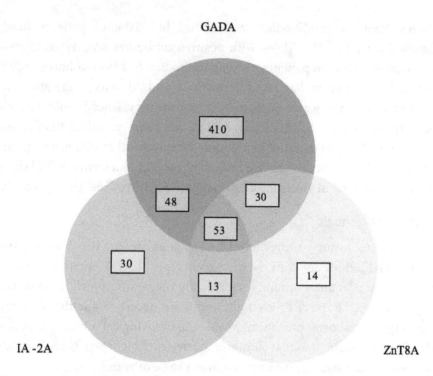

Figure 6.1—Autoantibodies in autoimmune diabetes (n = 598).

Venn diagram of numbers of patients with GADA, IA-2A, or ZnT8A; n = 598 of 6,156 (9.8%). Of the autoantibody-positive samples, GADA was identified in n = 541(90.5%) of the samples when an autoantibody was detected, with IA-2A and ZnT8A accounting for the remaining 9.5% of the autoantibodies detected. GADA, n = 541 (8.8%); IA-2A, n = 144 (2.3%); and ZnT8A, n = 110 (1.8%). *Source*: Adapted from Hawa et al.[12]

DQB1*0201/*0302 and limited HLA protection by HLA-DQB1*0602/X and 0603/X. Interestingly, HLA DQB1*0201/*0302 is observed more often in patients with classic T1D than in those presenting as LADA, whereas the protective genotype HLA-DQB1*0602/X is more common in LADA than in T1D.[21–23]

The insulin gene variable number of tandem repeats (INS VNTR) is located on chromosome 11 and has two general Classes—short (Class I: 26-63 repeats) and long (Class III: 141-209 repeats). The UKPDS cohorts showed that Class I has strong susceptibility to both T1DM and LADA.[24,25] The protein tyrosine phosphatase nonreceptor type 22 (PTPN22) gene on chromosome 1 also contributes to the genetic risk of both T1D and LADA.[26] Studies showed that a single nucleotide polymorphism (SNP) in the PTPN22 gene is associated with increased risk of T1D.[27] A meta-analysis in 2014 suggested that the same SNP in the PTPN22 gene also contributes to susceptibility to LADA.[28]

Transcription factor TCF genes have been shown to be associated with different subtypes of diabetes.[29-31] Of these genes, T2D and LADA share the transcription factor 7-like 2 (TCF7L2) gene,[2] which is not associated with T1D.[32] These relationships were confirmed in a Swedish cohort with a statistically significant increased frequency of TCF7L2 in both T2D 54.1% and LADA 52.8% when compared to T1D 43.3% and control subjects 44.8%.[2] The frequencies of the various risk genotypes for T1D, LADA, and T2D are shown in Figure 6.2.

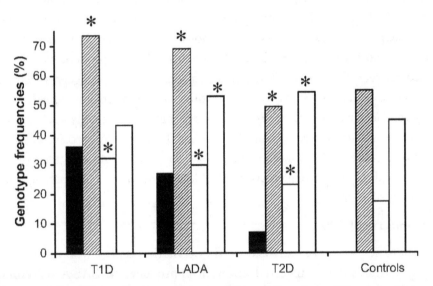

Figure 6.2—Risk genotype frequencies of the four different susceptibility loci in type 1 diabetes, LADA, and type 2 diabetes. HLA-DQB1 was not genotyped in control subjects. *Significant association to diabetes ($P < 0.05$).

■, HLA-DQB1 (*0201/*0302);

▨, INS VNTR-rs689 (AA genotype);

☐, PTPN22-rs2476601 (CT/TT genotypes)

▤, TCF7L2-rs7903146 (CT/TT genotypes).

T1D, type 1 diabetes; T2D, type 2 diabetes

Source: Adapted from Cervin et al[2] with permission.

Clinical and Metabolic Features

LADA shares autoimmune and insulin deficiency characteristics with T1D; however, other phenotypic features overlap with T2D cohorts. When compared to T2D patient cohorts, LADA patients tend to be leaner, have more symptoms including polyuria and polydipsia, have more pronounced unintentional weight loss, and have more organ-specific autoimmune diseases.[33] But, since LADA is diagnosed in adulthood, some patients will be overweight or obese, and some will have metabolic syndrome characteristics such as hypertension and hyperlipidemia.[12] When compared to autoantibody-negative patients with diabetes (presumed T2D), autoantibody positivity (T1D and LADA) was significantly associated with female gender, younger age at onset of diabetes, lower BMI, lower waist-to-hip ratio (WHR), lower waist circumference, lower systolic blood pressure (SBP), higher high-density lipoprotein (HDL), lower triglycerides (TG), and greater use of insulin. These associations were observed regardless of the number of positive autoantibodies.[12] But when similar comparisons were investigated between T1D and LADA, T1D was associated with younger age of onset of diabetes, greater use of insulin, shorter time to insulin use, lower BMI, lower WHR, and lower waist circumference. Other metabolic characteristics, including HDL, SBP, and TG levels were similar between T1D and LADA cohorts. These comparisons are depicted in Table 6.1, which shows autoantibody-positive versus autoantibody-negative patients, and Table 6.2, which compares patients with T1D versus LADA.[12]

Screening for LADA

There are no universally accepted criteria that define when to test for LADA. Studies have suggested different approaches to LADA screening, incorporating age of onset, BMI, hemoglobin A1C (HbA_{1c}), and C-peptide levels among other criteria. Newly diagnosed adult patients with diabetes should be considered for antibody testing if they have the following features: 1) age of onset <50 years, 2) acute symptoms, 3) BMI <25 kg/m^2, 4) personal history of autoimmune disease, and 5) family history of autoimmune disease. These features put together the LADA clinical risk score. The presence of two or more criteria (LADA clinical risk score ≥2) had a 90% sensitivity and 71% specificity for identifying patients positive for anti-GAD antibodies. The presence of only one feature or none had a negative predictive value of 99%.[33]

Table 6.1—Features of Any Autoantibody-Positive (GADA, IA-2A, or ZnT8A), LADA Patients, versus Autoantibody-Negative Presumed T2D Patients

	Autoantibody Positive	Autoantibody Negative	P
Cases	598	5,558	
Females, n (%)*	299 (50.0)	2,260 (40.7)	<0.001
Males, n (%)	294 (49.0)	3,298 (59.3)	
Age (years)	49.0 (10.7)	54.9 (9.4)	<0.001
Age at onset (years)	47.4 (11.7)	52.5 (10.6)	<0.001
Duration of disease (years)	2.2 (1.6)	2.3 (1.6)	>0.50
BMI (kg/m²)	27.2 (6.2)	30.9 (6.5)	<0.001
Subjects on insulin	279/564 (49.5)	728/5,508 (13.2)	<0.001
Time to insulin (years)	0.61 (1.03)	0.87 (1.4)	0.180
WHR	0.90 (0.1)	0.95 (0.09)	<0.001
Waist circumference (cm)	93.7 (16.1)	103.8 (14.6)	<0.001
HDL cholesterol (mmol/L)	1.44 (0.4)	1.29 (0.39)	<0.001
LDL cholesterol (mmol/L)	2.05 (0.95)	1.60 (0.82)	>0.50
Systolic BP (mmHg)	116.6 (29.1)	122 (31.0)	<0.001
TG (mmol/L)	1.5 (1.4)	1.97 (1.5)	<0.001

Data are n, means (SD), or n/n (%) unless otherwise indicated. More autoantibody-positive patients were receiving insulin (49.5 vs. 13.2% autoantibody-negative patients; P < 0.001), younger (49.6 vs. 54.9 years old), and leaner (27.2 vs. 30.9 kg/m²). BP, blood pressure; TG, triglyceride. *Information for sex was missing in five autoantibody cases.

Table 6.2—Features of Type 1 Diabetes versus LADA Patients

	Type 1 Diabetes	LADA	P
Cases	114	377	
Females, n (%)	55 (48.2)	187 (49.6)	
Males, n (%)	59 (51.8)	190 (50.4)	>0.50
Mean age (years)	44.1 (9.9)	51.9 (10.5)	<0.001
Age at onset (years)	41.8 (15.2)	49.7 (12.3)	<0.001
Duration of disease (years)	1.93 (1.7)	2.37 (1.6)	0.005
Subjects on insulin	114/114 (100)	152/377 (40.3)	<0.001
Time to insulin (years)	0.04 (0.08)	1.85 (1.1)	<0.001

(Continued)

Table 6.2—(Continued)

	Type 1 Diabetes	LADA	P
Multiple autoantibodies (GADA/IA-2A and ZnT8A)	15/114 (13.2)	34/377 (9.0)	0.17
GADA high titer	91/114 (79.8)	296/377 (78.5)	0.43
BMI (kg/m^2)	25.6 (5.0)	28.6 (6.6)	<0.001
WHR	0.87 (0.08)	0.90 (0.1)	<0.001
Waist circumference (cm)	88.3 (12.7)	96.8 (16.6)	<0.001
HDL cholesterol (mmol/L)	1.4 (0.4)	1.5 (0.5)	>0.5
LDL cholesterol (mmol/L)	2.8 (1.0)	2.2 (1.0)	0.013
Systolic BP (mmHg)	120 (25)	119 (26)	>0.5
TG (mmol/L)	1.2 (0.5)	1.6 (1.5)	0.16

Data are n, means (SD), or n/n (%) unless otherwise indicated. BP, blood pressure; TG, triglyceride.
Source: Hawa M et al.[12]

Natural History of LADA

LADA patients tend to be started on insulin later than in T1D but sooner than in T2D. It is possible that the early insulin use in LADA is driven by insulin deficiency rather than insulin resistance. This is supported by the following points:[34]

1. Insulin-treated LADA patients have higher GAD antibody titers than LADA patients not treated with insulin.
2. Insulin-treated LADA patients show a strong negative correlation between the GAD antibody titer and levels of C-peptide. This suggests more destruction of β-cells by the ongoing autoimmune process.
3. When compared to non-insulin-treated LADA patients, insulin-treated LADA patients did not have higher rates of adiposity, hypertension, dyslipidemia, or any other parameters associated with metabolic syndrome. Obesity was also observed in similar rates and extent in both groups. These observations make insulin resistance a less likely cause for the early use of insulin in LADA. To further support this point, obesity was more marked in T2D patients with a perceived need for insulin treatment.

An interesting, and unexplained, conundrum of diabetes antibody positivity is that the ability of GADA to predict progression to insulin treatment declines with age. In insulin-naïve patients, GADA predict more rapid progression to insulin treatment in those diagnosed under 45 years of age as compared with those diagnosed later (see Figure 6.3).[6] More relevant clinically is the negative predictive value of autoantibodies, which is the likelihood that patients with initially non–insulin-requiring diabetes without GADA will not progress to insulin treatment. In the UKPDS, only 5.7% without GADA went on to require insulin, with a high negative predictive value of 94%.[35]

Autoimmune Disease Association in LADA

LADA is associated with increased risk of thyroid and gastrointestinal autoimmunity.[36] About 25% of patients with adult-onset autoimmune diabetes have serological evidence of autoimmune thyroiditis, but there are no reports on the frequency of clinical thyroid disease.[5,37] About 19% of patients

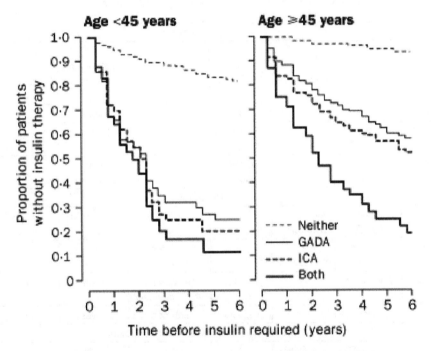

Figure 6.3—Kaplan-Meier plots of proportion of patients with and without islet-cell antibodies (ICA) and GADA requiring insulin therapy during 6 years' follow-up.

Source: Turner R et al.[6]

with LADA were reported to have antibodies to gliadin, but the prevalence of biopsy-confirmed celiac disease is unknown.[38] LADA has been noted to have increased frequency of antibodies to 21-hydroxylase and 17-hydroxylase, which are markers of autoimmune adrenal failure (Addison's disease).[39]

Table 6.3 summarizes the pathogenic characteristics, phenotypes, and genotypes of T1D, LADA, and T2D. Clearly additional work needs to be done to better understand the autoimmune disease burden in LADA.

Diabetes Complications in LADA

Table 6.4 shows comparisons of diabetes complications among T1D, LADA, and T2D.

Table 6.3—Pathogenesis, Phenotypic, and Genotype Comparisons: T1D, LADA, and T2D

	Pathogenesis					
	Beta Cell Destruction	Insulin Resistance	T Cell Mediated	Autoantibodies	Autoimmune Nature	Association with Autoimmune Disease
T1D	Complete	No	+	Present	Autoimmune	+++
LADA	Ongoing	+/-	+ less than T1	Present	Autoimmune	++?
T2D	No	Yes	Minimal or None	Not present	Non autoimmune	+
	Phenotype					
	Age at Onset	Metabolic Syndrome	BMI	Insulin Use	A1c at Dx	Family History
T1D	Youngest	+	Lowest	Immediate diagnosis	Highest	++
LADA	Adulthood	++	Variable	6+ months after diagnosis	High	High ++
T2D	Oldest	+++	Highest	Later on	Lowest	+++
	Genotype and Genetic Susceptibility					
	HLA-DQB1 *0201/*0302 Risk Factor	HLA-DQB1 *0602 Protective	PTPN22 gene	TCF7L2	INS VNTR	
T1D	+	+	+	-	++	
LADA	+	++	+	+	++	
T2D	-	-	+	+	+	

Table 6.4—Comparison of Diabetes Complications among T1D, LADA, and T2D

	Microvascular			Macrovascular	Comorbidities			
	Retinopathy	Nephropathy	Neuropathy	CHD	HTN	HLD	Obesity	Ketoacidosis
T1D	+++	++	+	+				++++
LADA	++	++	+ ↑ with duration of disease	++ ↑ with duration of disease	+	+	+	+/-
T2D	++	++	+++	+++	+++	+++	+++	+/---

Source: Kobayashi T et al.[14]

Patients with T1D have a higher frequency of retinopathy than patients diagnosed with either LADA or T2D. This is likely related to younger age of onset and longer duration of diabetes, and possibly more years in poor control.[40] Macrovascular complications were similar in patient cohorts with LADA and T2D despite the fact that hypertension, hyperlipidemia, and obesity are less common in LADA.[41]

Treatment and Management of LADA

Like T1D and T2D, treatment goals in LADA should be directed to achieve optimal glycemic control, preserve β-cell function, and decrease micro- and macrovascular complications while being safe and practical for everyday use. β-cell secretory function can be measured by fasting or stimulated C-peptide levels. There are no clear guidelines for treatment of patients with LADA. However, since patients with LADA have relative and possibly progressive insulin deficiency, early use of insulin seems prudent.

Diet and lifestyle changes are important in the management of LADA and should be tailored to the individual, taking into consideration phenotypic, ethnic, and social characteristics. LADA patients who are obese will benefit from caloric restriction and increased physical activity.[42,43]

All of the major European LADA studies showed that LADA patients progress to insulin treatment more rapidly than those with T2D.[6,12,36,44] However, many LADA patients can be managed successfully without insulin therapy. In one study, 44% of LADA patients were still not on insulin after 11.8 years of disease, perhaps reflecting lower GADA titers and less β-cell destruction.[45] LADA patients with higher autoantibody titers or lower C-peptide levels should be started on insulin therapy without delay to avoid prolonged periods of poor control and potentially to preserve β-cell function. Incretin-based therapy or potentially a combination of insulin plus incretin therapy has been postulated to preserve β-cell function, but this has not been proven.[46]

Insulin secretagogues such as sulfonylureas and glinides should probably be avoided, because patients treated with sulfonylureas have a faster loss of insulin secretory capacity than when treated with insulin. A Cochrane database systematic review of randomized controlled trials and controlled clinical trials showed that sulfonylureas did not only lead to earlier insulin dependence but also poorer metabolic control measured by HbA_{1c} when prescribed for patients with LADA compared to insulin alone.[47] Metformin and thiazolidinediones may provide a safe and efficacious adjunctive therapy to insulin when treating LADA. These agents are potentially interesting for LADA because they improve insulin content and secretion in β-cells; preserve β-cell mass, facilitate its proliferation, and protect it from oxidative stress and apoptosis; and have anti-inflammatory effects.[48-51] None of these effects have been shown to have clinical relevance in a LADA patient population, however. Metformin should be used carefully as there is a potential risk of lactic acidosis in patients who progress toward complete insulin deficiency.[52,53]

Incretin mimetics have demonstrated potential in the treatment of LADA.[51,54-57] Exenatide, a glucagon-like peptide (GLP)-1 agonist with glucoregulatory actions similar to the incretin hormones, has a potential beneficial effect on preservation/augmentation of β-cell mass by modifying the susceptibility to apoptotic injury, stimulating β-cell proliferation, and promoting islet neogenesis from precursor cells.[53,58] Dipeptidyl peptidase 4 (DPP-4) inhibitors increase incretin levels. A randomized controlled study evaluating the use of DPP-4 inhibitors showed the addition of sitagliptin to insulin in LADA patients maintained β-cell function when compared to insulin alone.[59] Sodium-glucose cotransporter 2 inhibitors are used to treat T2D. There is a growing body of evidence suggesting that they may be beneficial as adjunctive to insulin treatment in patients with T1D.[60] This group of drugs may potentially be useful in LADA patients. A cautionary note is the association of DKA with these agents, which could put both T1D and LADA patients at risk.

Immune modulation is a new horizon in the treatment of the autoimmune forms of diabetes, including T1D and LADA. A number of immune modulators have been studied in adults with new-onset immune-mediated diabetes, including heat shock protein,[51] diamyd, an alum-formulated human recombinant GAD65, otelixizumab, and others. None have shown efficacy in preserving C-peptide in randomized controlled trials.[42,61–64] Better understanding of the natural history of LADA is needed to develop study protocols for this population. The role of preserving C-peptide for both diabetes control and avoidance of complications needs further study.

Conclusion

LADA is a common disorder that merits awareness, accurate diagnosis, and appropriate treatment to ensure optimal outcomes. Given a broad phenotype and rate of loss of β-cell function, treatment should be tailored to individual patient needs. Preservation of C-peptide is a goal of both treating physicians and researchers. The best approach may be to use current therapies to achieve excellent glucose control. Further study is clearly needed to define screening and treatment guidelines, as well as to test the efficacy of immune modulating therapies.

Stiff Person Syndrome

Stiff person syndrome (SPS) is a rare neurologic disorder characterized by progressive muscle rigidity and stiffness. First described in 1924, the index patient was a 49-year-old Iowa farmer who over four years developed an insidious disability, including painful muscle spasms, difficulty walking, and stiffness in his trunk, who might "fall as a wooden man." He and another 13 patients were described in the seminal case series of SPS by Drs. Frederick Moersch and Henry Woltman of Mayo Clinic in 1956.[65] Initially nicknamed "stiff man syndrome," the disease has since been renamed to incorporate the other demographics affected.

SPS has a strong immunologic basis and is recognized as an autoimmune disease.[66] The majority of patients have high levels of autoantibodies in their serum or CSF against glutamic acid decarboxylase (GAD), the rate-limiting enzyme for the synthesis of the neurotransmitter gamma aminobutyric acid (GABA).[66,67] Not only are anti-GAD antibodies a strong marker of disease, they are also implicated in the pathophysiology of SPS as they inhibit GAD activity and GABA synthesis,[68] and antibody titers correlate with the severity of neurologic disease. Other antibodies described include anti-amphiphysin and antigephyrin, which are associated with the paraneoplastic variant of SPS.[69,70]

Classic SPS is characterized by excessive rigidity that affects the trunk, lumbar, and proximal limb muscles. It usually presents with comorbid autoimmune conditions, most commonly T1D, which shares the same autoantigen GAD, albeit the autoantibodies in each case recognize different GAD epitopes.[71,72] GAD65 antibody titers tend to be 5–10 fold higher in SPS than typically seen in T1D; these antibodies not only act as a marker for the disease but also the likely source for the neuropathy itself, as GAD antibodies target GABAergic neurons and their nerve terminals. In contrast, anti-GAD autoantibodies in T1D are not necessarily pathogenic. Also, distinct from T1D but similar to other autoimmune diseases, SPS shows a strong female predominance, and its clinical presentation is often modified by emotional stress or anxiety. Other associated autoimmune conditions include Graves' disease, celiac sprue, vitiligo, and rheumatologic diseases.[73–75] SPS is also found in certain malignancies and postulated to be due to altered humoral immunity from paraneoplastic syndromes.[76,77]

The diagnosis of SPS is based on both clinical and neurophysiologic features. An electromyogram usually shows abnormal contractions of antagonistic muscles and continuous motor unit activity that can be abolished by diazepam, sleep, and anesthesia.[78] Notable differential diagnoses include tetany, restless leg syndrome, startle disease, and progressive encephalomyelitis with rigidity and myoclonus. In addition, due to the strong emotional component in SPS attacks and the fact that these patients often suffer psychiatric comorbidities including anxiety and depression, SPS is unfortunately sometimes misdiagnosed as a factitious disorder, conversion disorder, or even malingering.

Treatment for SPS is twofold: symptomatic control with antispasmodics, and immunosuppressive therapy. Diazepam has long been used in the management of SPS, as benzodiazepines can potentiate GABA activity. Baclofen is another GABA-modulating drug that can be used with or instead of benzodiazepines. When the disease is severe, immunosuppressive therapy is also considered, generally with high-dose glucocorticoids or IVIG. Plasmapheresis is reserved for patients with respiratory compromise. Anecdotal use of the β-cell depleting agent rituximab has been reported with some success.[79]

Although the majority of SPS cases are autoimmune in nature, there exist other subtypes including the paraneoplastic and idiopathic variants. Paraneoplastic markers such as anti-amphiphysin antibodies have been observed in SPS, predominantly in patients with carcinoma. Therefore, an extensive paraneoplastic workup is often required before deferring to the diagnosis of SPS.

Anti-Insulin Receptor Antibody–Related Diabetes

Anti-insulin receptor antibodies cause a rare, but well-described form of immune-mediated diabetes that was first reported by Flier et al. in 1975 in a small cohort of six women.[80] The cause of the syndrome was determined to be an autoantibody or antibodies directed against the cell surface insulin receptor.[80-82] The term type B insulin resistance (TBIR) syndrome was proposed by Kahn et al. in 1976, and additional cases were noted.[82,83] The initial cohorts were middle-aged women with other autoimmune diseases, typically systemic lupus erythematosus (SLE); however, later reports have included men and patients across the age spectrum.[84-86] The presentation is usually moderate to severe hyperglycemia with accompanying weight loss and symptomatic polyuria and polydipsia. Extreme insulin resistance is determined by measurement of elevated insulin and C-peptide levels, and poor response to exogenous insulin, even when it is given in supraphysiologic doses. While the etiology of the syndrome is clearly the presence of anti-insulin receptor antibodies (AIRA), assays of AIRA are not available through commercial labs; thus the diagnosis of the disorder is based on clinical signs and symptoms.

TBIR is an uncommon disorder, and despite a plethora of case reports, the exact prevalence is unknown. The largest case series was published in 2002, and reflected over 25 years of experience with TBIR syndrome at the National Institutes of Health (NIH): 24 patients were included with follow-up of 0–28 years.[87] The majority of the patients were female (20/24, 83%) and 88% were African American, including all of the men. Acanthosis nigricans was present in 21 of the 24 patients and involved the axilla, groin, and neck but also the face in a distinctive distribution around the lips and eyes. Other physical findings included low or reduced BMI in patients presenting with hyperglycemia, but higher BMI in those presenting with hypoglycemia. Hyperandrogenism and enlarged ovaries were common in females, including one prepubertal girl.[87,88] In addition to hyperglycemia and elevated HbA$_{1c}$, typical laboratory findings in TBIR syndrome include markedly elevated fasting insulin concentrations, hyperadiponectinemia, and low to normal fasting triglycerides.[87,89] Proteinuria, indicating immune-mediated glomerular disease, was present in half of the patients and has been subsequently described in a patient with SLE.[87,90] While the most common presentation in the NIH series was rapid development of severe hyperglycemia and weight loss, patients have also presented with hypoglycemia.[87,91–93]

SLE is the most common autoimmune disease associated with TBIR syndrome and generally precedes the metabolic disorder.[87–90] Other autoimmune diseases have been reported in patients with TBIR syndrome, including primary biliary cirrhosis, thyroiditis, progressive systemic sclerosis, Sjogren syndrome, autoimmune thrombocytopenia, and interstitial lung disease.[87,88,94–98] Rarely, patients with malignancies such as Hodgkin's disease develop antibodies to the insulin receptor and either hyper- or hypoglycemia.[99] The diagnosis of TBIR syndrome is often recognized when steroid treatment of the underlying autoimmune disease improves the hyperglycemia in these insulin-resistant patients rather than worsening it, suggesting an autoimmune cause for the metabolic disorder.

Anti-insulin receptor antibodies are polyclonal, are primarily from the IgG class, and may bind to cells constitutively causing unremitting insulin resistance or hypoglycemia.[80,85,90,95,100,101] The clinical course of this antibody-mediated disease is highly variable, but it tends to parallel the antibody levels in cases in which they have been measured serially.[87,101–103] In the NIH series, one-third of patients had spontaneous remission of their insulin resistance, acanthosis nigricans, hyperandrogenism, and diabetes over months to years.[87] Spontaneous remission of all symptoms has been reported similarly by others.[86,101–103] Treatment of hyperglycemia in TBIR syndrome varies from the use of typical oral agents only in mild cases or those in remission to insulin in doses up to thousands of units daily.[87,104] Use of concentrated insulin, either by injection or via an insulin pump has provided glycemic control in some cases.[104] Insulin-like growth factor (IGF-1) has also been used with some success, but it is no longer available.[105]

In the majority of cases, the inability to control hyperglycemia with extraordinarily high doses of insulin or the presence of persistent hypoglycemia has prompted the use of immune-modulating treatments.[8] Corticosteroids are often the mainstay of treatment, but side effects from high-dose steroids and incomplete response can be problematic.[87,100] Cyclosporine has been used successfully alone or in combination with plasmapheresis and cyclosporine A.[87,97,106] Other regimens have included azathioprine, mycophenolate mofetil, rituximab, intravenous immunoglobulin therapy, or a combination of these agents.[87,98,107–110] In the NIH cohort, half of the patients in whom spontaneous remission did not occur responded to immune-modulating therapy and had euglycemia restored, while the other half had persistent hyperglycemia that was treatment resistant.[87] A few patients in the follow-up study, and in other reports, experience a transition from hyperglycemia to hypoglycemia as their dominant symptom, which may increase the risk of mortality.[87,111]

TBIR syndrome is a rare condition most often seen in middle-aged African-American women with underlying SLE or other systemic autoimmune disease. Autoantibodies to the insulin receptor have uncertain behavior, causing either extreme insulin resistance or hypoglycemia. Spontaneous remission occurs in about one-third of patients, and another third respond to immune modulating therapies. Persistence of treatment-resistant hyper- or hypoglycemia may herald increased mortality in this syndrome.

References

1. Leslie RD, Kolb H, Schloot NC, et al. Diabetes classification: grey zones, sound, and smoke: action LADA 1. *Diabetes Metab Res Rev* 2008;24:511–519

2. Cervin C, Lyssenko V, Bakhtadze E, et al. Genetic similarities between latent autoimmune diabetes in adults, type 1 diabetes, and type 2 diabetes. *Diabetes* 2008;57:1433–1437

3. Alberti KG, Zimmet PZ. Definition, diagnosis and classification of diabetes mellitus and its complications. Part 1: diagnosis and classification of diabetes mellitus provisional report of a WHO consultation. *Diabet Med* 1998:15;539–553

4. Groop L, Tuomi T, Rowley M, Zimmet P, Mackay IR. Latent autoimmune diabetes in adults (LADA)—more than a name. *Diabetologia* 2006;49:1996–1998

5. Fourlanos S, Dotta F, Greenbaum CJ, et al. Latent autoimmune diabetes in adults (LADA) should be less latent. *Diabetologia* 2005;48:2206–2212

6. Turner R, Stratton I, Horton V, et al. UKPDS 25: autoantibodies to islet-cell cytoplasm and glutamic acid decarboxylase for prediction of insulin requirement in type 2 diabetes. U.K. Prospective Diabetes Study Group. *Lancet* 1997;350:1288–1293

7. Hosszúfalusi N, Vatay A, Rajczy K, et al. Similar genetic features and different islet cell autoantibody pattern of latent autoimmune diabetes in adults (LADA) compared with adult-onset type 1 diabetes with rapid progression. *Diabetes Care* 2003;26;452–457

8. Cosentino A, Gambelunghe G, Tortoioli C, Falorni A. CTLA-4 gene polymorphism contributes to the genetic risk for latent autoimmune diabetes in adults. *Ann N Y Acad Sci* 2002;958:337–340

9. Kahn R, Alperin P, Eddy D, et al. Age at initiation and frequency of screening to detect type 2 diabetes: a cost-effectiveness analysis. *Lancet* 2010;375:1365–1374

10. American Diabetes Association. 2. Classification and diagnosis of diabetes. *Diabetes Care* 2016;39(Suppl. 1):S13–S22

11. Leslie RD, Williams R, Pozzilli P. Clinical review: type 1 diabetes and latent autoimmune diabetes in adults: one end of the rainbow. *J Clin Endocrinol Metab* 2006;91:1654–1659

12. Hawa MI, Kolb H, Schloot N, et al. Adult-onset autoimmune diabetes in Europe is prevalent with a broad clinical phenotype. *Diabetes Care* 2013;36:908–913

13. Biesenbach G, Auinger M, Clodi M, et al. Prevalence of LADA and frequency of GAD antibodies in diabetic patients with end-stage renal disease and dialysis treatment in Austria. *Nephrol Dial Transplant* 2005;20:559–565

14. Kobayashi T, Tamemoto K, Nakanishi K, et al. Immunogenetic and clinical characterization of slowly progressive IDDM. *Diabetes Care* 1993;16:780–788

15. Kanungo A, Sanjeevi CB. IA-2 autoantibodies are predominant in latent autoimmune diabetes in adults patients from eastern India. *Ann N Y Acad Sci* 2003;1005:390–394

16. Kulmala P, Rahko J, Savola K, et al. Beta-cell autoimmunity, genetic susceptibility, and progression to type 1 diabetes in unaffected schoolchildren. *Diabetes Care* 2001;24:171–173

17. Strebelow M, Schlosser M, Ziegler B, Rjasanowski I, Ziegler M. Karlsburg type I diabetes risk study of a general population: frequencies and interactions of the four major type I diabetes-associated autoantibodies studied in 9419 schoolchildren. *Diabetologia* 1999;42:661–670

18. Atkinson MA, Eisenbarth GS, Michels AW. Type 1 diabetes. *Lancet* 2014;383: 69–82

19. Kahn SE, Cooper ME, Del Prato S. Pathophysiology and treatment of type 2 diabetes: perspectives on the past, present, and future. *Lancet* 2014;383:1068–1083

20. Kantárová D, Buc M. Genetic susceptibility to type 1 diabetes mellitus in humans. *Physiol Res* 2007;56:255–266

21. Tuomi T, Carlsson A, Li H, et al. Clinical and genetic characteristics of type 2 diabetes with and without GAD antibodies. *Diabetes* 1999;48:150–157

22. Greenbaum CJ, Schatz DA, Cuthbertson D, et al. Islet cell antibody-positive relatives with human leukocyte antigen DQA1*0102, DQB1*0602: identification by the Diabetes Prevention Trial-type 1. *J Clin Endocrinol Metab* 2000;85:1255–1260

23. Sabbah E, Savola K, Ebeling T, et al. Genetic, autoimmune, and clinical characteristics of childhood- and adult-onset type 1 diabetes. *Diabetes Care* 2002;23:1326–1332

24. Bennett ST, Todd JA. Human type 1 diabetes and the insulin gene: principles of mapping polygenes. *Annu Rev Genet* 1996;30:343–370

25. Desai M, Zeggini E, Horton VA, et al. The variable number of tandem repeats upstream of the insulin gene is a susceptibility locus for latent autoimmune diabetes in adults. *Diabetes* 2006;55:1890–1894

26. Bottini N, Musumeci L, Alonso A, et al. A functional variant of lymphoid tyrosine phosphatase is associated with type I diabetes. *Nat Genet* 2004;36:337–338

27. Smyth D, Cooper JD, Collins JE, Replication of an association between the lymphoid tyrosine phosphatase locus (LYP/PTPN22) with type 1 diabetes, and evidence for its role as a general autoimmunity locus. *Diabetes* 2004;53:3020–3023

28. Dong F, Yang G, Pan H-W, et al. The association of PTPN22 rs2476601 polymorphism and CTLA-4 rs231775 polymorphism with LADA risks: a systematic review and meta-analysis. *Acta Diabetol* 2014;51:691–703

29. Grant SF, Thorleifsson G, Reynisdottir I, et al. Variant of transcription factor 7-like 2 (TCF7L2) gene confers risk of type 2 diabetes. *Nat Genet* 2006;38:320–323

30. Saxena R, Gianniny L, Burtt NP, et al. Common single nucleotide polymorphisms in TCF7L2 are reproducibly associated with type 2 diabetes and reduce the insulin response to glucose in nondiabetic individuals. *Diabetes* 2006;55:2890–2895

31. Noble JA, White AM, Lazzeroni LC, et al. A polymorphism in the TCF7 gene, C883A, is associated with type 1 diabetes. *Diabetes* 2003;52:1579–1582

32. Field SF, Howson JMM, Smyth DJ, Walker NM, Todd JA. Analysis of the type 2 diabetes gene, TCF7L2, in 13,795 type 1 diabetes cases and control subjects. *Diabetologia* 2007;50:212–213

33. Fourlanos S, Perry C, Stein MS, et al. A clinical screening tool identifies autoimmune diabetes in adults. *Diabetes Care* 2006;29:970–975

34. Radtke MA, Midthjell K, Nilsen TIL, Grill V. Heterogeneity of patients with latent autoimmune diabetes in adults: linkage to autoimmunity is apparent only in those with perceived need for insulin treatment: results from the Nord-Trøndelag Health (HUNT) study. *Diabetes Care* 2009;32:245–250

35. Bottazzo GF, Bosi E, Cull CA, et al. IA-2 antibody prevalence and risk assessment of early insulin requirement in subjects presenting with type 2 diabetes (UKPDS 71). *Diabetologia* 2005;48:703–708

36. Zampetti S, Capizzi M, Spoletini M, et al. GADA titer-related risk for organ-specific autoimmunity in LADA subjects subdivided according to gender (NIRAD study 6). *J Clin Endocrinol Metab* 2012;97:3759–3765

37. Jin P, Huang G, Lin J, et al. High titre of antiglutamic acid decarboxylase autoantibody is a strong predictor of the development of thyroid autoimmunity in patients with type 1 diabetes and latent autoimmune diabetes in adults. *Clin Endocrinol (Oxf)* 2011;74:587–592

38. Kucera P, Nováková D, Behanová M, et al. Gliadin, endomysial, and thyroid antibodies in patients with latent autoimmune diabetes of adults (LADA). *Clin Exp Immunol* 2003;133:139–143

39. Gambelunghe G, Forini F, Laureti S, et al. Increased risk for endocrine autoimmunity in Italian type 2 diabetic patients with GAD65 autoantibodies. *Clin Endocrinol (Oxf)* 2000;52:565–573

40. The Diabetes Control and Complications Trial Research Group. Effect of intensive therapy on residual beta-cell function in patients with type 1 diabetes in the Diabetes Control and Complications Trial. A randomized, controlled trial. *Ann Intern Med* 1998;128:517–523

41. Isomaa B, Almgren P, Henricsson M, et al. Chronic complications in patients with slowly progressing autoimmune type 1 diabetes (LADA). *Diabetes Care* 1999;22:1347–1353

42. Pozzilli P, Guglielmi C. Immunomodulation for the prevention of SPIDDM and LADA. *Ann N Y Acad Sci* 2006;1079:90–98

43. Davis TM, Wright AD, Mehta ZM, et al. Islet autoantibodies in clinically diagnosed type 2 diabetes: prevalence and relationship with metabolic control (UKPDS 70). *Diabetologia* 2005;48:695–702

44. Andersen CD, Bennet L, Nyström L, et al. Worse glycaemic control in LADA patients than in those with type 2 diabetes, despite a longer time on insulin therapy. *Diabetologia* 2013;56:252–258

45. Hawa MI, Buchan AP, Ola T, et al. LADA and CARDS: a prospective study of clinical outcome in established adult-onset autoimmune diabetes. *Diabetes Care* 2014;37:1643–1649

46. Leslie RD, Palmer J, Schloot NC, Lernmark A. Diabetes at the crossroads: relevance of disease classification to pathophysiology and treatment. *Diabetologia* 2016;59:13–20

47. Brophy S, Davies H, Mannan S, Brunt H, Williams R. Interventions for latent autoimmune diabetes (LADA) in adults. *Cochrane Database Syst Rev* 2011;7:CD006165

48. Hanefeld M. Pioglitazone and sulfonylureas: effectively treating type 2 diabetes. *Int J Clin Pract Suppl* 2007;61:20–27

49. Finegood DT, McArthur MD, Kojwang D, et al. Beta-cell mass dynamics in Zucker diabetic fatty rats. Rosiglitazone prevents the rise in net cell death. *Diabetes* 2001;50:1021–1029

50. Diani AR, Sawada G, Wyse B, Murray FT, Khan M. Pioglitazone preserves pancreatic islet structure and insulin secretory function in three murine models of type 2 diabetes. *Am J Physiol Endocrinol Metab* 2004;286:E116–E122

51. Guglielmi C, Palermo A, Pozzilli P. Latent autoimmune diabetes in the adults (LADA) in Asia: from pathogenesis and epidemiology to therapy. *Diabetes Metab Res Rev* 2012;28(Suppl. 2):40–46

52. Pozzilli P, Di Mario U. Autoimmune diabetes not requiring insulin at diagnosis (latent autoimmune diabetes of the adult). *Diabetes Care* 2001;24:1460–1467

53. Cernea S, Buzzetti R, Pozzilli P. β-cell protection and therapy for latent autoimmune diabetes in adults. *Diabetes Care* 2009;32:S246–S252

54. Ghazi T, Rink L, Sherr JL, Herold KC. Acute metabolic effects of exenatide in patients with type 1 diabetes with and without residual insulin to oral and intravenous glucose challenges. *Diabetes Care* 2014;37:210–216

55. Lebovitz HE. Adjunct therapy for type 1 diabetes mellitus. *Nat Rev Endocrinol* 2010;6:326–334

56. Munir KM, Davis SN. The treatment of type 1 diabetes mellitus with agents approved for type 2 diabetes mellitus. *Expert Opin Pharmacother* 2015;16:2331–2341

57. Renukuntla VS, Ramchandani N, Trast J, Cantwell M, Heptulla RA. Role of glucagon-like peptide-1 analogue versus amylin as an adjuvant therapy in type 1 diabetes in a closed loop setting with ePID algorithm. *J Diabetes Sci Technol* 2014;8:1011–1017

58. Xu G, Stoffers DA, Habener JF, Bonner-Weir S. Exendin-4 stimulates both beta-cell replication and neogenesis, resulting in increased beta-cell mass and improved glucose tolerance in diabetic rats. *Diabetes* 1999;48:2270–2276

59. Zhao Y, Yang L, Xiang Y, et al. Dipeptidyl peptidase 4 inhibitor sitagliptin maintains β-cell function in patients with recent-onset latent autoimmune diabetes in adults: one year prospective study. *J Clin Endocrinol Metab* 2014;99:E876–E880

60. Perkins BA, Cherney DZ, Partridge H, et al. Sodium-glucose cotransporter 2 inhibition and glycemic control in type 1 diabetes: results of an 8-week open-label proof-of-concept trial. *Diabetes Care* 2014;37:1480–1483

61. Birk OS, Elias D, Weiss AS, et al. NOD mouse diabetes: the ubiquitous mouse hsp60 is a beta-cell target antigen of autoimmune T cells. *J Autoimmun* 1996;9:159–166

62. Raz I, Elias D, Avron A, et al. Beta-cell function in new-onset type 1 diabetes and immunomodulation with a heat-shock protein peptide (DiaPep277): a randomised, double-blind, phase II trial. *Lancet* 2001;358:1749–1753

63. Raz I, Avron A, Tamir M, et al. Treatment of new-onset type 1 diabetes with peptide DiaPep277 is safe and associated with preserved beta-cell function: extension of a randomized, double-blind, phase II trial. *Diabetes Metab Res Rev* 2007;23:292–298

64. Agardh CD, Cilio CM, Lethagen A, et al. Clinical evidence for the safety of GAD65 immunomodulation in adult-onset autoimmune diabetes. *J Diabetes Complications* 2005;19:238–246

65. Moersch FP, Woltman HW. Progressive fluctuating muscular rigidity and spasm ("stiff-man" syndrome); report of a case and some observations in 13 other cases. *Proc Staff Meet Mayo Clin* 1956;31:421–427

66. Blum P, Jankovic J. Stiff-person syndrome: an autoimmune disease. *Mov Disord* 1991;6:12–20

67. Butler MH, Solimena M, Dirkx R, Hayday A, De Camilli P. Identification of a dominant epitope of glutamic acid decarboxylase (GAD-65) recognized by auto-antibodies in stiff-man syndrome. *J Exp Med* 1993;178:2097–2106

68. Ali F, Rowley M, Jayakrishnan B, et al. Stiff-person syndrome (SPS) and anti-GAD-related CNS degenerations: protean additions to the autoimmune central neuropathies. *J Autoimmun* 2011;37:79–87

69. De Camilli P, Thomas A, Cofiell R, et al. The synaptic vesicle-associated protein amphiphysin is the 128-kD autoantigen of stiff-man syndrome with breast cancer. *J Exp Med* 1993;178:2219–2223

70. Butler MH, Hayashi A, Ohkoshi N, et al. Autoimmunity to gephyrin in stiff-man syndrome. *Neuron* 2000;26:307–312

71. Solimena M, Folli F, Aparisi R, Pozza G, De Camilli, P. Autoantibodies to GABA-ergic neurons and pancreatic β-cells in stiff-man syndrome. *N Engl J Med.* 1990;322:1555–1560

72. Kim J, Namchuk M, Bugawan T, et al. Higher autoantibody levels and recognition of a linear NH2-terminal epitope in the autoantigen GAD65, distinguish stiff-man syndrome from insulin-dependent diabetes mellitus. *J Exp Med* 1994; 180:595–606

73. O'Sullivan EP, Behan LA, King TFJ, Hardiman O, Smith D. A case of stiff-person syndrome, type 1 diabetes, celiac disease and dermatitis herpetiformis. *Clin Neurol Neurosurg* 2009;111:384–386

74. George TM, Burke JM, Sobotka PA, Greenberg HS, Vinik AI. Resolution of stiff-man syndrome with cortisol replacement in a patient with deficiencies of ACTH, growth hormone, and prolactin. *N Engl J Med* 1984;310:1511–1513

75. Orija IB, Gupta M, Zimmerman RS. Graves' disease and stiff-person (stiff-man) syndrome: case report and literature review. *Endocr Pract* 2005;11:259–264

76. Grimaldi LM, Martino G, Braghi S, et al. Heterogeneity of autoantibodies in stiff-man syndrome. *Ann Neurol* 1993;34:57–64

77. Ariño H, Höftberger R, Gress-Arribas N, et al. Paraneoplastic neurological syndromes and glutamic acid decarboxylase antibodies. *JAMA Neurol* 2015;72:874–881

78. Lorish TR, Thorsteinsson G, Howard FM. Stiff-man syndrome updated. *Mayo Clin Proc* 1989;64:629–636

79. Baker MR, Das M, Isaacs, J, Fawcett P, Bates D. Treatment of stiff person syndrome with rituximab. *J Neurol Neurosurg Psychiatry* 2005;76:999–1001

80. Flier JS, Kahn CR, Roth J, Bar RS. Antibodies that impair insulin receptor binding in an unusual diabetic syndrome with severe insulin resistance. *Science* 1975;190:63–65

81. Carnegie PR, Mackay IR. Vulnerability of cell-surface receptors to autoimmune reactions. *Lancet* 1975;2:684–687

82. Pulini M, Raff SB, Chase R, Gordon EE. Insulin resistance and acanthosis nigricans. Report of a case with antibodies to insulin receptors. *Ann Intern Med* 1976;85:749–751

83. Kahn CR, Flier JS, Bar RS, et al. The syndromes of insulin resistance and acanthosis nigricans. Insulin-receptor disorders in man. *N Engl J Med* 1976;294:739–745

84. Wilkin TJ. Receptor autoimmunity in endocrine disorders. *N Engl J Med* 1990;323:1318–1324

85. Baldwin D, Winston E, Hoshizaki RJ, et al. Insulin-resistant diabetes with insulin receptor autoantibodies in a male patient without acanthosis nigricans. *Diabetes Care* 1979;2:275–277

86. Esperanza LE, Fenske NA. Hyperandrogenism, insulin resistance, and acanthosis nigricans (HAIR-AN) syndrome: spontaneous remission in a 15-year-old girl. *J Am Acad Dermatol* 1996;34:892–897

87. Arioglu E, Andewelt A, Diabo C, et al. Clinical course of the syndrome of autoantibodies to the insulin receptor (type B insulin resistance): a 28-year perspective. *Medicine (Baltimore)* 2002;81:87–100

88. Kellett HA, Collier A, Taylor R, et al. Hyperandrogenism, insulin resistance, acanthosis nigricans, and systemic lupus erythematosis associated with insulin receptor antibodies. *Metabolism* 1988;37:656–659

89. Willard DL, Stevenson M, Steenkamp D. Type B insulin resistance syndrome. *Curr Opin Endocrinol Diabetes Obes* 2016;23:318–323

90. De Pirro RD, Borboni P, Lauro R, et al. Tissue-specific antibodies against the fibroblast insulin receptor in a patient with lupus nephritis and hypoglycemia. *Diabetes* 1985;34:1088–1091

91. Taylor SI, Grunberger G, Marcus-Samuels B, et al. Hypoglycemia associated with antibodies to the insulin receptor. *N Engl J Med* 1982;307:1422–1426

92. Varga J, Lopatin M, Boden G. Hypoglycemia due to antiinsulin receptor antibodies in systemic lupus erythematosus. *J Rheumatol* 1990;17:1226–1229

93. Tardella L, Rossetti L, De Pirro R, et al. Circulating anti-insulin receptor antibodies in a patient suffering from lupus nephritis and hypoinsulinemic hypoglycaemia. *J Clin Lab Immunol* 1983;12:159–165

94. Selinger S, Tsai J, Pulini M, Saperstein A, Taylor S. Autoimmune thrombocytopenia and primary biliary cirrhosis with hypoglycemia and insulin receptor autoantibodies. A case report. *Ann Intern Med* 1987;107:686–688

95. Bloise W, Wajchenberg BL, Moncada VY, Marcus-Samuels B, Taylor SI. Atypical antiinsulin receptor antibodies in a patient with type B insulin resistance and scleroderma. *J Clin Endocrinol Metab* 1989;68:227–231

96. Kinoshita O, Kubo K, Kusama S. A case of insulin resistant diabetes mellitus due to insulin-receptor autoantibodies with Sjögren syndrome. *Nihon Naika Gakkai Zasshi* 1988;77:1572–1575

97. Kramer N, Rosenstein ED, Schneider G. Refractory hyperglycemia complicating an evolving connective tissue disease: response to cyclosporine. *J Rheumatol* 1998;25:816–818.

98. Page KA, Dejardin S, Kahn CR, et al. A patient with type B insulin resistance syndrome, responsive to immune therapy. *Nat Clin Pract Endocrinol Metab* 2007;3:835–840

99. Braund WJ, Naylor BA, Williamson DH, et al. Autoimmunity to insulin receptor and hypoglycaemia in patient with Hodgkin's disease. *Lancet* 1987;1:237–240

100. Rodriguez O, Collier E, Arakaki R, Gorden P. Characterization of purified autoantibodies to the insulin receptor from six patients with type B insulin resistance. *Metabolism* 1992;41:325–331

101. Auclair M, Vigouroux C, Desbois-Mouthon C, et al. Antiinsulin receptor autoantibodies induce insulin receptors to constitutively associate with insulin receptor substrate-1 and -2 and cause severe cell resistance to both insulin and insulin-like growth factor I. *J Clin Endocrinol Metab* 1999;84:3197–3206

102. Flier JS, Bar RS, Muggeo M, et al. The evolving clinical course of patients with insulin receptor autoantibodies: spontaneous remission or receptor proliferation with hypoglycemia. *J Clin Endocrinol Metab* 1978;47:985–995

103. Fareau GG, Maldonado M, Oral E, Balasubramanyam A. Regression of acanthosis nigricans correlates with disappearance of anti-insulin receptor autoantibodies and achievement of euglycemia in type B insulin resistance syndrome. *Metabolism* 2007;56:670–675

104. Lalej-Bennis D, Selam JL, Fluteau-Nadler S, et al. Extreme insulin resistance: clinical management by external subcutaneous insulin infusion. *Diabetes Metab* 1997;23:533–536

105. Kuzuya H, Matsuura N, Sakamoto M, et al. Trial of insulinlike growth factor I therapy for patients with extreme insulin resistance syndromes. *Diabetes* 1993;42:696–705

106. Eriksson JW, Bremell T, Eliasson B, et al. Successful treatment with plasmapheresis, cyclophosphamide, and cyclosporin A in type B syndrome of insulin resistance. Case report. *Diabetes Care* 1998;21:1217–1220

107. Gehi A, Webb A, Nolte M, Davis J. Treatment of systemic lupus erythematosus-associated type B insulin resistance syndrome with cyclophosphamide and mycophenolate mofetil. *Arthritis Rheum* 2003;48:1067–1070

108. Manikas ED, Isaac I, Semple RK, et al. Successful treatment of type B insulin resistance with rituximab. *J Clin Endocrinol Metab* 2015;100:1719–1722

109. Zhang S, Wang G, Wang J. Type B insulin resistance syndrome induced by systemic lupus erythematosus and successfully treated with intravenous immunoglobulin: case report and systematic review. *Clin Rheumatol* 2013;32:181–188

110. Malek R, Chong AY, Lupsa BC, et al. Treatment of type B insulin resistance: a novel approach to reduce insulin receptor autoantibodies. *J Clin Endocrinol Metab* 2010;95:3641–3647

111. Di Paolo S, Giorgino R. Insulin resistance and hypoglycemia in a patient with systemic lupus erythematosus: description of antiinsulin receptor antibodies that enhance insulin binding and inhibit insulin action. *J Clin Endocrinol Metab* 1991;73:650–657

7
Diabetes of Unknown Cause

Yusra Azhar, MBBS;[1] Chelsea A. Baker, MS, PA-C;[1] and Neda Rasouli, MD[1]

Introduction

According to the American Diabetes Association (ADA), diabetes is defined as "a group of metabolic diseases characterized by hyperglycemia resulting from defects in insulin secretion, insulin action, or both."[1] In 1997, the ADA revised the classification of diabetes into four categories based on pathophysiology (rather than treatment): type 1 diabetes, type 2 diabetes, other specific types, and gestational diabetes.[2]

Type 1 diabetes is caused by β-cell destruction resulting in complete insulin deficiency. Type 1 diabetes is further subclassified as either immune-mediated (type 1A diabetes) or idiopathic (type 1B diabetes). In type 1A patients, the presence of autoantibodies to islet cells, insulin, glutamic acid decarboxylase (GAD), or tyrosine phosphatase IA-2 and IA-2b indicates autoimmunity to β-cells. Furthermore, the presence of minimal levels of plasma C-peptide confirms little or no insulin secretion. This presentation of autoimmune diabetes is usually in childhood and adolescence but can occur in any decade of

[1]University of Colorado School of Medicine, Division of Endocrinology, Metabolism and Diabetes, Aurora, CO, and VA Eastern Colorado Health Care System, Denver, CO

DOI: 10.2337/9781580406666.07

life. However, patients with the idiopathic subtype lack the autoantibodies but do have insulin deficiency. This form of diabetes is more prevalent in African and Asian ethnicities. Patients with type 1 diabetes often present with diabetic ketoacidosis (DKA) and are at risk of ketoacidosis when they skip insulin treatment. They are at increased risk for autoimmune disorders and typically do not have the phenotype of metabolic syndrome.[3]

Type 2 diabetes is the most prevalent type of diabetes, accounting for 90–95% of individuals with diabetes. Such individuals have insulin resistance with inadequate β-cell compensation resulting in hyperglycemia. They lack the autoantibodies, tend to be obese with a strong family history of diabetes, and rarely experience unprovoked ketoacidosis.[1]

Despite this distinction between type 1 and type 2 diabetes, there are subtypes of diabetes that do not fit in either category and thus form a continuum between types 1 and 2 diabetes. It has been proposed that this spectrum of diabetes subtypes is essentially a product of varying severities of immune and metabolic dysfunction modified by genetic and nongenetic factors.[4] One of the examples of these subtypes is ketosis-prone diabetes (KPD), also described in literature as atypical diabetes. This form of diabetes is most commonly observed among African Americans but is also seen with increasing frequency among other ethnicities worldwide.[5] Patients with KPD often present with hyperglycemic crisis or DKA (resembling type 1 diabetes), but have a distinct natural history of β-cell dysfunction.[5-8] One of the unique characteristics of this type of diabetes is the restoration of β-cell function and ultimately β-cell remission shortly after resolution of hyperglycemic crisis.[8,9] In addition to atypical diabetes or KPD, this form of diabetes has been referred to as type 1.5, idiopathic, or Flatbush diabetes.[6,7]

Since there are increasing reports of this emerging form of diabetes worldwide, a comprehensive review is appropriate to fully understand this atypical form of diabetes. This chapter focuses on the history, pathophysiology, detailed classification, and the importance of the management of KPD.

History of Ketosis-Prone Diabetes

Cases of KPD have been emerging since the late 1960s.[5] Winter et al.[10] described this unique presentation in obese African-American children who first presented with hyperglycemia, polyuria, polydipsia, weight loss, and keto-acidosis. They lacked autoantibodies and did not require insulin for indefinite periods after initial treatment for DKA.

Banerji et al.[6,11] first used the term "Flatbush Diabetes" with reference to the area surrounding the hospital where this atypical presentation of diabetes was the most prevalent among African Americans. They described patients initially presenting with DKA with the absence of autoantibodies and a clinical course resembling non–insulin-dependent diabetes. Most of these patients did not require long-term insulin therapy and maintained glycemic control using oral agents or diet restrictions. The long-term normoglycemic remission in this population could not be explained by weight loss and was related to a significant improvement in β-cell function as evidenced by increased C-peptide levels.[9,12]

Similarly, Umpierrez et al.[9] described a subgroup of obese African Americans who presented with DKA and lacked autoantibodies. Intensive glycemic control in this cohort resulted in regaining of β-cell function and not requiring insulin treatment long-term. Several other case series have further identified patients from vast ethnic and geographic backgrounds presenting with unprovoked ketosis, absence of autoantibodies, and normoglycemic remission.[5,8,9] It is noteworthy that after a period of near-normoglycemic remission, relapses of hyperglycemic crisis and ketosis are common with unpredictable outcomes of either remission or insulin dependence. The severity of hyperglycemia at presentation increases the risk of DKA. This type of diabetes is more common in men with older age and higher BMI as compared to patients with type 1 diabetes.[8]

Due to the unique and distinct course of KPD, it is important to adopt a classification system to accurately predict the prognosis of diabetes and also to treat optimally. There are different systems available for classification of diabetes in patients presenting with DKA including the ADA classification, the BMI-based system, the modified ADA classification, and the Aβ system.[5]

According to the ADA classification, the KPD patients fall under the category of type 1B diabetes.[1] They present with unprovoked DKA and also lack the autoantibodies. However, in contrast to type 1 diabetes, they do not remain insulin dependent.[5,13] The BMI-based classification described by Umpierrez et al.[14] suggests that lean patients presenting with DKA are predicted to be similar to type 1, and obese patients with ketosis are likely to be similar to type 2. According to this scheme, obese patients who present with DKA have a greater β-cell functional reserve than lean patients, leading to insulin independence. Mauvais-Jarvis et al.[8] proposed the modified ADA classification in which patients who were antibody positive were classified as type 1A and those who were antibody negative were classified further into ketosis-prone diabetes non–insulin-dependent (KPD-NID) or ketosis-prone diabetes insulin-dependent (KPD-ID). KPD-ID patients behaved as type 1 diabetes, and KPD-NID behaved as type 2 diabetes with some β-cell functional reserve.

The Aβ classification designed by Maldonado et al.[15] and adopted by the collaborative group at the Baylor College of Medicine and University of Washington divided patients who presented with DKA into four subgroups on the basis of presence or absence of autoantibodies and β-cell reserve. The following are the four subgroups:[5,15]

1. A+β−: autoantibodies present and β-cell function absent
2. A−β−: autoantibodies absent and β-cell function absent
3. A+β+: autoantibodies present and β-cell function present
4. A−β+: autoantibodies absent and β-cell function present

The β-cell functional reserve was defined as β+ with the fasting serum C-peptide >1 ng/mL or the peak serum C-peptide after glucagon administration >1.5 ng/ml.[15] The glucagon stimulation test was performed using 1 mg IV glucagon injection followed by the measurements of C-peptide at 0, 5, and 10 min. Patients with the presence of the two antibodies GAD and IA-2 above the 99th ethnic-specific percentile were classified as A+ and those below the 99th percentile as A−.[5,15] In the Aβ classification, groups 1 and 2 behave as type 1 diabetes, requiring insulin for management of hyperglycemia; inadequate insulin therapy will predispose them to an unprovoked ketosis. Groups 3 and 4 behave more like type 2 diabetes as they have some degree of preserved β-cell function and are not dependent on insulin therapy to prevent ketosis. A+β− group classically presents as type 1 diabetes whereas A+β+ may be similar to LADA (latent autoimmune diabetes of adults). However, LADA patients do not require insulin initially whereas A+β+ KPD patients present with insulin deficiency and therefore require insulin at presentation.[5]

Maldonado et al.[16] further described that insulin discontinuation relies most heavily upon being newly diagnosed with diabetes and having a higher β-cell reserve. The A−β+ subgroup, which was the largest in the cohort, consisted of the greatest number with new-onset diabetes and had similar characteristics to patients with KPD. The Aβ classification has been further supported to be the most accurate in predicting the β-cell function reserve and the prognosis of diabetes over a period of 12 months after initial presentation with DKA.[17,18]

Pathophysiology of Atypical Ketosis-Prone Diabetes

The mechanisms underlying severe, permanent β-cell dysfunction in some subgroups of KPD and marked, sustained improvement in β-cell function in other subgroups remain unclear. Investigating factors related to humoral autoimmunity in A+ subgroups showed a significant association between β-cell reserve and GAD antibody specific for the epitope DPD.[19,20] To further investigate this association, the levels of overt as well as masked antibodies were investigated in KPD patients.[19] The presence of anti-idiotypic antibodies can interfere with GAD antibody detection in standard antibody tests (masked GAD). Therefore, additional steps are needed to measure masked GAD antibody.[21] Investigating the A– subgroup of KPD (negative overt GAD) showed that 80% of these patients indeed had masked GAD (DPD) antibody and the presence of masked GAD antibody was associated with preserved β-cell function.[19] In addition, it has been reported that there is a small but significant increase in the prevalence of susceptibility alleles in the autoantibody-positive (A+ vs A–) as well as a higher prevalence of resistance alleles in the groups with preserved β-cell function (β+ vs β–) groups.[19,22]

Absence of GAD or IA2 antibodies and susceptibility alleles are characteristics of the A-β–phenotype, and the pathophysiology of β-cell dysfunction remains unclear in this subgroup.[5,15,22] It seems that temporary β-cell "desensitization" leads to insulin deficiency and that this damage is reversible as evidenced by near-normoglycemic remission in this population.[8,9,12] Glucotoxicity, lipotoxicity, or glucolipotoxicity have been proposed as the cause for transient β-cell failure; however, data supporting this hypothesis remain inconsistent.[23] Once diabetes is diagnosed, hyperglycemia and hyperlipidemia could have additional transient effects on β-cell dysfunction and might even lead to permanent β-cell failure.[24] To investigate effects of glucotoxicity and lipotoxicity on the pathogenesis of hyperglycemic crisis/ketosis in this population, Umpierrez et al.[25] exposed patients who had presented with KPD to hyperglycemia and intralipid infusion 48 hours after resolution of DKA and 1 week after their near-normoglycemic remission. African-American obese women had decreased C-peptide levels after glucose infusion, but not in response to intralipid infusion, suggesting that hyperglycemia but not lipotoxicity leads to β-cell dysfunction.

Effects of lipotoxicity and hyperglycemia on β-cell function were more extensively studied in obese African Americans who had presented with hyperglycemic crisis, with a history of unprovoked DKA compared to controls.[26,27]

β-cell function was measured using a glucose-potentiated arginine–stimulated test. When given with glucose, arginine has synergistic effects on insulin secretion.[28] These studies[26,27] showed that short-term intralipid or glucose infusion did not reduce insulin secretion, suggesting that lipotoxicity or glucotoxicity might not play a role in the pathogenesis of transient β-cell failure in this group. It is not clear whether dose or duration of lipotoxicity/glucotoxicity played a role. It is also possible that both lipotoxicity and glucotoxicity are required to impair β-cell function.

Metabolomics with targeted kinetic measurements was used to investigate the pathophysiology of A–β+ KPD subgroup. It showed a shift in fuel metabolism in A–β+ KPD patients described as an "impaired ketone oxidation and fatty acid utilization for energy, leading to accelerated leucine catabolism and transamination of α-ketoglutarate to glutamate, with impaired tricarboxylic acid anaplerosis of glutamate carbon."[29] More recently, a study on the previously reported relationship between KPD and G6PD (Glucose-6-phosphate dehydrogenase) deficiency[30] concluded that hyperglycemia did not explain G6PD deficiency in the absence of G6PD gene mutation.[31] Other proposed causes predisposing to A–β+ KPD include PAX4 gene (paired box gene 4) variations and human herpesvirus 8 infection.[32,33]

Management of KPD

KPD has a complex course, different from type 1 and type 2 diabetes. Patients present with acute hyperglycemic crisis or DKA but undergo a relatively quick recovery phase of β-cell function resulting in near-normoglycemic remission.[9,12] Recurrence of DKA or hyperglycemic crisis is also common.[8] Therefore, the management of diabetes should be appropriate for different phases of the disease. We can divide KPD management into three phases, consisting of acute management of DKA, outpatient management after resolution of DKA, and long-term management.[5] Acute management of DKA is followed by the standard inpatient protocols that include aggressive fluid replacement, insulin therapy, managing precipitating factors, resolution of hyperglycemia, electrolyte disorders, ketoacidosis, and transition from IV insulin to SC insulin.[34,35] All KPD patients presenting with DKA should be treated universally regardless of the phenotype and should be discharged from the hospital on an insulin regimen.[5]

In an outpatient setting, intensive glycemic control leads to improved β-cell function and near-normoglycemic remission.[36] Basal-bolus regimen might be the ideal treatment unless the patient is not a great candidate due to factors such as lack of compliance to the treatment or increased risk of hypoglycemia. Due to a higher chance of β-cell function remission in this population and increased risk of hypoglycemia, the transition of care plays an important role.

Ideally, the first follow-up outpatient visit should be performed 1–3 weeks after hospital discharge. During this period, patients should be evaluated for β-cell function and autoimmunity (if not done previously). Evaluation of β-cell function during hospitalization is not valuable or recommended. However, it is recommended to be performed about 3 weeks after resolution of DKA, to help with the classification of diabetes and formulating a plan for management.[5]

For patients with sustained β-cell dysfunction or β– subgroup, insulin should not be discontinued regardless of their antibody status. However, insulin dose should be adjusted based on self-monitored blood glucose monitoring results.[5] In patients with preserved β-cell function or β+ subgroup, typically, insulin requirement rapidly decreases and they will no longer need prandial insulin. The dose of insulin could be decreased by 50% if the fasting or random blood glucose values meet the ADA recommendations. Insulin should be stopped if the patient starts experiencing hypoglycemia or when glucose levels are maintained at target on a low dose of insulin (<10 units per day). Other antihyperglycemic agents can be added if glucose levels remain elevated. If the patient develops ketosis on insulin dose reduction, the insulin regimen is readjusted and no further attempts are made to discontinue insulin. This outpatient management in assessing insulin withdrawal and patient stability takes approximately 3 months or longer.[5]

The glycemic target (A1C) for these patients is personalized as with other patients with diabetes based on ADA recommendations. Counselling by a diabetes educator and/or dietitian, increased physical activity, and smoking cessation are all encouraged. Patients should also be screened for diabetes microvascular and macrovascular complications. Patients might present with recurrence of unprovoked DKA or hyperglycemic crisis after several months of near normoglycemic remission. Therefore, regular follow-up and patient education are important in prevention/early detection of the crisis and optimally managing the disease.

Conclusion

KPD is a distinct type of diabetes that presents with severe hyperglycemic crisis with ketosis. This acute phase is followed by remission and recovery of β-cell function in some patients. The cause of acute onset of hyperglycemia and the events leading to remission remain unknown. The management of diabetes in these patients is intriguing and requires different approaches in each phase of the disease.

KPD suggests that diabetes is not a single homogeneous disease but runs a gamut of pathologies that have hyperglycemia as a common denominator. Therefore, in the era of precision medicine, there is a need for improved classification of diabetes to predict disease progression and therapeutic responses based on multiple factors including genetic, immune, and metabolic features. In fact, some diabetologists suggest changes in the current classification of diabetes to be more β-cell-centric[37] or based on multiple factors including autoimmunity, genotyping, and endogenous insulin production.[38] The new classification might enhance the management of diabetes.

References

1. American Diabetes Association. Diagnosis and classification of diabetes mellitus. *Diabetes Care* 2014;37(Suppl. 1):S81–S90

2. American Diabetes Association. Report of the Expert Committee on the diagnosis and classification of diabetes mellitus. *Diabetes Care* 1997;20:1183–1197

3. American Diabetes Association. Classification and diagnosis of diabetes mellitus. *Diabetes Care* 2017;40(Suppl. 1):S11–S24

4. Leslie RD, Kolb H, Schloot NC, Buzzetti R, Mauricio D, De Leiva A, Yderstraede K, Sarti C, Thivolet C, Hadden D, Hunter S, Schernthaner G, Scherbaum W, Williams R, Pozzilli P. Diabetes classification: grey zones, sound and smoke: action LADA 1. *Diabetes Metab Res Rev* 2008;24:511–519

5. Balasubramanyam A, Nalini R, Hampe CS, Maldonado M. Syndromes of ketosis-prone diabetes mellitus. *Endocr Rev* 2008;29:292–302

6. Banerji MA, Chaiken RL, Huey H, Tuomi T, Norin AJ, Mackay IR, Rowley MJ, Zimmet PZ, Lebovitz HE. GAD antibody negative NIDDM in adult black subjects with diabetic ketoacidosis and increased frequency of human leukocyte antigen DR3 and DR4: Flatbush diabetes. *Diabetes* 1994;43:741–745

7. Xie XJ, Hu Y, Cheng C, Feng TT, He K, Mao XM. Should diabetic ketosis without acidosis be included in ketosis-prone type 2 diabetes mellitus? *Diabetes Metab Res Rev* 2014;30:54–59

8. Mauvais-Jarvis F, Sobngwi E, Porcher R, Riveline JP, Kevorkian JP, Vaisse C, Charpentier G, Guillausseau PJ, Vexiau P, Gautier JF. Ketosis-prone type 2 diabetes in patients of sub-Saharan African origin: clinical pathophysiology and natural history of beta-cell dysfunction and insulin resistance. *Diabetes* 2004;53:645–653

9. Umpierrez GE, Casals MM, Gebhart SP, Mixon PS, Clark WS, Lawrence S. Phillips. Diabetic ketoacidosis in obese African-Americans. *Diabetes* 1995;44:790–795

10. Winter WE, Maclaren NK, Riley WJ, Clarke DW, Kappy MS, Spillar RP. Maturity-onset diabetes of youth in black Americans. *N Engl J Med* 1987;316:285–291

11. Banerji MA. Diabetes in African Americans: unique pathophysiologic features. *Curr Diab Rep* 2004;4:219–223

12. Banerji MA, Chaiken RL, Lebovitz HE. Long-term normoglycemic remission in black newly diagnosed NIDDM subjects. *Diabetes* 1996;45:337–341

13. Piñero-Piloña A, Litonjua P, Aviles-Santa L, Raskin P. Idiopathic type 1 diabetes in Dallas, Texas: a 5-year experience. *Diabetes Care* 2001;24:1014–1018

14. Umpierrez GE, Woo W, Hagopian WA, Isaacs SD, Palmer JP, Gaur LK, Nepom GT, Clark WS, Mixon PS, Kitabchi AE. Immunogenetic analysis suggests different pathogenesis for obese and lean African-Americans with diabetic ketoacidosis. *Diabetes Care* 1999;22:1517–1523

15. Maldonado M, Hampe CS, Gaur LK, et al. Ketosis-prone diabetes: dissection of a heterogeneous syndrome using an immunogenetic and beta-cell functional classification, prospective analysis, and clinical outcomes. *J Clin Endocrinol Metab* 2003;88:5090–5098

16. Maldonado MR, Otiniano ME, Cheema F, Rodriguez L, Balasubramanyam A. Factors associated with insulin discontinuation in subjects with ketosis-prone diabetes but preserved beta-cell function. *Diabet Med* 2005;22:1744–1750

17. Balasubramanyam A, Garza G, Rodriguez L, Hampe CS, Gaur L, Lernmark A, Maldonado MR. Accuracy and predictive value of classification schemes for ketosis-prone diabetes. *Diabetes Care* 2006;29:2575–2579

18. Banerji MA, Dham S. A comparison of classification schemes for ketosis-prone diabetes. *Nat Clin Pract Endocrinol Metab.* 2007;3:506–507

19. Oak S, Gaur LK, Radtke J, Patel R, Iyer D, Ram N, Gaba R, Balasubramanyam A, Hampe CS. Masked and overt autoantibodies specific to the DPD epitope of

65-kDa glutamate decarboxylase (GAD65-DPD) are associated with preserved β-cell functional reserve in ketosis-prone diabetes. *J Clin Endocrinol Metab* 2014;99:E1040–E1044

20. Hampe CS, Nalini R, Maldonado MR, et al. Association of amino-terminal-specific anti-glutamate decarboxylase (GAD65) autoantibodies with β-cell functional reserve and a milder clinical phenotype in patients with GAD65 antibodies and ketosis prone diabetes mellitus. *J Clin Endocrinol Metab* 2007;92:462–467

21. Oak S, Gilliam LK, Landin-Olsson M, et al. The lack of anti-idiotypic antibodies, not the presence of the corresponding autoantibodies to glutamate decarboxylase, defines type 1 diabetes. *Proc Natl Acad Sci U S A* 2008;105:5471–5476

22. Nalini R, Gaur LK, Maldonado M, Hampe CS, Rodriguez L, Garza G, Lernmark A, Balasubramanyam A. HLA class II alleles specify phenotypes of ketosis-prone diabetes. *Diabetes Care* 2008;31:1195–1200

23. Poitout V, Robertson RP. Glucolipotoxicity: fuel excess and beta-cell dysfunction. *Endocr Rev* 2008;29:351–366

24. Kim JW, Yoon KH. Glucolipotoxicity in pancreatic β-cells. *Diabetes Metab J* 2011;35:444–450

25. Umpierrez GE, Smiley D, Gosmanov A, Thomason D. Ketosis-prone type 2 diabetes: effect of hyperglycemia on β-cell function and skeletal muscle insulin signaling. *Endocr Pract* 2007;13:283–290

26. Umpierrez GE, Smiley D, Robalino G, Peng L, Gosmanov AR, Kitabchi AE. Lack of lipotoxicity effect on {beta}-cell dysfunction in ketosis-prone type 2 diabetes. *Diabetes Care* 2010;33:626–631

27. Gosmanov AR, Smiley D, Robalino G, Siqueira JM, Peng L, Kitabchi AE, Umpierrez GE. Effects of intravenous glucose load on insulin secretion in patients with ketosis-prone diabetes during near-normoglycemia remission. *Diabetes Care* 2010;33:854–860

28. Ward WK, Bolgiano DC, McKnight B, Halter JB, Porte D Jr. Diminished B cell secretory capacity in patients with noninsulin-dependent diabetes mellitus. *J Clin Invest* 1984;74:1318–1328

29. Patel SG, Hsu JW, Jahoor F, Coraza I, Bain JR, Stevens RD, Iyer D, Nalini R, Ozer K, Hampe CS, Newgard CB, Balasubramanyam A. Pathogenesis of A⁻β⁺ ketosis-prone diabetes. *Diabetes* 2013;62:912–922

30. Sobngwi E, Gautier JF, Kevorkian JP, Villette JM, Riveline JP, Zhang S, Vexiau P, Leal SM, Vaisse C, Mauvais-Jarvis F. High prevalence of glucose-6-phosphate dehydrogenase deficiency without gene mutation suggests a novel genetic mechanism predisposing to ketosis-prone diabetes. *J Clin Endocrinol Metab* 2005;90:4446–4451

31. Choukem SP, Sobngwi E, Garnier JP, Letellier S, Mauvais-Jarvis F, Calvo F, Gautier JF. Hyperglycaemia per se does not affect erythrocyte glucose-6-phosphate dehydrogenase activity in ketosis-prone diabetes. *Diabetes Metab* 2015;41:326–330

32. Mauvais-Jarvis F, Smith SB, Le May C, Leal SM, Gautier JF, Molokhia M, Riveline JP, Rajan AS, Kevorkian JP, Zhang S, Vexiau P, German MS, Vaisse C. PAX4 gene variations predispose to ketosis-prone diabetes. *Hum Mol Genet* 2004;13:3151–3159

33. Sobngwi E, Choukem SP, Agbalika F, Blondeau B, Fetita LS, Lebbe C, Thiam D, Cattan P, Larghero J, Foufelle F, Ferre P, Vexiau P, Calvo F, Gautier JF. Ketosis-prone type 2 diabetes mellitus and human herpesvirus 8 infection in sub-Saharan Africans. *JAMA* 2008;299:2770–2776

34. Umpierrez GE, Smiley D, Kitabchi AE. Narrative review: ketosis-prone type 2 diabetes mellitus. *Ann Intern Med* 2006;144:350–357

35. Kitabchi AE, Umpierrez GE, Murphy MB, Barrett EJ, Kreisberg RA, Malone JI, Wall BM. Management of hyperglycemic crises in patients with diabetes. *Diabetes Care* 2001;24:131–153

36. Rasouli N, Elbein SC. Improved glycemic control in subjects with atypical diabetes results from restored insulin secretion, but not improved insulin sensitivity. *J Clin Endocrinol Metab* 2004;89:6331–6335

37. Schwartz SS, Epstein S, Corkey BE, Grant SFA, Gavin JR 3rd, Aguilar RB. The time is right for a new classification system for diabetes: rationale and implications of the β-cell–centric classification schema. *Diabetes Care* 2016;39:179–186

38. Leslie RD, Palmer J, Schloot NC, Lernmark A. Diabetes at the crossroads: relevance of disease classification to pathophysiology and treatment. *Diabetologia* 2016;59:13–20

8
Genetic Syndromes Associated with Diabetes

Aurelia C.H. Wood, MD;[1] Damien Abreu, MD;[1] Amy L. Clark, DO;[1] Marjorie A. Malbas, MD;[1] Jennifer E. Sprague, MD, PhD;[1] and Janet B. McGill, MD[1]

Introduction

Diabetes that occurs in patients with genetic syndromes falls under the classification of "specific types" in the most recent American Diabetes Association (ADA) position statement of the diagnosis and classification of diabetes.[1] The genetic syndromes discussed in this chapter are listed under the subsection, "Other genetic syndromes sometimes associated with diabetes." Clearly, this is a broad category. The types of gene defects vary greatly, as do the characteristics of diabetes found in patients with the syndromes. The syndromes associated with chromosomal abnormalities such as Down syndrome, Klinefelter syndrome, and Turner syndrome have increased rates of immune-mediated diabetes during childhood, but in the case of Klinefelter syndrome, patients may have obesity and the metabolic syndrome in adulthood, predisposing them to type 2 diabetes (T2D). Diabetes in these syndromes follows the typical disease courses of type 1 diabetes (T1D) or T2D, and this nomenclature is used by investigators who have studied diabetes in the syndromes, which we will do also.

High rates of diabetes are also found in the basepair repeat syndromes such as Friedreich's ataxia, Huntington's disease, the myotonic dystrophies, and

---

[1] Division of Endocrinology, Metabolism and Lipid Research, Washington University School of Medicine, St. Louis, MO

DOI: 10.2337/9781580406666.08

the severe obesity syndromes like Bardet-Biedl and Prader-Willi. The disease course is variable, and not typical of classic T1D or T2D in most of the syndromes. Some patients may have features of insulin deficiency and insulin resistance concomitantly. The etiology of diabetes is best understood in Bardet-Biedl, where insulin receptors may be defective; however, the exact pathogenesis is not clear in the other base-pair repeat syndromes.[2] Wolfram syndrome patients present very much like T1D patients, but the insulin-deficient diabetes that characterizes the syndrome is caused by endoplasmic reticulum dysfunction and is not immune-mediated; therefore diabetes has somewhat different characteristics.[3]

Diabetes is just one of the many challenges faced by persons with genetic syndromes. Other manifestations of the underlying disorder such as cognitive dysfunction, neuropsychiatric symptoms, metabolic derangements, and physical limitations can impact diabetes treatment and outcomes in patients with complex genetic disorders.

Down Syndrome

Down syndrome (DS), also known as Trisomy 21, is one of the most common chromosomal disorders in humans, with a well-described phenotype consisting of characteristic facial features, intellectual disability, and congenital anomalies. Penetrance of all symptoms is variable and the constellation of symptoms and severity varies by patient. The disorder affects 1 in 800 newborns and there are approximately 5,300 affected infants born in the United States each year, and over 200,000 adults live with the condition.[4] About 94% of cases are not typically inherited, but due to a sporadic nondisjunction event during cell division, which results in three copies of chromosome 21 in nearly all tissues.[5] Other causes of Trisomy 21, more rarely, include mosaicism, in which only some body tissues have cells with Trisomy 21 while the remaining cells are unaffected. There is translocation in which, rather than having a separate chromosome 21, all or part is attached to another chromosome.[5] Medical advancements resulting in improvements in screening and treatment have improved life expectancy to the mid-50s from the 30s in prior years.[6]

Characteristic physical findings include short stature, upward slanting eyes, palpebral fissures, circumferential lesions around the iris known as Brushfield spots, a flat facial profile with a short nasal bridge, macroglossia, and fifth finger clinodactyly.[6] Trisomy 21 is universally associated with some degree of cognitive and developmental delay, and many patients also suffer from behavioral disruptions. Common clinical findings include central hypotonia, atlantoaxial hypermobility, GI malformations including duodenal atresia and Hirschsprung's disease, congenital cardiac septal defects, and early onset of dementia and Alzheimer's disease.[6]

Patients with Trisomy 21 are at risk for both immune dysfunction and autoimmune disease, specifically leukemoid reactions, leukemia, celiac disease, autoimmune thyroid disease, and T1D.[7] The prevalence of T1D in patients with Trisomy 21 is 2% as compared to 0.1–0.5% in the general population, a fourfold increase.[7,8] The average age of onset is 8 years; however, the onset of T1D in patients with DS has a bimodal appearance, with 22% being diagnosed before age 2 and another peak in adolescence.[9,10] A similar finding was observed by Alexander et al.[11] in a study of the incidence of morbidities and prevalence of medical prescriptions in a large DS population in the United Kingdom. While the overall incidence rate ratio (IRR) was 1.3 (1.1; 1.6) vs controls, a higher incidence rate for diabetes was observed among young adults (IRR 5.4; 2.7–11.0, $p < 0.001$ for 18–30y).[11] This study did not differentiate between T1D and T2D, but given the young age of the cohort, the most likely increase was in T1D.

Studies have also shown there is an increased prevalence of diabetes autoantibodies in DS patients without T1D compared to healthy controls.[9] Diabetes associated HLA haplotypes are more prevalent in patients with DS and T1D than in DS controls, but with reduced prevalence of the highest-risk haplotypes, suggesting that chromosome 21 harbors genes that potentiate the penetrance of T1D and organ-specific autoimmunity.[9,12] Patients with DS and T1D have an increased prevalence of thyroid disease and celiac disease, 74% and 14% respectively.[10] In the study by Alexander et al., the IRR for hypothyroidism was 13.1 (11.2; 15.2) compared to controls.[11]

Obesity is more common in DS than controls at all ages (IRR 2.6 (2.4; 2.8).[14] Despite significantly increased BMI compared with controls (29.1 +/− 5.0 vs 24.9 +/− 3.8, $p < 0.001$), adults with DS had lower blood pressure and heart rate but no difference in the rates of dyslipidemia or T2D in a Spanish study.[13] Compared to controls, DS patients had a higher prevalence of congenital heart disease, cardiac arrhythmia, dementia, pulmonary hypertension, diabetes, and sleep apnea, and a greater risk of incident cerebrovascular events (Risk Ratio, RR 2.70, 95% CI 2.08–3.52).[15] Insulin resistance increased with age, weight, and pubertal status in obese children with DS, but glucose intolerance was not detected.[6]

Interestingly, although the incidence of T1D is increased modestly in children with DS, there are no reports of latent autoimmune diabetes in adults with DS. Given the low prevalence of T2D in these patients, testing for autoimmune diabetes may be appropriate in patients with DS who develop diabetes as adolescents or adults, especially if hyperglycemia is pronounced or is accompanied by weight loss. As patients with DS are living longer, the risk for T2D may increase as it does in the general population, so routine screening should be performed. Treatment of either T1D or T2D in DS is not different from those without the syndrome. Glucose control can typically be achieved with standard approaches, given a less complex lifestyle and caretaker contributions. Patient-specific plans must be crafted in order to provide optimal care due to comorbidities associated with Trisomy 21.[6]

Diabetes-related complications are not well studied in DS, due in part to early mortality from dementia and other neurologic problems. Patients with DS have multiple ocular disorders, among them myopia that may be protective from retinopathy.[16] Rates of kidney disease are not known, and patients with DS have low incidences of cardiovascular events. The demographics of the DS population are changing, however, so standards of care for the treatment of T1D or T2D apply to these complex patients.[6]

Klinefelter Syndrome

Klinefelter syndrome (KS), also known as 47,XXY, is the most common sex chromosome disorder in males, and is estimated to occur in about 1 in 600 to 700 male infants.[17] This disorder is characterized by the presence of hypergonadotrophic hypogonadism, infertility, gynecomastia, learning disabilities, accelerated growth, and tall stature, as well as multiple metabolic and psychosocial comorbidities.[18] KS features are thought to be due to the presence of the additional X-chromosome, which though inactivated, hosts other genes that remain active, 10% of which are expressed in the testes.[18] At present, the exact role of each of these genes is unknown; however, tall stature noted in the syndrome is attributed to the presence of an additional SHOX gene (short-stature homeobox-containing gene on chromosome X).[19]

Common physical findings include tall stature, small testes, abdominal obesity, and female-pattern body fat distribution.[18] Suggestive clinical findings include speech delay, learning difficulties, and psychiatric disturbances including ADHD, autism spectrum disorders, depression, and schizophrenia. At present, there is no widely accepted standard for clinical diagnosis; therefore, genetic testing should always be performed and utilized in making the diagnosis.[17] Given that these findings do not become apparent until early adolescence or adult years, an estimated 75% of patients go undiagnosed until adulthood.[17,18]

Some, but not all, autoimmune diseases show increased prevalence in patients with KS. The risk ratio for T1D is 6.1 (95% CI 4.4–8.3) in KS compared to males of similar ages.[20] A similar study from the Danish National Register of Patients also reported an increased risk for T1D among persons with KS, HR 2.21 (1.18–4.14), based on hospital admission data.[21] In contrast to T1D, the other diseases with increased prevalence among men with KS are those that affect females more than males, including thyroid disease, Addison's disease, multiple sclerosis, rheumatoid arthritis, Sjogren's syndrome, and systemic lupus erythematosus.[22] The etiology of this predominance is unknown; however, it is postulated that the location of genes encoding immune factors on the X chromosome is contributory. A study of organ-specific humoral immunity showed increased diabetes associated antibodies, but no increase in thyroid or celiac immune markers in patients with KS compared to unaffected controls.[23] Interestingly, 1.9% of children with T1D seen at a clinic in India had KS, which presented management problems because of behavioral problems.[24]

As men with KS age, obesity and the metabolic syndrome become common problems, affecting 30–46% of adults with the syndrome.[25,26] In a metabolic study of KS adults, the occurrence of the metabolic syndrome correlated with BMI, body fat, waist circumference, insulin resistance, and increased LDL and CRP levels in KS patients, irrespective of testosterone therapy.[26] All measures typically associated with insulin resistance were pathologically altered: fasting serum insulin, fasting plasma glucose, total cholesterol, LDL cholesterol, and triglycerides were higher than controls while HDL and insulin sensitivity (HOMA2%S) were significantly reduced.[26] Interestingly, blood pressure and adiponectin levels were normal and not different from controls.[26] The role of lifelong hypogonadism in the altered metabolic profile of KS patients is not completely understood, but testosterone replacement has been associated with reductions in fat mass, improved body composition, and a more favorable metabolic profile.[27] Elevated body fat mass is apparent in prepubertal children with

KS despite normal lean body mass, suggesting that the genetic defects in KS may play a role independent of testosterone in body composition.[27,28]

It is estimated that 39% of patients with KS are diagnosed with T2D during their lifetime. The hazard ratio for T2D in a national survey of KS in Denmark was 3.71 (2.14–6.40) compared to age-matched controls.[21] In a Chinese cohort of 39 KS patients, the overall prevalence of diabetes was 20.5% with a mean age of onset of 27.1 +/–4.5 years, but varied by karyotype.[25] The incidence of diagnosed diabetes was 12.5% in patients with 47XXY karyotype but 57.1% in patients with atypical karyotypes, such as 46XY/47XXY chimera.[25] The increased risk for T2D appears to be multifactorial, and attributed to obesity, decreased insulin sensitivity, increased fasting insulin levels, hypogonadism, and low testosterone in the Chinese study.[25] Routine screening for diabetes should begin at earlier ages than in persons without the KS genetic disorder and treatment should commence if diabetes is diagnosed. Screening for cardiac risk factors is also recommended.[29]

KS is associated with a decrease in life expectancy of about 2 years, due to osteoporosis, obesity, metabolic syndrome, diabetes, and cardiovascular disease.[17,29] The cause-specific mortality for patients with KS due to diabetes is greatly increased at all ages, RR 7.07 (2.60– 15.42), much greater than the overall RR of 1.63 (1.40–1.91).[30] A subsequent study of 4,806 KS patients in the U.K. determined that the all-cause standardized mortality rate (SMR) was 1.5 (95% CI, 1.4–1.7); but that the risk of death from diabetes was even greater (SMR 5.8; 95% CI 3.4 – 9.3).[31] There are no clear evidence-based treatment guidelines for KS, but testosterone replacement and lifestyle management may have an impact on the adverse metabolic profiles observed in untreated hypogonadal adults with KS. While much new knowledge has been acquired in recent years, much remains to be explored to guide earlier diagnosis and treatment standards for KS.

Turner Syndrome

Turner syndrome (TS), also known as 45 X, is the most common sex chromosome abnormality in females and is associated with short stature and poor growth, gonadal dysgenesis, classic physical features, and multiple congenital defects. The syndrome affects 1 in 2,500 live-born female infants; however, the diagnosis is associated with 15% of all miscarriages, and therefore only 1% of fetuses with TS survive to term.[32,33]

TS occurs as a result of genetic defects related to the X chromosome. About half of affected patients only have one X chromosome in each cell in the body due to sporadic nondisjunction, known as monosomy X. Mosaicism is found in the majority of the remaining cases, and other mechanisms such as partial absence of an X-chromosome, translocation of an X-chromosome, and deletion of part of an X-chromosome can also result in the syndrome.[34] Short stature, a cardinal feature of TS patients, is due to deletion or rearrangement of the SHOX gene, located on the pseudoautosomal region, Xp22 of Yp11.3, of human sex chromosomes.[35] The diagnosis of TS is made on the basis of clinical findings plus karyotype confirmation.[32]

Common physical findings include short stature, increased nuchal folds, neck webbing, low posterior hairline, high arched palate, lymphedema, and a broad chest with widely spaced nipples. Girls with TS have slow linear growth during childhood and then show growth arrest during adolescence.[32] Congenital heart defects affect one-third of girls with TS, the most common being bicuspid aortic valves and coarctation of the aorta. Renal anomalies such as a horseshoe kidney, malrotation, and collecting duct anomalies occur in up to 20% of patients, and hypertension, hyperlipidemia, and obesity are also common.[32] Gonadal dysgenesis resulting in hypergonadotrophic hypogonadism occurs in nearly 90% of patients with TS, though up to 30% will show spontaneous pubertal development. Only 2–5% will start menses and may have the potential to achieve pregnancy.[32]

Patients with TS are at increased risk for autoimmune diseases; however, the prevalence and risks vary across studies and populations. In a landmark study of Danish women with TS, Gravholt and colleagues found an increase in the risk of T1D (RR 11.56, CI 5.29–21.95) and a non-significant increase in thyroid diseases (RR 2.0, CI 0.96–3.69).[36] A similar increased risk of T1D was also found in a U.K. population (RR 8.2, 95% CI 6.4–10.3).[37] In the U.S. NIH cohort 224 patients with TS, a nonsignificant increase of T1D was observed, prevalence 0.9% compared to 0.38% in the U.S. female population (RR 2.37, 95% CI 0.40–9.9); however, a high rate of Hashimoto's thyroiditis was found in this cohort (RR 7.2, 95% CI 5.85–8.7), suggesting that the ethnic background of the population may play a role in the risk of T1D, with higher risk in northern European populations than in populations with mixed ethnicity.[38] Interestingly, in a clinic cohort of 260 patients with T1D, 3.5% had TS.[24] The incidence of positive GAD-65 autoantibodies and anti-TPO antibodies is increased in patients with TS, especially in those with isochromosomal karyotypes, in which two copies of the q-arm are duplicated.[39] A number of hypotheses have been suggested to explain the increase in autoimmunity with inactivation or loss of an X-chromosome: loss of mosaicism, reactivation of genes in T cells, and haploinsufficiency of X-genes from pseudoautosomal regions in B and T cells.[40] Autoimmunity may increase with age, suggesting that screening for the highest-risk condition, hypothyroidism, should continue into adulthood. Screening for the other autoimmune disorders, such as T1D, may not be cost-effective.

Insulin resistance and T2D are both very common in patients with TS. There is a 2–4 times increased risk of T2D, with over half of patients showing abnormal findings on an oral glucose tolerance test as compared to the general population.[41] Studies have shown insulin resistance and β-cell dysfunction begins as young as childhood, independent of BMI, or concomitant medication usage.[42] However, once it develops, T2D typically has a mild phenotype that responds well to lifestyle modifications and/or monotherapy. Given the increased risk, it is recommended that fasting blood glucose be obtained every one to two years in patients with TS.[43]

Mainstays of therapy for TS include hormone replacement therapy for induction of puberty and menarche, growth hormone (GH) therapy to attain acceptable final adult height and management of associated comorbidities. Human growth hormone (hGH) therapy is associated with hyperglycemia and increased risk of insulin resistance, though evidence is conflicting as to whether this effect occurs in patients with TS.[44] Given the average height predication for women with TS is 4'8", the benefit typically outweighs the risk. Long-term follow-up has not demonstrated an association between prior hGH treatment and impaired glucose tolerance or diabetes.[45] In addition to the above, adult patients with TS are at increased risk of obesity, chronic liver disease, ulcerative colitis and Crohn's disease, colon cancer, gonadoblastoma, ischemic heart disease, and other serious cardiovascular complications such as aortic dilation and aortic dissection.[32]

Wolfram Syndrome

Wolfram syndrome (previously referenced in Chapter 1) is an autosomal recessive, progressive neurodegenerative disorder resulting from mutations in the Wolfram syndrome 1 (WFS1) gene.[46] The carrier frequency of Wolfram syndrome is 1 in 350, with an estimated prevalence of 1 in 770,000 children.[47,48] Wolfram and Wagener first described the syndrome in 1938 in four siblings with T1D and optic nerve atrophy, which prompted the original definition as a syndrome of juvenile-onset diabetes with optic nerve atrophy.[49] Since that time, many more conditions have been found to be associated with Wolfram syndrome. As such, Wolfram syndrome has also been coined DIDMOAD syndrome due to its frequent clinical presentation as a constellation of diabetes insipidus, diabetes mellitus, optic nerve atrophy, and deafness.[50,51]

Diabetes of nonimmune origin is typically the first manifestation of this disorder, occurring within the first decade of life.[3,48,52] Optic nerve atrophy with loss of color vision and peripheral vision loss typically ensues within the second decade, followed by diabetes insipidus and/or deafness in the following years.[3,53] Additional symptoms such as ataxia, hypogonadism, and neurogenic bladder have also been reported, along with a predisposition to psychiatric disease.[48,54–56]

Elegant research has shown that Wolfram syndrome is a disease resulting from endoplasmic reticulum (ER) stress-induced cell death.[57,58] Proper folding of secretory proteins and degradation of misfolded proteins is a key function of the ER. Accumulation of unfolded or misfolded proteins by perturbations in ER function leads to a cellular response known as the ER stress or unfolded protein response (UPR).[59] The WFS1 is protective from ER stress by negatively regulating a transcription factor involved in ER stress signaling, activating transcription factor 6α (ATF6α). β-cells from WFS1-deficient mice and lymphocytes from Wolfram syndrome patients exhibited dysregulated ER stress signaling, which led to inadequate UPR and ultimately β-cell apoptosis.[59] Similar processes have been shown to cause the neurodegeneration that characterizes the syndrome.[58]

In addition to β-cell failure, Wolfram syndrome patients develop severe neurologic manifestations in the first two decades of life, most commonly presenting as hearing loss and problems with balance and coordination beginning in adolescence and progressing to life-threatening brainstem atrophy.[3,54] Neuroimaging studies have shown that Wolfram patients have a smaller intracranial volume with specific abnormalities in the brainstem and the cerebellum, even before the neurologic symptoms are apparent.[60,61] This progressive neurodegeneration leads to a mortality of ~65% before the age of 35, largely due to respiratory failure secondary to brainstem atrophy.[56]

Diabetes in patients with Wolfram syndrome typically develops in the first decade of life, presenting in a manner similar to T1D. The standard of care for diabetes management in Wolfram syndrome is the same as for patients with T1D; however, studies suggest that patients with Wolfram syndrome may have a milder form of diabetes. Specifically, when compared with a cohort of T1D patients, Wolfram syndrome patients had better glycemic control and required lower daily doses of insulin.[62] Nevertheless, diabetes care in the setting of Wolfram syndrome is often complicated by the visual and neurologic impairments associated with the disorder. When compared to age and duration of disease-matched patients with T1D, Wolfram syndrome patients had a lower incidence of diabetic complications and diabetic ketoacidosis.[63] Clinical suspicion for Wolfram syndrome should arise in any patient with insulin-dependent diabetes who manifests hearing loss, vision loss, coordination problems, or other symptoms of Wolfram syndrome. Patients with suspected Wolfram syndrome should undergo genetic testing, which is available both commercially and via the International Wolfram Syndrome Registry (http://wolframsyndromedom.wustl.edu). There is currently no cure for the disease, but research efforts into novel therapies to delay disease progression are ongoing.[56,58] Indeed, Washington University in St. Louis launched the first interventional clinical trial for Wolfram syndrome in July 2016 to assess the safety and tolerability of dantrolene sodium as a treatment for Wolfram patients (NCT02829268).

Friedreich's Ataxia

Friedreich's ataxia (FRDA) is a progressive neurodegenerative disorder that begins in childhood and results in ataxia, weakness, spasticity, dysarthria, sensory loss, cardiomyopathy, bladder dysfunction, and diabetes in up to 30% of patients.[64] It is caused by autosomal recessive mutations in the frataxin (FXN) gene located on chromosome 9q21.11. The diagnosis is confirmed by the detection of pathogenic, abnormally expanded GAA repeats in intron 1 of the FXN gene. Penetrance is determined by the size of the expanded GAA repeat, which also relates to the clinical severity of the syndrome. GAA expansions may decrease the level of frataxin protein because of decreased mRNA transcription, leading to mitochondrial dysfunction.[64]

Diabetes or impaired fasting glucose is diagnosed in 10–40% of patients with FRDA.[65] Physiologic studies, including oral or intravenous glucose tolerance testing, homeostatic model assessment of insulin resistance, and β-cell function have shown that insulin resistance is prominent in some patients, but others show evidence of β-cell failure.[65] Both age and GAA length have been shown to predict abnormal glucose metabolism. Interestingly, some patients with FRDA present with insulin-requiring diabetes in childhood, and in general insulin levels in children with FRDA are lower than in age-and weight-matched controls.[66] A more typical presentation is progressive hyperglycemia, which develops during or after puberty. Higher BMI, older age, and longer GAA repeat length were associated with higher risk for developing glucose intolerance and progression to diabetes. Incident diabetes was not related to neurological or cardiac manifestations or severity in patients with FRDA.[67]

Examination of post-mortem pancreas samples from patients with FRDA showed a decrease in islet β-cells, but normal alpha cells.[66] In an in vitro model of β-cell frataxin deficiency, both functional defects and sensitivity to ER stressors were demonstrated.[66] Mitochondrial dysfunction and metabolic/ER stress–induced β-cell apoptosis may be prevented by the incretins GLP-1 and GIP, though clinical data are lacking. Treatment of diabetes in FRDA depends on the clinical picture; however, exogenous insulin will be needed in the majority of cases.[68] Various therapies have been aimed at reducing cardiac hypertrophy, including coenzyme Q10, vitamin E, and idebenone, a benzoquinone related to coenzyme Q10. None of these agents has a reported effect on β-cell function or diabetes, though clinical trials are underway.[68]

Huntington's Disease

Huntington's disease (HD) is a progressive neurologic disorder of CAG repeats in the Huntington gene on chromosome 4p16.3.[69] Polyglutamine segments encoded by the CAG repeats are incorporated in multiple parts of the cell, including the nucleus, though the exact mechanism of cell toxicity, and in particular neurotoxicity, is not known. The numbers of CAG repeats correlate with both age of onset and severity of disease in HD.[67,69]

Older studies suggested an increased prevalence of diabetes among those affected by HD, though more recent prevalence data are conflicting.[67,70] A survey of 340 U.S. nursing home residents with HD, from a pool of 249,811 residents overall, showed that only 0.3% of HD patients had either diabetes or cancer.[71] Studies of glucose homeostasis in cohorts of patients with HD have shown reduced insulin sensitivity and lower acute insulin response despite normal glucose tolerance,[72] or no difference between patients with HD and controls.[70] The same authors found that insulin release from β-cells expressing the HD gene was normal when the polyglutamine lengths were within the range of adults with HD.[71] When pancreatic tissue sections from HD patients were examined, the pattern of insulin immunostaining, islet β-cell area, and levels of insulin transcripts were similar to controls.[73] Transgenic mouse models have been shown to develop intranuclear inclusions in pancreatic β-cells, which are temporally associated with impaired expression of regulatory proteins necessary for insulin gene transcription. Reductions in insulin mRNA preceded the development of hyperglycemia in this HD transgenic mouse model.[74]

Clinical chorea-ballism, hemilateral or bilateral, has been described during periods of severe hyperglycemia in older patients with T2D and rarely in patients with T1D during episodes of diabetic ketoacidosis (DKA). A case report of an occurrence during an episode of DKA that improved but did not resolve thereafter resulted in the diagnosis of HD in a 40-year-old woman.[75] Depletion of gamma-aminobutyric acid in the basal ganglia is the putative mechanism for exacerbation of choreoathetosis in susceptible patients during hyperglycemia, including patients with HD.

Myotonic Dystrophy Disorders

Myotonic dystrophy type 1 (DM1) is caused by a dominantly inherited CTG repeat expansion on a noncoding region of the dystrophia myotonica protein kinase (DMPK) gene on chromosome 19q13.3.[76] The CTG expansions vary in different tissues and over time in DM1. While the pathogenic disease mechanism is not clear in every tissue, it appears that the mutant DMPK gene alters normal RNA metabolism resulting in disruption of mRNA translation, alternative splicing, and stability.[76,77] Congenital DM1, a severe form with >1,000 repeats, can present prenatally with polyhydramnios and decreased fetal movements in the neonatal period as hypotonia or failure to thrive.[78] Children with the syndrome may have intellectual disability, facial weakness, and dysarthria, in addition to generalized weakness. Adults typically present with early cataracts, have myotonia and muscle weakness in the third or fourth decades, and experience progressive cognitive impairment and other neuropsychiatric disorders with age. The number of CTG repeats influences the age of onset and severity; however, the correlation is not entirely predictive and may change over time.[78]

Physiologic studies of insulin sensitivity in adult patients with DM1 showed that whole-body glucose disposal was reduced by 15–25% during a hyperinsulinemic clamp procedure compared to controls, even when controlled for differences in muscle mass.[79] In a similar study of forearm muscle, glucose uptake was reduced by 70%.[80] Alternative splicing of the insulin receptor pre-mRNA was found to be aberrantly regulated in skeletal muscle biopsies, causing increased expression of the nonmuscle isoform, insulin receptor A (IR-A).[81] Testing of the muscle tissue in culture showed decreased metabolic response to insulin, confirming skeletal muscle insulin resistance.[81] Further studies of DMPK using a Dmpk $^{-/-}$ knockout mouse model showed impaired insulin signaling in muscle tissues, but not in adipocytes or liver.[82] Dmpk $^{-/-}$ mice displayed abnormal glucose tolerance, reduced glucose uptake, and impaired insulin-dependent GLUT4 trafficking in muscle. DMPK was also shown to be responsible for intracellular trafficking of insulin and IGF-1 receptors.[82]

Patients with DM1 have a high prevalence of endocrine dysfunction, in particular hypogonadism, diabetes, and hyperparathyroidism. In a Danish cohort of 68 patients with DM1 who were followed for 8 years with final average age of 43, an oral glucose tolerance test (OGTT) showed impaired glucose tolerance in 11, and impaired fasting glucose in 2 patients.[83] Four of the 68 patients had developed diabetes, and one of the patients with an abnormal OGTT had an A1C >6.5%. The majority of the patients had a BMI <25 kg/m², only a few had a BMI between 25–27 kg/m², and none were >27 kg/m².[83] In a euglycemic clamp study of young DM1 patients, preserved insulin sensitivity despite lower lean muscle mass but increased proinsulin secretion in both fasting and poststimulus states were found.[84] Treatment of this unusual form of diabetes has not been established, but response to pioglitazone has been reported in two cases.[85] The prevalence and severity of diabetes, hypogonadism, and hyperparathyroidism has been shown to increase over time, but the endocrine disorders did not correlate with muscle dysfunction in patients with DM1.[83]

Myotonic dystrophy type 2 (DM2 [OMIM 602668]) is the most common form of adult-onset muscular dystrophy, and affects approximately 1 in 8,000 in northern European populations or descendants.[86] DM2 is an autosomal dominant, multisystem disorder characterized by myotonia or muscle weakness, stiffness and pain (90%), iridescent posterior subcapsular cataracts (36–78%), insulin insensitivity (25–75%), testicular failure (29–65%), and cardiac conduction defects (19%).[87] Myotonia, or involuntary muscle contraction and delayed relaxation such as inability to loosen a hand grip, is the first symptom and typically presents in the third decade. The muscle stiffness and pain symptoms are variable among patients and fluctuate over time in the same patient, making DM2 a challenging diagnosis.[88] The other manifestations occur at later ages and increase in prevalence and severity with age.[87]

DM2 is caused by an untranslated CCTG tetranucleotide repeat expansion in intron 1 of the zinc finger protein 9 (ZNF9) gene on chromosome 3q21.3.[89] DM2 poses diagnostic challenges for geneticists, since the CCTG repeats are unstable and vary between generations.[87] Similar to DM1, the CCUG repeat-containing RNA accumulates in ribonuclear inclusions of affected DM2 tissues. Insulin-sensitive muscle is one such tissue.[90] Muscle from DM2 subjects expressed altered insulin receptor splicing, with reductions in exon 11 inclusion and reduced expression of the insulin sensitive IR-B isoform, leading to insulin insensitivity. The insulin receptor (IR) defects and other pathogenic splicing alterations appeared in histologically normal muscle, prior to clinical evidence of dystrophic changes of evidence of insulin resistance and glucose intolerance. Patients who had repeated muscle biopsies over several years showed progressive loss of IR-B due to alternative splicing.[90] Insulin-insensitive diabetes is one of the hallmarks of DM2, with incidence and severity increasing with age. Reports of treatment success or failure are lacking in patient series in DM2 and diabetes.

Bardet-Biedl Syndrome

Bardet-Biedl syndrome (BBS) is an autosomal recessive disorder with cardinal manifestations of retinal degeneration, obesity, polydactyly, learning disabilities, and urogenital defects.[2] The prevalence of BBS is 1 in 125,000–160,000 in Europe, and 1 in 65,000 in the Middle East.[2,91] The genotype and phenotypes vary, as the syndrome is caused by mutations in any of at least 18 genes (BBS1-18).[91] The diagnosis is made by the presence of at least four of the major manifestations, including retinal dystrophy, obesity, polydactyly, genital anomalies, cognitive difficulties, and renal anomalies. The anatomic anomalies are present at birth and often identify affected persons. Vision loss and obesity begin in childhood, along with developmental delay, speech delay, learning difficulties, hearing loss, and anosmia/hyposmia.[2]

The pathogenesis of BBS is complex and rests on the accumulation of complexes of eight BBS proteins, collectively known as the BBSome.[92] The BBSome is required for ciliogenesis and cilium function, and disruption of this protein complex may prevent critical cell–cell communication, cell-environment interaction, and vesicular transport.[92] BBS proteins are necessary for the sorting and cell surface expression of the IR.[93] Loss of BBS proteins leads to a reduction of IR at the cell surface, which manifests as insulin resistance, blunted insulin-induced activation of IR signaling in insulin-sensitive tissues (liver, skeletal muscle, and adipose tissue), and hyperglycemia.[93] Insulin resistance is independent from obesity in mice that lack the BBS proteins, though this is less clear in humans. BBS knockout mice are hyperphagic, which causes obesity, but have increased adiposity and decreased energy expenditure despite pair feeding.[94]

Obesity is a common feature of BBS, occurring in 72–92% of patients, and nearly 100% of those carrying homozygous mutations.[2] Compared to non-BBS subjects with similar BMI, patients with BBS have greater adiposity, more abdominal visceral fat, and lower lean body mass.[95] Obesity has been linked to leptin resistance, which may have defective action in the POMC region of the hypothalamus, leading to poor response to changes in energy balance.[96] Diabetes is considered a secondary or minor feature and occurs in 6–48% of patients with BBS.[2] Diabetes is characterized by hyperinsulinemia and insulin resistance. In a population cohort of 46 patients with BBS, T2D was diagnosed in 22 (48%), while impaired glucose tolerance occurred in 4 additional patients.[97] The median age of onset of diabetes was 43 years, and there was no difference among groups with different genotypes.[97] Treatment of diabetes in BBS should follow usual care guidelines. Insulin may be required but is likely to be less effective than in insulin-deficient patients.

Laurence-Moon Syndrome

Laurence-Moon syndrome (LMS [OMIM 245800]) has a number of similarities with BBS. It was first described in 1866 by Laurence and Moon, who identified retinitis pigmentosa in four siblings with "general imperfections of development" that included hypogenitalism.[98] Persons with LMS present with early neurological changes, including spasticity and ataxia, in addition to short stature and retinal dystrophy. Vision loss is progressive during childhood due to pigmentary retinal degeneration and choroidal atrophy. Nystagmus is also a prominent feature. Neurologic findings include ataxia with or without spasticity, peripheral neuropathy, intellectual disability, and hypopituitarism manifesting as hypothyroidism and hypogonadotrophic hypogonadism, all presenting in childhood. Obesity is present in some, but not all patients with LMS; and none have polydactyly.[99]

LMS is inherited as an autosomal recessive disorder, with mutations occurring in the PNPLA6 gene, chromosome 19p13.2, which encodes for neuropathy target esterase (NTE) that is critical for phosphatidylcholine metabolism, membrane phospholipids, and axonal integrity.[100] NTE impairments cause Oliver-McFarlane syndrome and LMS.[100] Mutations in the PNPLA6 gene are associated with other neurodegenerative conditions, but only LMS manifests infantile or childhood onset pituitary dysfunction, smaller anterior pituitary size, short stature, and hypogonadism. Significant heterogeneity is seen between families with LMS and similar syndromes.[100] Neuroimaging shows cerebellar atrophy in nearly 90% of affected individuals, and small pituitary in 20–30% of persons with mutations in PNPLA6.[101]

Prior to identification of the spectrum of PNPLA6 gene defects, LMS and BBS were considered to be overlapping syndromes due to the early vision loss, obesity, and neurologic disorders that are similar between the two disorders, and BBS patients without polydactyly were often considered to have LMS, but on genetic testing have been found to have one of the variants of BBS.[97] Because of the confusion between these syndromes, and the relative rarity of LMS compared to BBS, the prevalence of obesity and of diabetes are not known. Childhood onset and severe adult obesity are considered typical for Laurence-Moon-Bardet-Biedl syndrome,[101] but prevalence has not been reported for genetically confirmed LMS patients with PNPLA6 gene defects. In the original report by Laurence and Moon, the siblings were obese, which set the stage for many descriptions of inherited obesity syndromes to follow.[102]

Prader-Willi

Prader-Willi syndrome (PWS) is the most common cause of syndromic obesity. Prevalence from epidemiologic data widely varies and has been cited at 1 in 8,000 in a Swedish county.[103] Given a birth incidence of 1:29,000 but increased mean mortality, Whittington et al. concluded that the prevalence of PSW in the United Kingdom was 1:45,000 to 1:52,000 population.[104] PSW occurs equally in males and females. The genetic basis of the disease has been identified as an error in genomic imprinting from loss of expression of paternally derived genes in chromosome 15q11-q13, resulting from microdeletion, imprinting defects, or uniparental dismay.[105] Other genetic causes are maternal chromosome 15 disomies, mutations of an imprinting locus, and chromosomal translocations, which account for the non-deletion cases of PWS.[105]

PWS is a complex, multisystem disorder with a well-described phenotype that varies strikingly with age.[106] Infants present with hypotonia, poor suck, failure to thrive, and global developmental delay in the first two years of life. Hyperphagia from lack of satiety and progressive weight gain begins in childhood and continues into adulthood. Growth hormone deficiency and hypogonadotropic hypogonadism stem from hypothalamic dysfunction, which can also produce central hypothyroidism or central adrenal insufficiency.[107] Other notable features of PWS include short stature, sleep apnea, lymphedema, and stereotypical behavioral disorders (anxiety, obsessive compulsive behaviors, learning disabilities, temper tantrums, and chronic skin picking). Characteristic physical traits, in addition to short stature, include hypopigmented skin, hair, or eyes, short stature, narrow face, prominent forehead, almond-shaped eyes, and thin upper lip with downtrend corners of the mouth. Diagnosis can be made clinically using Holm criteria[107,108] and confirmed by molecular genetic testing.[106,108]

Obesity, a prominent feature of PWS if food is not strictly regulated, is a strong risk factor for T2D, similar to the general population. The prevalence of T2D in adults with PWS, reported at 25%, is fivefold higher than the age-matched unaffected population prevalence of 5–7%.[109] The mean age of onset of diabetes has been reported to be 20 years old, and it is relatively uncommon in prepubertal children with PWS.[110] In a large cohort of 274 patients with PWS in Italy, a higher incidence of altered glucose metabolism (impaired fasting glucose, impaired glucose tolerance, and T2D) was observed, more commonly among the obese and adult patients.[111] Higher intra-abdominal visceral fat area among PWS subjects may increase the risk of obesity-related complications, including diabetes, compared to PWS subjects without increased visceral fat.[112] Additional contributory risk factors for diabetes in PWS include sedentary lifestyle and positive family history.

The relationship between morbid obesity and diabetes in PWS is complex as some studies have observed hypoinsulinemia and greater insulin sensitivity in children and adults with PWS compared to weight-matched non-PWS patients.[113,114] When compared to nonsyndromic persons with obesity, young adult patients with PWS had a similar rate of T2D (23.8%), lower weight but higher BMI due to short stature, but higher fat mass percentage, lower insulin levels, and HOMA-IR.[114] Adipocyte size relative to body fat was higher in PWS versus controls, and metabolic syndrome characteristics were reduced relative to obese controls.[114] Treatment with recombinant hGH has been shown to improve body composition, growth velocity, and adaptive functioning. GH therapy has been continued into adulthood with ongoing effects of improved ratio of lean mass to fat mass.[115] The effects on glucose metabolism have been conflicting, and GH therapy is contraindicated in uncontrolled diabetes and severe obesity.[115]

Treatment of diabetes follows the conventional standard of care and includes dietary and lifestyle modification, weight loss, exercise, metformin, sulfonylurea, and insulin. GLP-1 analogs, in particular liraglutide and exenatide, have been used with some degree of success in several cases to control appetite, decrease body weight, and improve glycemic control in PWS. These have been well tolerated and promising.[110] Larger prospective studies are needed to further characterize the efficacy and safety of GLP-1 agonist in PWS.

PWS is associated with increased mortality, with the average age of death 29 years +/− 16 years.[116] Mortality was due to cardiac and obesity-related complications such as respiratory insufficiency.[117] Weight control through strict management of food availability and exercise as possible are the key interventions for management of PWS and may prevent diabetes and obesity-related morbidity and mortality. With early diagnosis and timely behavioral interventions, and advances in medical care, the mortality rate has decreased from estimated 3% per year across age range and 7% per year above age of 30[104] to 1.25%.[117] With increased life expectancy, diabetes and other comorbidities of obesity, such as hypertension, hyperlipidemia, and cardiovascular disease are commonplace among aging PWS population and have important implications in treatment.

References

1.   American Diabetes Association. Standards of medical care in diabetes—2017. *Diabetes Care* 2017;40(Suppl. 1):S11–S25

2.   M'hamdi O, Ouertani I, Chaabouni-Bouhamed H. Update on the genetics of Bardet-Biedl syndrome. *Mol Syndromol* 2014;5:51–56

3.   Marshall BA, Permutt MA, Paciorkowski AR, et al. Phenotypic characteristics of early Wolfram syndrome. *Orphanet J Rare Dis* 2013;8:64

4.   Parker SE, Mai CT, Canfield MA, et al. Updated national birth prevalence estimates for selected birth defects in the United States, 2004–2006. *Birth Defects Res A Clin Mol Teratol* 2010;88:1008–1016

5. Papavassiliou P, Charalsawadi C, Rafferty K, Jackson-Cook C. Mosaicism for trisomy 21: a review. *Am J Med Genet A* 2015;167A:26–39

6. Smith DS. Health care management of adults with Down syndrome. *Am Fam Physician* 2001;64:1031–1038

7. Goldacre MJ, Wotton CJ, Seagroatt V, Yeates D. Cancers and immune related diseases associated with Down's syndrome: a record linkage study. *Arch Dis Child* 2004;89:1014–1017

8. Anwar AJ, Walker JD, Frier BM. Type 1 diabetes mellitus and Down's syndrome: prevalence, management and diabetic complications. *Diabet Med* 1998;15:160–163

9. Aitken RJ, Mehers KL, Williams AJ, et al. Early-onset, coexisting autoimmunity and decreased HLA-mediated susceptibility are the characteristics of diabetes in Down syndrome. *Diabetes Care* 2013;36:1181–1185

10. Rohrer TR, Hennes P, Thon A, et al. Down's syndrome in diabetic patients aged <20 years: an analysis of metabolic status, glycaemic control and autoimmunity in comparison with type 1 diabetes. *Diabetologia* 2010;53:1070–1075

11. Alexander M, Petri H, Ding Y, Wandel C, Khwaja O, Foskett N. Morbidity and medication in a large population of individuals with Down syndrome compared to the general population. *Dev Med Child Neurol* 2016;58:246–254

12. Gillespie KM, Dix RJ, Williams AJK, et al. Islet autoimmunity in children with Down's syndrome. *Diabetes* 2006;55:3185–3188

13. Real de Asua D, Quero M, Moldenhauer F, Suarez C. Clinical profile and main comorbidities of Spanish adults with Down syndrome. *Eur J Intern Med* 2015;26:385–391

14. Sobey CG, Judkins CP, Sundararajan V, Phan TG, Drummond GR, Srikanth VK. Risk of major cardiovascular events in people with Down syndrome. *PloS One* 2015;10:e0137093

15. Fonseca CT, Amaral DM, Ribeiro MG, Beserra ICR, Guimaraes MM. Insulin resistance in adolescents with Down syndrome: a cross-sectional study. *BMC Endocr Disord* 2005;5:6

16. Fulcher T, Griffin M, Crowley S, Firth R, Acheson R, O'Meara N. Diabetic retinopathy in Down's syndrome. *Br J Ophthalmol* 1998;82:407–409

17. Groth KA, Skakkebæk A, Høst C, Gravholt CH, Bojesen A. Clinical review: Klinefelter syndrome–a clinical update. *J Clin Endocrinol Metab* 2013;98:20–30

18. Lanfranco F, Kamischke A, Zitzmann M, Nieschlag E. Klinefelter's syndrome. *Lancet* 2004;364:273–283

19. Ottesen AM, Aksglaede L, Garn I, et al. Increased number of sex chromosomes affects height in a nonlinear fashion: a study of 305 patients with sex chromosome aneuploidy. *Am J Med Genet A* 2010;152A:1206–1212

20. Seminog OO, Seminog AB, Yeates D, Goldacre MJ. Associations between Klinefelter's syndrome and autoimmune diseases: English national record linkage studies. *Autoimmunity* 2015;48:125–128

21. Bojesen A, Juul S, Birkebæk NH, Gravholt CH. Morbidity in Klinefelter syndrome: a Danish register study based on hospital discharge diagnoses. *J Clin Endocrinol Metab* 2006;91:1254–1260

22. Sawalha AH, Harley JB, Scofield RH. Autoimmunity and Klinefelter's syndrome: when men have two X chromosomes. *J Autoimmun* 2009;33:31–34

23. Panimolle F, Tiberti C, Granato S, et al. Screening of endocrine organ-specific humoral autoimmunity in 47,XXY Klinefelter's syndrome reveals a significant increase in diabetes-specific immunoreactivity in comparison with healthy control men. *Endocrine* 2016;52:157–164

24. Kota SK, Meher LK, Jammula S, Kota SK, Modi KD. Clinical profile of coexisting conditions in type 1 diabetes mellitus patients. *Diabetes Metab Syndr* 2012;6:70–76

25. Jiang-Feng M, Hong-Li X, Xue-Yan W, et al. Prevalence and risk factors of diabetes in patients with Klinefelter syndrome: a longitudinal observational study. *Fertil Steril* 2012;98:1331–1335

26. Bojesen A, Kristensen K, Birkebaek NH, et al. The metabolic syndrome is frequent in Klinefelter's syndrome and is associated with abdominal obesity and hypogonadism. *Diabetes Care* 2006;29:1591–1598

27. Bojesen A, Høst C, Gravholt CH. Klinefelter's syndrome, type 2 diabetes and the metabolic syndrome: the impact of body composition. *Mol Hum Reprod* 2010;16:396–401

28. Aksglaede L, Molgaard C, Skakkebaek NE, Juul A. Normal bone mineral content but unfavourable muscle/fat ratio in Klinefelter syndrome. *Arch Dis Child* 2008;93:30–34

29. Salzano A, Arcopinto M, Marra AM, et al. Klinefelter syndrome, cardiovascular system, and thromboembolic disease: review of literature and clinical perspectives. *Eur J Endocrinol* 2016;175:R27–40

30. Swerdlow AJ, Hermon C, Jacobs PA, et al. Mortality and cancer incidence in persons with numerical sex chromosome abnormalities: a cohort study. *Ann Hum Genet* 2001;65:177–188

31. Swerdlow AJ, Higgins CD, Schoemaker MJ, Wright AF, Jacobs PA, United Kingdom Clinical Cytogenetics Group. Mortality in patients with Klinefelter syndrome in Britain: a cohort study. *J Clin Endocrinol Metab* 2005;90:6516–6522

32. Bondy CA, Turner Syndrome Study Group. Care of girls and women with Turner syndrome: a guideline of the Turner Syndrome Study Group. *J Clin Endocrinol Metab* 2007;92:10–25

33. Gravholt CH, Juul S, Naeraa RW, Hansen J. Prenatal and postnatal prevalence of Turner's syndrome: a registry study. *BMJ* 1996;312:16–21

34. Gravholt CH. Clinical practice in Turner syndrome. *Nat Clin Pract Endocrinol Metab* 2005;1:41–52

35. Rao E, Weiss B, Fukami M, et al. Pseudoautosomal deletions encompassing a novel homeobox gene cause growth failure in idiopathic short stature and Turner syndrome. *Nat Genet* 1997;16:54–63

36. Gravholt CH, Juul S, Naeraa RW, Hansen J. Morbidity in Turner syndrome. *J Clin Epidemiol* 1998;51:147–158

37. Goldacre MJ, Seminog OO. Turner syndrome and autoimmune diseases: record-linkage study. *Arch Dis Child* 2014;99:71–73

38. Bakalov VK, Gutin L, Cheng CM, et al. Autoimmune disorders in women with Turner syndrome and women with karyotypically normal primary ovarian insufficiency. *J Autoimmun* 2012;38:315–321

39. Mortensen KH, Cleemann L, Hjerrild BE, et al. Increased prevalence of autoimmunity in Turner syndrome—influence of age. *Clin Exp Immunol* 2009;156: 205–210

40. Libert C, Dejager L, Pinheiro I. The X chromosome in immune functions: when a chromosome makes the difference. *Nat Rev Immunol* 2010;10:594–604

41. Gravholt CH, Naeraa RW, Nyholm B, et al. Glucose metabolism, lipid metabolism, and cardiovascular risk factors in adult Turner's syndrome. The impact of sex hormone replacement. *Diabetes Care* 1998;21:1062–1070

42. Holl RW, Kunze D, Etzrodt H, Teller W, Heinze E. Turner syndrome: final height, glucose tolerance, bone density and psychosocial status in 25 adult patients. *Eur J Pediatr* 1994;153:11–16

43. Elsheikh M, Dunger DB, Conway GS, Wass JA. Turner's syndrome in adulthood. *Endocr Rev* 2002;23:120–140

44. Mazzanti L, Bergamaschi R, Castiglioni L, Zappulla F, Pirazzoli P, Cicognani A. Turner syndrome, insulin sensitivity and growth hormone treatment. *Horm Res* 2005;64(Suppl. 3):51–57

45. Wilson DM, Frane JW, Sherman B, Johanson AJ, Hintz RL, Rosenfeld RG. Carbohydrate and lipid metabolism in Turner syndrome: effect of therapy with growth hormone, oxandrolone, and a combination of both. *J Pediatr* 1988;112:210–217

46. Inoue H, Tanizawa Y, Wasson J, et al. A gene encoding a transmembrane protein is mutated in patients with diabetes mellitus and optic atrophy (Wolfram syndrome). *Nat Genet* 1998;20:143–148

47. Aloi C, Salina A, Pasquali L, et al. Wolfram syndrome: new mutations, different phenotype. *PloS One* 2012;7:e29150

48. Barrett TG, Bundey SE, Macleod AF. Neurodegeneration and diabetes: UK nationwide study of Wolfram (DIDMOAD) syndrome. *Lancet* 1995;346:1458–1463

49. Wolfram DJ, Wagener HP. Diabetes mellitus and simple optic atrophy among siblings: report of four cases. *Mayo Clin Proc* 1938;13:715–718

50. Richardson JE, Hamilton W. Diabetes insipidus, diabetes mellitus, optic atrophy, and deafness. 3 cases of "DIDMOAD" syndrome. *Arch Dis Child* 1977;52:796–798

51. Raiti S, Plotkin S, Newns GH. Diabetes mellitus and insipidus in two sisters. *BMJ* 1963;2:1625–1629

52. Karasik A, O'Hara C, Srikanta S, et al. Genetically programmed selective islet beta-cell loss in diabetic subjects with Wolfram's syndrome. *Diabetes Care* 1989;12:135–138

53. Hardy C, Khanim F, Torres R, et al. Clinical and molecular genetic analysis of 19 Wolfram syndrome kindreds demonstrating a wide spectrum of mutations in WFS1. *Am J Hum Genet* 1999;65:1279–1290

54. Chaussenot A, Bannwarth S, Rouzier C, et al. Neurologic features and genotype-phenotype correlation in Wolfram syndrome. *Ann Neurol* 2011;69:501–508

55. Lessell S, Rosman NP. Juvenile diabetes mellitus and optic atrophy. *Arch Neurol* 1977;34:759–765

56. Urano F. Wolfram syndrome: diagnosis, management, and treatment. *Curr Diab Rep* 2016;16:6

57. Fonseca SG, Fukuma M, Lipson KL, et al. WFS1 is a novel component of the unfolded protein response and maintains homeostasis of the endoplasmic reticulum in pancreatic beta-cells. *J Biol Chem* 2005;280:39609–39615

58. Lu S, Kanekura K, Hara T, et al. A calcium-dependent protease as a potential therapeutic target for Wolfram syndrome. *Proc Natl Acad Sci U S A* 2014;111:E5292–E5301

59. Yamada T, Ishihara H, Tamura A, et al. WFS1-deficiency increases endoplasmic reticulum stress, impairs cell cycle progression and triggers the apoptotic pathway specifically in pancreatic beta-cells. *Hum Mol Genet* 2006;15:1600–1609

60. Bischoff AN, Reiersen AM, Buttlaire A, et al. Selective cognitive and psychiatric manifestations in Wolfram syndrome. *Orphanet J Rare Dis* 2015;10:66

61. Hershey T, Lugar HM, Shimony JS, et al. Early brain vulnerability in Wolfram syndrome. *PloS One* 2012;7:e40604

62. Cano A, Molines L, Valéro R, et al. Microvascular diabetes complications in Wolfram syndrome (diabetes insipidus, diabetes mellitus, optic atrophy, and deafness [DIDMOAD]): an age- and duration-matched comparison with common type 1 diabetes. *Diabetes Care* 2007;30:2327–2330

63. Kinsley BT, Swift M, Dumont RH, Swift RG. Morbidity and mortality in the Wolfram syndrome. *Diabetes Care* 1995;18:1566–1570

64. Bidichandani SI, Delatycki MB. Friedreich Ataxia. In *GeneReviews* [Internet]. Pagon RA, Adam MP, Ardinger HH, et al., Eds. Seattle, WA, University of Washington, Seattle, 1993–2016

65. Greeley NR, Regner S, Willi S, Lynch DR. Cross-sectional analysis of glucose metabolism in Friedreich ataxia. *J Neurol Sci* 2014;342:29–35

66. Cnop M, Igoillo-Esteve M, Rai M, et al. Central role and mechanisms of β-cell dysfunction and death in Friedreich ataxia-associated diabetes. *Ann Neurol* 2012;72:971–982

67. Farrer LA. Diabetes mellitus in Huntington disease. *Clin Genet* 1985;27:62–67

68. Schulz JB, Boesch S, Bürk K, et al. Diagnosis and treatment of Friedreich ataxia: a European perspective. *Nat Rev Neurol* 2009;5:222–234

69. Huntington Study Group PHAROS Investigators, Biglan KM, Shoulson I, et al. Clinical-genetic associations in the Prospective Huntington at Risk Observational

Study (PHAROS): implications for clinical trials. *JAMA Neurol.* 2016;73: 102–110

70. Boesgaard TW, Nielsen TT, Josefsen K, et al. Huntington's disease does not appear to increase the risk of diabetes mellitus. *J Neuroendocrinol* 2009;21:770–776

71. Zarowitz BJ, O'Shea T, Nance M. Clinical, demographic, and pharmacologic features of nursing home residents with Huntington's disease. *J Am Med Dir Assoc* 2014;15:423–428

72. Lalić NM, Marić J, Svetel M, et al. Glucose homeostasis in Huntington disease: abnormalities in insulin sensitivity and early-phase insulin secretion. *Arch Neurol* 2008;65:476–480

73. Bacos K, Björkqvist M, Petersén A, et al. Islet beta-cell area and hormone expression are unaltered in Huntington's disease. *Histochem Cell Biol* 2008;129:623–629

74. Andreassen OA, Dedeoglu A, Stanojevic V, et al. Huntington's disease of the endocrine pancreas: insulin deficiency and diabetes mellitus due to impaired insulin gene expression. *Neurobiol Dis* 2002;11:410–424

75. Hashimoto K, Ito Y, Tanahashi H, Hayashi M, Yamakita N, Yasuda K. Hyperglycemic chorea-ballism or acute exacerbation of Huntington's chorea? Huntington's disease unmasked by diabetic ketoacidosis in type 1 diabetes mellitus. *J Clin Endocrinol Metab* 2012;97:3016–3020

76. Ranum LPW, Day JW. Myotonic dystrophy: RNA pathogenesis comes into focus. *Am J Hum Genet* 2004;74:793–804

77. Morrone A, Pegoraro E, Angelini C, Zammarchi E, Marconi G, Hoffman EP. RNA metabolism in myotonic dystrophy: patient muscle shows decreased insulin receptor RNA and protein consistent with abnormal insulin resistance. *J Clin Invest* 1997;99:1691–1698

78. Smith CA, Gutmann L. Myotonic dystrophy type 1 management and therapeutics. *Curr Treat Options Neurol* 2016;18:52

79. Moxley RT, Corbett AJ, Minaker KL, Rowe JW. Whole body insulin resistance in myotonic dystrophy. *Ann Neurol* 1984;15:157–162

80. Moxley RT, Griggs RC, Goldblatt D, VanGelder V, Herr BE, Thiel R. Decreased insulin sensitivity of forearm muscle in myotonic dystrophy. *J Clin Invest* 1978;62:857–867

81. Savkur RS, Philips AV, Cooper TA. Aberrant regulation of insulin receptor alternative splicing is associated with insulin resistance in myotonic dystrophy. *Nat Genet* 2001;29:40–47

82. Llagostera E, Catalucci D, Marti L, et al. Role of myotonic dystrophy protein kinase (DMPK) in glucose homeostasis and muscle insulin action. *PloS One* 2007;2:e1134

83. Dahlqvist JR, Ørngreen MC, Witting N, Vissing J. Endocrine function over time in patients with myotonic dystrophy type 1. *Eur J Neurol* 2015;22:116–122

84. Perseghin G, Caumo A, Arcelloni C, et al. Contribution of abnormal insulin secretion and insulin resistance to the pathogenesis of type 2 diabetes in myotonic dystrophy. *Diabetes Care* 2003;26:2112–2118

85. Abe H, Mita T, Kudo K, et al. Dramatic improvement of blood glucose control after pioglitazone treatment in poorly controlled over-weight diabetic patients with myotonic dystrophy. *Endocr J* 2009;56:911–913

86. Bachinski LL, Udd B, Meola G, et al. Confirmation of the type 2 myotonic dystrophy (CCTG)n expansion mutation in patients with proximal myotonic myopathy/proximal myotonic dystrophy of different European origins: a single shared haplotype indicates an ancestral founder effect. *Am J Hum Genet* 2003;73:835–848

87. Day JW, Ricker K, Jacobsen JF, et al. Myotonic dystrophy type 2: molecular, diagnostic and clinical spectrum. *Neurology* 2003;60:657–664

88. Meola G, Moxley RT. Myotonic dystrophy type 2 and related myotonic disorders. *J Neurol* 2004;251:1173–1182

89. Liquori CL, Ricker K, Moseley ML, et al. Myotonic dystrophy type 2 caused by a CCTG expansion in intron 1 of ZNF9. *Science* 2001;293:864–867

90. Savkur RS, Philips AV, Cooper TA, et al. Insulin receptor splicing alteration in myotonic dystrophy type 2. *Am J Hum Genet* 2004;74:1309–1313

91. Zaghloul NA, Katsanis N. Mechanistic insights into Bardet-Biedl syndrome, a model ciliopathy. *J Clin Invest* 2009;119:428–437

92. Nachury MV, Loktev AV, Zhang Q, et al. A core complex of BBS proteins cooperates with the GTPase Rab8 to promote ciliary membrane biogenesis. *Cell* 2007;129:1201–1213

93. Starks RD, Beyer AM, Guo DF, et al. Regulation of insulin receptor trafficking by Bardet Biedl syndrome proteins. *PLoS Genet* 2015;11:e1005311

94. Rahmouni K, Fath MA, Seo S, et al. Leptin resistance contributes to obesity and hypertension in mouse models of Bardet-Biedl syndrome. *J Clin Invest* 2008;118:1458–1467

95. Feuillan PP, Ng D, Han JC, et al. Patients with Bardet-Biedl syndrome have hyperleptinemia suggestive of leptin resistance. *J Clin Endocrinol Metab* 2011;96:E528–E535

96. Seo S, Guo D-F, Bugge K, Morgan DA, Rahmouni K, Sheffield VC. Requirement of Bardet-Biedl syndrome proteins for leptin receptor signaling. *Hum Mol Genet* 2009;18:1323–1331

97. Moore SJ, Green JS, Fan Y, et al. Clinical and genetic epidemiology of Bardet-Biedl syndrome in Newfoundland: a 22-year prospective, population-based, cohort study. *Am J Med Genet A* 2005;132A:352–360

98. Laurence JZ, Moon RC. Four cases of "retinitis pigmentosa" occurring in the same family, and accompanied by general imperfections of development. 1866. *Obes Res* 1995;3:400–403

99. Synofzik M, Hufnagel RB, Züchner S. PNPLA6-related disorders. In *GeneReviews* [Internet]. Pagon RA, Adam MP, Ardinger HH, et al., Eds. Seattle, WA, University of Washington, Seattle, 1993–2016

100. Hufnagel RB, Arno G, Hein ND, et al. Neuropathy target esterase impairments cause Oliver-McFarlane and Laurence-Moon syndromes. *J Med Genet* 2015;52:85–94

101. Rainier S, Albers JW, Dyck PJ, et al. Motor neuron disease due to neuropathy target esterase gene mutation: clinical features of the index families. *Muscle Nerve* 2011;43:19–25

102. Bray GA. Laurence, Moon, Bardet, and Biedl: reflections on a syndrome. *Obes Res* 1995;3:383–386

103. Akefeldt A, Gillberg C, Larsson C. Prader-Willi syndrome in a Swedish rural county: epidemiological aspects. *Dev Med Child Neurol* 1991;33:715–721

104. Whittington JE, Holland AJ, Webb T, Butler J, Clarke D, Boer H. Population prevalence and estimated birth incidence and mortality rate for people with Prader-Willi syndrome in one UK Health Region. *J Med Genet* 2001;38:792–798

105. Nicholls RD, Saitoh S, Horsthemke B. Imprinting in Prader-Willi and Angelman syndromes. *Trends Genet TIG.* 1998;14:194–200

106. Cassidy SB, Schwartz S, Miller JL, Driscoll DJ. Prader-Willi syndrome. *Genet Med* 2012;14:10–26

107. Holm VA, Cassidy SB, Butler MG, et al. Prader-Willi syndrome: consensus diagnostic criteria. *Pediatrics* 1993;91:398–402

108. Gunay-Aygun M, Schwartz S, Heeger S, O'Riordan MA, Cassidy SB. The changing purpose of Prader-Willi syndrome clinical diagnostic criteria and proposed revised criteria. *Pediatrics.* 2001;108:E92

109. Butler JV, Whittington JE, Holland AJ, Boer H, Clarke D, Webb T. Prevalence of, and risk factors for, physical ill-health in people with Prader-Willi syndrome: a population-based study. *Dev Med Child Neurol* 2002;44:248–255

110. Fintini D, Grugni G, Bocchini S, et al. Disorders of glucose metabolism in Prader-Willi syndrome: results of a multicenter Italian cohort study. *Nutr Metab Cardiovasc Dis* 2016;26:842–847

111. Talebizadeh Z, Butler MG. Insulin resistance and obesity-related factors in Prader-Willi syndrome: comparison with obese subjects. *Clin Genet* 2005;67:230–239

112. Haqq AM, Muehlbauer MJ, Newgard CB, Grambow S, Freemark M. The metabolic phenotype of Prader-Willi syndrome (PWS) in childhood: heightened insulin sensitivity relative to body mass index. *J Clin Endocrinol Metab* 2011;96:E225–E232

113. Höybye C, Hilding A, Jacobsson H, Thorén M. Metabolic profile and body composition in adults with Prader-Willi syndrome and severe obesity. *J Clin Endocrinol Metab* 2002;87:3590–3597

114. Lacroix D, Moutel S, Coupaye M, et al. Metabolic and adipose tissue signatures in adults with Prader-Willi syndrome: a model of extreme adiposity. *J Clin Endocrinol Metab* 2015;100:850–859

115. Deal CL, Tony M, Höybye C, et al. Growth Hormone Research Society workshop summary: consensus guidelines for recombinant human growth hormone therapy in Prader-Willi syndrome. *J Clin Endocrinol Metab* 2013;98:E1072–E1087

116. Butler MG, Manzardo AM, Heinemann J, Loker C, Loker J. Causes of death in Prader-Willi syndrome: Prader-Willi Syndrome Association (USA) 40-year mortality survey. *Genet Med.* 17 November 2016 [Epub ahead of print]

117. Whittington JE, Holland AJ, Webb T. Ageing in people with Prader-Willi syndrome: mortality in the UK population cohort and morbidity in an older sample of adults. *Psychol Med* 2015;45:615–621

Part III
Case Studies

Introduction

The following 21 cases of atypical diabetes highlight clinical presentation of diabetes in patients with endocrinopathies, immune-mediated pathogenesis of diabetes, diabetes of unknown cause, and diabetes arising in patients with other genetic diseases. Cases 44 through 49 spotlight frequent development of diabetes in patients with other endocrine diseases, such as acromegaly, Cushing's syndrome, pheochromocytoma, and glucagonoma. Successful therapy of the underlying disease in these cases usually dramatically improves or completely normalizes glycemic control. Patients with latent autoimmune diabetes of adults (LADA) represent a distinct group of individuals with diabetes that is often initially mistaken for type 2 (Cases 50–53). Once an appropriate diagnosis is made, insulin therapy is instituted and these patients are managed similarly to those with type 1 diabetes. Other examples of immune-mediated diabetes are presented by cases 54–57. They include Type B insulin resistance, polyglandular failure, and stiff person syndrome. An unusual entity of ketosis-prone diabetes is illustrated by cases 58–60. This form of diabetes appears to be not as rare as was originally thought, and many diabetologists have seen these atypical cases of diabetes in their practices. Finally, there are other genetic syndromes associated with diabetes and they are depicted by cases 61–64.

Chapters 5 through 8 of Part III of this volume offer in-depth discussion of these conditions as well as extensive lists of references to aid practitioners to diagnose and manage atypical cases of diabetes they might encounter in their offices.

Case 44:
Acromegaly and Diabetic Ketoacidosis

Padmaja Akkireddy, MD;[1] and Andjela Drincic, MD[1]

Case

A previously healthy 43-year-old Caucasian female presented with altered mental status after experiencing two weeks of polyuria, polydipsia, weakness, and fatigue. Diagnosis of new-onset diabetes with diabetic ketoacidosis (DKA) was made based on the following laboratory data: random plasma glucose of 545 mg/dL, serum bicarbonate level of 9 mmol/L, positive serum beta-hydroxyl butyrate, and arterial pH of 6.99. Her HbA$_{1c}$ level was 13.7%. Computerized tomography (CT) of her head obtained at presentation showed a 3 cm pituitary adenoma.

Additional history was obtained after patient's mental status improved following treatment of DKA. Family history was negative for diabetes or other endocrinopathies. Review of systems was positive for excessive sweating and excess facial and body hair. Her wedding ring increased by two sizes over the past ten years, and she had been wearing flip-flops most of the time as her shoes were not fitting her. She denied headaches or visual difficulties, and her menstrual periods had been regular.

On physical examination, she weighed 73 kg with a BMI of 25.6 kg/m^2. She had coarse facial features with frontal bossing, a widened and thickened nose, periorbital puffiness (Figure C44.1), excess facial and body hair with Ferriman-Gallwey score of 15, widened and thickened hands and feet,

---

[1]Division of Diabetes, Endocrinology, and Metabolism, University of Nebraska Medical Center, Omaha, NE

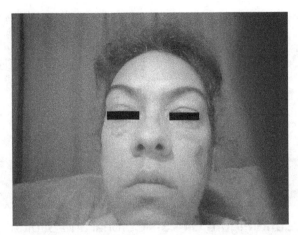

Figure C44.1—Patient's face showing coarsening of features, frontal bossing, periorbital edema, prognathism, thickened lips, and wide nasal bridge.

hidradenitis, and acanthosis nigricans. Ophthalmologic examination was normal without any visual field defects.

Laboratory evaluation showed: prolactin 16.2 ng/mL (3.3–26.7 ng/mL), TSH 1.150 mcIU/mL (0.4–5.0 mcIU/mL), Free T4 0.6 ng/dL (0.6–1.5 ng/dL), 8 A.M. cortisol 24.6 mcg/dL (6.7–22.6 mcg/dL), ACTH 43 pg/mL (0–46 pg/mL), estradiol 124 pg/mL (27–294 pg/mL) with normal gonadotrophins. Her insulin-like growth factor 1 (IGF-1) level was normal at 258 ng/mL (normal range for age/sex 118–298 ng/mL). Antibodies to glutamic acid decarboxylase were negative. MRI of the sella showed 3.1 cm pituitary adenoma with bilateral cavernous sinus invasion with the optic chiasm displaced superiorly (Figure C44.2 and Figure C44.3).

Three weeks after her discharge, when blood glucose levels were well controlled, a repeat IGF-1 was elevated at 713 ng/L and a random growth hormone (GH) was elevated at >80 ng/mL (<7.1 ng/mL). The diagnosis of acromegaly with secondary diabetes was made, and patient underwent transphenoidal resection of pituitary adenoma. Surgical pathology confirmed somatotroph adenoma, strongly immunoreactive for GH, and negative for prolactin, TSH, ACTH, and p53. Total daily insulin dose prior to surgery was 60 units, falling to 25 units after the surgery (Table C44.1).

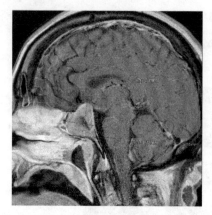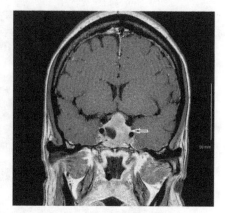

Figure C44.2 and Figure C44.3—Coronal and Sagittal MR images showing pituitary adenoma with cavernous sinus invasion and displacement of optic chiasm.

Table C44.1—Variation of Serum IGF-1 Levels and Insulin Doses from the Time of Presentation

Days from Presentation	Day 2	Day 4	Day 21	Day 54, post op day 1	Day 75	Day 89
Mean glucose (mg/dL)	245	164	108	120	118	110
IGF-1 levels (ng/mL)	258	316	713	N/A	N/A	N/A
Total insulin dose (units/day)	96	74	63	45	30	25

Discussion

DKA as the presenting feature of acromegaly is rare with only a few reported cases in the literature, most of which had elevated IGF-1 at the time of diagnosis. Our case illustrates two important features of secondary diabetes associated with GH excess:

1. Insulin resistance in acromegaly can present as DKA.

2. In the setting of uncontrolled diabetes, IGF-1 may be unreliable for the diagnosis of acromegaly as it can be falsely low.

Acromegaly is a chronic disorder caused by GH hypersecretion in adults, most commonly arising from a pituitary tumor. Glucose intolerance is seen in nearly 50% of patients with acromegaly and overt diabetes in 10–20% of patients.[1]

Insulin resistance is the hallmark of diabetes in acromegaly, and therefore clinically it resembles type 2 diabetes. GH induces insulin resistance at several levels including the insulin receptor and its postreceptor signal transduction pathways. Consequently insulin action is reduced in both hepatic and extrahepatic tissues causing decrease in both insulin-dependent peripheral glucose uptake and gluconeogenesis leading to hyperglycemia.[2] The level of glycemia is to a degree dependent on balance between the activities of GH and IGF-1, since GH-stimulated IGF-1 has insulin-like actions. The French registry data showed that age at diagnosis of acromegaly, BMI, hypertension, and duration of evolution of acromegaly are significant independent risk factors associated with development of diabetes.[3] Presence of hypertension increased the risk of diabetes by 2.5% in acromegaly patients, and female acromegalic patients had a higher probability of developing diabetes than males.

DKA, conventionally regarded as the hallmark of type 1 diabetes, may also occur in patients with type 2 diabetes and other insulin-resistant states including acromegaly due to glucotoxicity-induced transient β-cell failure and relative insulin deficiency. GH also enhances lipolysis, where free fatty acid substrates can then act as a competitive energy source and inhibit glucose oxidation.[2]

IGF-1 is recommended to be the initial test for screening and monitoring of acromegaly and in selected circumstances may be diagnostic as it provides an assessment of integrated GH secretion. It is considered that a normal IGF-1 excludes acromegaly. However, falsely low IGF-1 levels can be seen in malnutrition, hepatic or renal failure, and uncontrolled diabetes.[4] The mechanism for low IGF-1 in patients with acromegaly and uncontrolled diabetes is poorly understood. Studies have shown that IGF-1 levels can be low in otherwise healthy patients with uncontrolled diabetes.[5,6]

Glucose tolerance and diabetes generally improve following successful treatment of acromegaly; those with a shorter duration of diabetes and lower levels of GH are more likely to undergo complete resolution. In the case discussed above, a diagnosis of acromegaly could have been missed based on normal IGF-1 measured during a DKA episode. In the setting of high clinical suspicion of acromegaly and uncontrolled diabetes, IGF-1 should be measured after hyperglycemia is controlled.[3]

References

1. Melmed S, Kleinberg D. Pituitary masses and tumors. In *Williams Textbook of Endocrinology*. 12th ed. Melmed S, Polonsky KS, Larsen PR, Kronenberg HM, Eds. Philadelphia, PA Elsevier Saunders, 2011, p. 229–290

2. Møller N, Jørgensen JO. Effects of growth hormone on glucose, lipid, and protein metabolism in human subjects. *Endocr Rev* 2009;30:152–177

3. Fieffe S, Morange I, Petrossians P, et al. Diabetes in acromegaly, prevalence, risk factors and evolution: data from French Acromegaly Registry. *Eur J Endocrinol* 2011;164: 877–884

4. Katznelson L, Atkinson JLD, Cook DM, Ezzat SZ, Hamrahian AH, Miller KK; American Assocation of Clinical Endocrinologists. American Association of Clinical Endocrinologists medical guidelines for clinical practice for the diagnosis and treatment of acromegaly - 2011 update. *Endocr Pract* 2011;17(Suppl. 4): 1–44

5. Clayton KL, Holly JM, Carlsson LM, et al. Loss of the normal relationships between growth hormone, growth hormone-binding protein and insulin-like growth factor-I in adolescents with insulin dependent diabetes mellitus. *Clin Endocrinol (Oxf)* 1994;41:517–524

6. Teppala S, Shankar A. Association between serum IGF-1 and diabetes among U.S. adults. *Diabetes Care* 2010;33:2257–2259

Case 45:
Cushing's Syndrome and Diabetes

Katherine Peicher, DO;[1] and Luigi Meneghini, MD, MBA[1]

Case

A 78-year-old lady with a past medical history of congestive heart failure, type 2 diabetes, coronary artery disease, hypertension, obstructive respiratory disorder of unknown etiology on home oxygen, and chronic kidney disease was hospitalized with shortness of breath, anasarca, and intermittent chest pain. Admission diagnoses included volume overload, hypokalemia, hypernatremia, metabolic alkalosis, and hypertension. Upon further questioning, she reported increased bruising, hirsutism, acne, subjective weight gain, as well as facial plethora over the past several months. She reported pain in her thighs upon standing but denied muscle weakness. On physical exam, she was afebrile with stable vital signs; blood pressure was 156/85 mmHg. She weighed 101.2 kg (BMI 40.9 kg/m²). She was initially quite lethargic and morbidly obese. Terminal hairs were present on her cheeks bilaterally and on her chin; moon facies were noted. Abdomen was morbidly obese, and no striae were noted. Lower extremities had 2+ pitting edema, and her skin was notable for multiple bruises on her upper extremities. Supraclavicular fat pads were present bilaterally.

Initial morning laboratory tests revealed an elevated ACTH level of 339 pg/mL (reference range 6–58 pg/mL) and serum cortisol level of 111.6 mcg/dL (reference range 5–23 mcg/dL), with a nighttime (22:25 P.M.)

---

[1]Division of Endocrinology, UT Southwestern Medical Center, Dallas, TX

serum cortisol level of 102.5 mcg/dL, highlighting a loss in diurnal variation. Eight milligrams of dexamethasone failed to suppress morning cortisol levels (115.6 mcg/dL); concomitant ACTH was 226 pg/mL. On subsequent 24-hour urinary collection, the urine cortisol was 1,406 mcg/24 hours (reference range 3.5–45 mcg/24 hours).

Pituitary MRI showed an ill-defined area of heterogeneous postcontrast enhancement within the pituitary gland measuring approximately 7 mm.

Chest CT displayed a 22 x 16 x 16 mm nodule with well-defined margins in the major fissure of the inferior right upper lobe.

Thyroid ultrasound showed multiple nodules, the largest measuring 2.5 cm in greatest dimension, but none with definite features worrisome for malignancy.

The patient and her family were offered inferior petrosal sinus sampling but refused. The patient was empirically started on ketoconazole 400 mg PO daily for medical management of hypercortisolemia, and the dose was subsequently increased due to persistently elevated serum cortisol levels (see Table C45.1). Given the ACTH-dependent nature of the hypercortisolism and chest CT findings, we suspected a small-cell carcinoma; however, we were unable to obtain a tissue biopsy due to surrounding vasculature and patient's respiratory condition. An empiric round of chemotherapy was discussed with oncology should there be evidence of rapid tumor growth, but the patient and family declined. The dose of ketoconazole eventually reached the maximum recommended dose of 1,600 mg p.o. daily, with improvement in serum cortisol (54 mcg/dL), blood glucose (BG) levels, and reduction in total daily dose (TDD) of insulin (85 units/day). After three weeks on treatment, ketoconazole had to be discontinued due to an increase in liver function tests to more than three times the upper limit of normal, with subsequent increase in the TDD of insulin to 111 units per day. Cabergoline 0.5 mg twice weekly was started with improvement in BG values and reduction in the TDD (103 units/day). As part of her workup, serum calcitonin levels were measured and found to be 850 pg/mL (reference range: 0.0–5.1 pg/mL). The patient and her family opted against pursuing the workup for possible medullary thyroid carcinoma. The patient was started on metyrapone 250 mg p.o. q.i.d., and within one day the patient's BG levels improved, allowing for a reduction in the TDD of insulin to 79 units/day, with further insulin dose decreases needed in the subsequent days (see Table C45.1). Unfortunately, the patient's clinical

Table C45.1 — Hospital Course and Response to Medical Treatment for Hypercortisolism. As the Cortisol Value Decreased, the Patient Required Less Daily Insulin and Experienced Improved Glycemic Control

Day	Home Dose	Day 3	Day 11	Day 13	Day 15	Day 17	Day 19	Day 24	Day 42	Day 44	Day 57	Day 63
Treatment for hypercortisolism	None	None	Ketoconazole	Ketoconazole	Ketoconazole	Ketoconazole	Ketoconazole	Ketoconazole	Ketoconazole stopped	Cabergoline	Metyrapone	Metyrapone
Dose of medication	N/A	N/A	400 mg PO q.d.	600 mg p.o. q.d.	800 mg p.o. q.d.	1,200 mg p.o. q.d.	1,400 mg p.o. q.d.	1,600 mg p.o. q.d.	N/A	0.5 mg p.o. twice weekly	1,000 mg p.o. q.d.	500 mg p.o. q.d.
ACTH (reference range: 6–58 pg/mL)	N/A	339	226	N/A	N/A	N/A	N/A	N/A	N/A	N/A	N/A	N/A
Cortisol (reference range: 5–23 mcg/dL)	N/A	110	116	121	107	75	52	54	110	N/A	65	33
TDD of insulin (units / day)	95	142	110	116	110	90	85	85	107	111	103	21
Daily BG (mg/dL)	N/A	92–359	89–309	95–188	86–171	59–146	99–207	132–319	191–283	94–203	106–162	117–223

course continued to deteriorate, and the patient's family elected for the patient to be discharged to hospice care.

Cushing's syndrome is a condition characterized by excessive cortisol production due to either ACTH-dependent mechanisms, as seen in pituitary adenomas or in ectopic tumors producing ACTH, or ACTH-independent conditions, as seen in adrenal adenomas or hyperplasia. The resulting hypercortisolemia can lead to central obesity, purple striae, proximal muscle weakness, hirsutism, acne, fatigue, osteoporosis, emotional liability, menstrual irregularities, impaired glucose tolerance, diabetes, and death.[1-4] The pathophysiology of diabetes in these patients is complex, arising from both pancreatic β-cell dysfunction, as well as increased insulin resistance.[2] Glucocorticoid excess can cause glucose intolerance with normal fasting blood glucose values, and the diagnosis can be missed without an oral glucose tolerance test.[1,2,4] Hypercortisolemia can exacerbate hyperglycemia in patients with established diabetes, and treatment of the underlying condition often leads to improvement in glycemic control.[1,4]

Hypercortisolemia can lead to hyperglycemia and diabetes by decreasing insulin sensitivity in the liver, skeletal muscles, and adipose tissues in the postprandial state.[1] ACTH-dependent Cushing's syndrome is most commonly due to an ACTH-producing pituitary tumor. In this case, the condition is termed Cushing's disease. However, the differential diagnosis includes ectopic tumors overproducing ACTH, primary adrenal malignancies, or very rarely ectopic corticotropin-releasing hormone secretion. Additionally, tumors such as various lung cancers, carcinoid tumors, medullary thyroid cancers, and pheochromocytomas can secrete ACTH, causing Cushing's syndrome.[3,4] The primary treatment is surgical, with some cases requiring a second surgery if the pituitary adenoma is large, or radiation therapy in the event of incomplete resection or recurrence.[4] In our case, surgery was not an option because of the patient's condition, the family's refusal for invasive interventions, and the lack of a definitively identified source of ACTH secretion. Several therapies can be considered for medical treatment of hypercortisolemia, although none of them curative. Medical therapies include ketoconazole, mitotane, metyrapone, and etomidate, which work to inhibit adrenal steroidogenesis. Mifepristone blocks the effects of cortisol and is approved for treatment of hyperglycemia due to Cushing's syndrome. Pasireotide and cabergoline work in Cushing's disease to decrease ACTH production from the pituitary gland.[3-5] When present, hyperglycemia needs to be properly addressed to mitigate associated risks of morbidity and mortality; treatment of hypercortisolemia will significantly improve, if not completely resolve, the hyperglycemia and/or diabetes.

References

1.   Mazziotti G, Gazzaruso C, Giustina A. Diabetes in Cushing syndrome: basic and clinical aspects. *Trends Endocrinol Metab* 2011;22:499–506

2.   Pivonello R, De Leo M, Vitale P, Cozzolino A, Simeoli C, De Martino MC, Lombardi G, Colao A. Pathophysiology of diabetes mellitus in Cushing's syndrome. *Neuroendocrinology* 2010;92(Suppl. 1):77–81

3.   Newell-Price J, Bertegna X, Grossman AB, Nieman LK. Cushing's syndrome. *Lancet* 2006;367:1605–1617

4.   Sharma S, Nieman L, Feelders R. Cushing's syndrome: epidemiology and developments in disease management. *Clin Epidemiol* 2015;7:281–293

5.   Fleseriu M. Recent advances in the medical treatment of Cushing's disease. *F1000Prime Rep* 2014;6:1–9

Case 46:
Pheochromocytoma and Diabetes

Katherine Modzelewski, MD;[1] and Devin Steenkamp, MD[1]

Case

A lean, 70-year-old woman (55 kg, BMI of 19.6 kg/m²) with poorly controlled type 2 diabetes, hypertension, and a known adrenal nodule was admitted to the hospital for abdominal pain, significant weight loss, and marked hyperglycemia. She had been diagnosed with type 2 diabetes at least seven years prior to hospitalization, at which time she weighed 96 kg and had a BMI of 36.1 kg/m². She initially demonstrated excellent glycemic control while being treated with pioglitazone, but for three years prior to hospitalization had progressive worsening of glycemic control. Metformin and glipizide were added without significant improvement, and she consistently declined insulin therapy.

Her admission laboratory data were notable for a blood glucose of 721 mg/dL (40 mmol/L), ketonuria, and an elevated anion gap, but she did not meet diagnostic criteria for diabetic ketoacidosis or hyperosmolar hyperglycemic state. Hemoglobin A1C (HbA$_{1c}$) was 15.8%. She was admitted to the medical intensive care unit and hyperglycemia was managed with an insulin infusion initially, but her blood glucose quickly improved and she was transitioned to basal-bolus insulin. At the time of hospital discharge, oral hypoglycemic agents were stopped, and she was discharged on 0.4 unit/kg of insulin per day.

---

[1]Section of Endocrinology, Diabetes and Nutrition, Boston Medical Center and Boston University School of Medicine, Boston, MA

During her hospital admission, she reported abdominal pain, constipation, and significant weight loss of over 40 kg over the course of two years. Abdominal computerized tomography (CT) without contrast revealed a right adrenal mass measuring 5.1 x 5.7 x 5.4 cm, increased in size from 4.6 x 4.9 x 5.3 cm on prior study five years earlier during the workup for ovarian mucinous adenocarcinoma (see Figure C46.1). The mass had previously been described as cystic, but on the current study it appeared solid with unenhanced CT attenuation of 36 Hounsfield units, concerning for malignancy, metastatic disease, or pheochromocytoma. Intravenous contrast washout was not performed on this study. Although this mass had been present for at least seven years, diagnostic workup with hormonal evaluation had never been completed.

On further history, she reported well-controlled hypertension treated with hydrochlorothiazide alone. She denied palpitations, headaches, sweating, or anxiety. Review of her medical record revealed that following

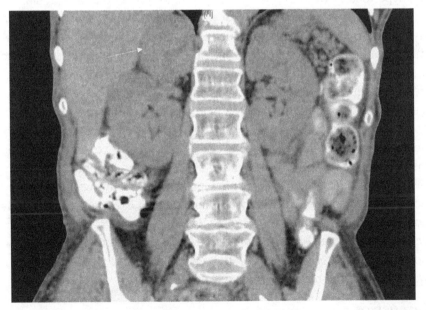

Figure C46.1—Right adrenal mass measuring 5.1 x 5.7 x 5.4 cm with unenhanced CT attenuation of 36 Hounsfield units. The mass had increased in size from 4.6 x 4.9 x 5.3 cm on CT abdomen obtained five years earlier.

a previous ovarian tumor resection, she had labile blood pressure, but this was thought to be secondary to medication noncompliance. Given the size, growth, and Hounsfield attenuation of the right adrenal mass, laboratory hormonal evaluation was performed and revealed markedly elevated plasma metanephrine concentrations of 1,298 pg/mL (normal range ≤57 pg/mL) with normal ACTH, cortisol, renin, and aldosterone concentrations. A presumptive diagnosis of pheochromocytoma was made based on the combination of hypertension, suggestive adrenal mass, and elevated plasma metanephrines. Confirmatory plasma metanephrine concentrations obtained at an outpatient visit two weeks later remained elevated at 2,438 pg/mL.

At follow-up, she reported checking blood glucose four times per day, and her glucose was consistently greater than 300 mg/dL despite compliance with insulin therapy. Prandial insulin doses were increased over the next month as a result of persistent postprandial hyperglycemia. She was referred to endocrine surgery for pheochromocytoma resection, and her antihypertensive was changed from hydrochlorothiazide to doxazosin.

She remained on doxazosin for three months while preparing for surgery, and soon after initiation of the alpha blockade she noted improvement in her glycemic control. Repeat HbA$_{1c}$ one week prior to surgery had improved to 7.5% with increase in total daily insulin dose to 0.6 unit/kg/day. Doxazosin was discontinued and she was transitioned onto phenoxybenzamine, titrated to maintain low-normal blood pressure without orthostatic hypotension. One week later, she underwent laparoscopic right adrenalectomy. Following surgery both antihypertensive and scheduled insulin therapy were discontinued and optimal glycemic control was maintained with minimal correction bolus insulin doses. She was discharged home without any insulin or diabetes medications. Surgical pathology was consistent with a 7.5 cm pheochromocytoma, and plasma metanephrines were undetectable at three months following surgical resection. At follow-up one month after surgery, her HbA$_{1c}$ was 7.3%, and six months later it was 6.2% without diabetes pharmacotherapy.

Discussion

The coexistence of pheochromocytoma and diabetes has been established since the early 1900s, though the understanding of the relationship between the two has evolved over time. Although initially managed as separate entities, it has been increasingly understood that treatment of pheochromocytoma, both medical and surgical, can lead to improvement or resolution of diabetes.[1] A possible causal relationship between pheochromocytoma and diabetes was first described by Duncan et al.[2] in 1944. They reported a male patient with long-standing diabetes who was subsequently noted to have uncontrolled hypertension, which ultimately led to the diagnosis of a pheochromocytoma. Preoperatively, he required as much as 1.6 units/kg/day of insulin, but within a few days of surgical resection required no further pharmacological diabetes treatment, suggesting that diabetes could be directly caused by pheochromocytoma and that subsequent resection of the pheochromocytoma could potentially result in diabetes remission.

It was initially suggested that hyperglycemia in pheochromocytoma-associated diabetes resulted from high levels of catecholamines stimulating excess hepatic gluconeogenesis via beta adrenergic receptors in the liver.[3] Subsequent studies suggested that catecholamine activity on pancreatic alpha cells results in inhibition of insulin secretion.[4] It was hypothesized that treatment with phenoxybenzamine, a potent, irreversible, nonselective alpha-blocking agent, would cure diabetes in pheochromocytoma. However, treatment with phenoxybenzamine preoperatively improved diabetes in only a select group of patients, suggesting a more complex mechanism that may be related to increasing metanephrine concentration leading to increased suppression of insulin release.[3,4]

Based on prior animal studies reporting that epinephrine impairs glycogenesis in the liver and glucose utilization in skeletal muscle, Wiesner et al.[5] performed a hyperinsulinemic euglycemic clamp study to assess insulin resistance in patients with pheochromocytoma. Hyperinsulinemic euglycemic clamps were performed before and after surgical resection in five patients with diabetes and five healthy controls. Glucose infusion rate needed to maintain euglycemia significantly increased in both groups after surgery, but to a greater extent in patients with diabetes. In addition, C-peptide and fasting insulin levels decreased after surgery in both groups, suggesting improved insulin sensitivity with lower circulating catecholamine concentrations. In our case, significantly more insulin was required to cover postprandial glucose excursions, with comparatively low basal insulin requirement. This suggests that peripheral insulin resistance and impaired glucose disposal in the muscle may have played a predominant role in the development of postprandial hyperglycemia. In our case, the diabetes diagnosis preceded the diagnosis of pheochromocytoma, although it is certainly conceivable that the long-standing growing adrenal mass contributed to progressive hyperglycemia.

This case highlights the need to maintain a high index of suspicion for possible secondary causes of hyperglycemia in individuals with an atypical diabetes phenotype. Pheochromocytoma is a very unusual etiology to consider, especially in an individual without the classic paroxysmal hypertension, sweating spells, or headaches. This case also directs our attention toward recognizing that an "incidental adrenal mass" may be functional and may contribute to diabetes, and that timely and thorough workup for abnormal hormonal secretion should not be delayed. Our case also strongly suggests that preoperative alpha blockade may improve glucose control in certain individuals with pheochromocytoma- associated diabetes, particularly at higher metanephrine concentrations. Our patient's HbA$_{1c}$ decreased from 15.8% to 7.5% preoperatively (see Figure C46.2) with minimal increases in her total daily insulin requirement, suggesting a direct alpha blockade-mediated improvement. However, blood glucose did not completely normalize until after pheochromocytoma resection, suggesting that complete removal of excess catecholamines was necessary to result in diabetes resolution.

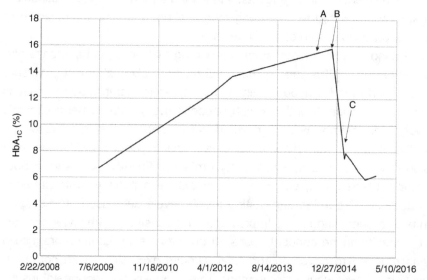

Figure C46.2—Hemoglobin A1C throughout follow-up period. A. Initiation of insulin therapy; B. initiation of doxazosin; C. surgical resection.

References

1. Stenström G, Sjöström L, Smith U. Diabetes mellitus in phaeochromocytoma: Fasting blood glucose levels before and after surgery in 60 patients with phaeochromocytoma. *Acta Endocrinol (Copenh)* 1984;106:511–515

2. Duncan LE, Semans JH, Howard JE. Adrenal medullary tumor (pheochromocytoma) and diabetes mellitus; disappearance of diabetes after removal of the tumor. *Ann Intern Med* 1944;20:815–821

3. Isles CG, Johnson JK. Phaeochromocytoma and diabetes mellitus: further evidence that α2 receptors inhibit insulin release in man. *Clin Endocrinol (Oxf)* 1983;18:37–41

4. Illig R, Ziegler WH. Glucose tolerance and immunoreactive insulin in patients with pheochromocytoma: the effect of α-receptor blocking agents. *Acta Endocrinol (Copenh)* 1971;66:368–378

5. Wiesner TD, Blüher M, Windgassen M, Paschke R. Improvement of insulin sensitivity after adrenalectomy in patients with pheochromocytoma. *J Clin Endocrinol Metab* 2003;88:3632–3636

Case 47: Hypertension plus Hyperglycemia May Be Equal to Pheochromocytoma

Licy L. Yanes Cardozo, MD;[1] Vishnu Garla, MD;[1] and Lillian F. Lien, MD[1]

Case

A 59-year-old woman with past medical history of hepatitis C, hypertension, and hypothyroidism presented to the ER due to worsening spells consisting of headaches, dizziness, and tinnitus that lasted for 15 minutes and then resolved spontaneously. No identified precipitating factors were noted. She reported multiple episodic spells during the day, occurring in the last 5 years and worsening in the last 6 months. She recalled that her blood pressure (BP) was low during her primary care visit, which prompted her primary care physician to prescribe pseudoephedrine, and her antihypertensive medications were discontinued in the past year. Review of systems was positive for an unintentional 15-pound weight loss, diffuse sweating, and back pain in the last 6 months.

On admission, BP was 152/89, heart rate was 90, and temperature was 98.1°F. Labile BP was noted from systolic of 110 to 200 mmHg and diastolic of 80 to 130 mmHg. On physical examination, she was a well-developed, well-nourished woman who appeared anxious. She was alert and fully oriented. No cushingoid features were noted. Facial flushing was present. Her musculoskeletal examination was positive for tenderness to palpation in the lumbar spine. Cardiac, pulmonary, and abdominal examinations were unremarkable. A laboratory evaluation during admission

[1]Division of Endocrinology, Metabolism, and Diabetes, University of Mississippi Medical Center, Jackson, MS

Table C47.1—Catecholamines and Metanephrines at Presentation

Determination	Value	Normal Range
Normetanephrines, free	26	<0.90 nmol/L
Metanephrines, free	1.3	<0.50 nmol/L
Epinephrine	244	<111 pg/mL
Norepinephrine	9,241	<750 pg/mL
Dopamine	80	<30 pg/mL
24-h urine normetanephrine	25,025	<900 mcg/24 h
24-h urine metaneprhine	3,086	<400 mcg/24 h

revealed a high level of plasma and 24-hour urine metanephrines and cat-echolamines (Table C47.1), and preoperative workup showed an abnormal fasting plasma glucose level of 149 mg/dL (8.3 mmol/L). Computerized tomography (CT) of abdomen showed a 6 cm heterogeneous lobulated enhancing mass in the right adrenal with ill-defined borders, invading the diaphragm (Figure C47.1). An I-metaiodobenzylguanidine scan showed avid uptake of tracer in the right adrenal mass (Figure C47.2) and multiple areas of metastasis (skull, pelvis, liver, lumbar, and thoracic spine).

After adequate alpha and beta blockade with doxazosin 16 mg daily and labetalol 400 mg daily for 4 weeks, adrenalectomy, liver wedge resection of metastasis and resection and repair of the inferior vena cava were performed without complications. On the morning of surgery, she had

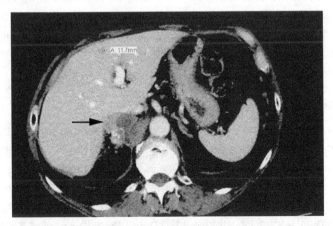

Figure C47.1—Right adrenal mass on abdomen CT (red arrow).

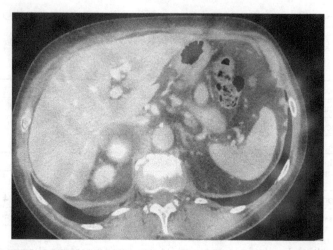

Figure C47.2—Avid uptake by right adrenal mass on MIBG scan.

point-of-care blood glucose levels of 163 mg/dL (9.1 mmol/L) and 227mg/dL (12.6 mmol/L). Postoperatively, fasting plasma glucose levels dropped from 140 mg/dL (7.8 mmol/L) on POD#1, to 113 mg/dL (6.3 mmol/L) on POD#2, and 99 mg/dL (5.5 mmol/L) on POD#3. She was discharged home after 5 days of hospitalization. Postoperatively, the dose of alpha blockade and beta blockade was titrated down to doxazosin 8 mg daily and labetalol 200 mg daily. Histological examination confirmed the diagnosis of pheochromocytoma. Genetic testing was negative for known possible pheochromocytoma-causing mutations. She is currently undergoing treatment with systemic chemotherapy for malignant pheochromocytoma with cyclophosphamide, vincristine, and dacarbazine. At her most recent visit, BP control has improved significantly, and she does not require alpha blockade to maintain normal BP. Levels of plasma metanephrines remain elevated.

Discussion

Pheochromocytoma is a rare endocrine disorder occurring in 0.2–0.6% of patients with hypertension. Derived from intra- or extra-adrenal chromaffin cells, the hallmark of the tumor is the ability to store, secrete, and metabolize catecholamines. 90% of them arise from the adrenal medulla and the rest (paragangliomas) from extra-adrenal sites. Pheochromocytomas are typically found in middle-aged patients, with a similar frequency in men and women.[1] New onset hyperglycemia or worsening of preexisting diabetes may be the presenting feature in some patients with pheochromocytoma. Very rarely, a patient with a pheochromocytoma may present in diabetic ketoacidosis. Epidemiological data on the prevalence and incidence of diabetes in patients with pheochromocytoma are rather limited. Abnormal glucose metabolism is found in 25 to 75% of patients with pheochromocytoma.[2] Diagnostic criteria for diabetes are the same used in non pheochromocytoma patients, such as a fasting plasma glucose value ≥126 mg/dL (7.0 mmol/L) or a 2-h plasma glucose value ≥200 mg/dL (11.1 mmol/L) during a 75 g oral glucose tolerance test or a random plasma glucose ≥200 mg/dL (11.1 mmol/L) in a symptomatic patient or HbA$_{1c}$ ≥6.5.

Catecholamine-induced impaired glucose metabolism results from a combination of effects upon carbohydrate metabolism via adrenergic receptors (β1-2 and α2). Catecholamines mediate inhibition of insulin release via α2 receptors. However, hyperinsulinemia in patients with pheochromocytoma has also been reported, suggesting insulin resistance. Gluconeogenesis takes place due to increased availability of the gluconeogenic precursors such as lactate, glycerol, and alanine generated by β-adrenergic-mediated adipose tissue lipolysis. β-2 adrenergic stimulation also induces insulin resistance at the level of muscle, resulting in reduced peripheral glucose utilization.[2] All these physiological effects result in hyperglycemia.

Unlike the normal adrenal medulla that predominantly secretes epinephrine, most pheochromocytomas, especially large and extra-adrenal tumors, secrete norepinephrine as the predominant catecholamine. The effect of norepinephrine seems to be less important in metabolic process than epinephrine.[3] Moreover, clinical manifestations may vary according to the number of receptors, postsignaling mechanisms, or the target organ metabolic capacity.[4] Other metabolic effects observed in patients with pheochromocytomas are weight loss with reduction of subcutaneous and visceral fat, a decrease in HDL, an increase in energy expenditure, and enhanced glucose oxidation.[5]

Workup for the diagnosis of pheochromocytoma in a patient with preexisting or newly detected diabetes is essentially the same as those for a patient without hyperglycemia. Recommended initial tests are 24-h urinary free catecholamine and fractionated metanephrines (high specificity), or plasma fractionated metanephrines (high sensitivity), or both. Contrast enhanced CT scan is the method of choice for tumor localization.[1-3] I- MIBG scan is specific for the detection of metastasis.[1]

Before surgery, alpha blockade with either selective or nonselective alpha blocker is recommended. Calcium channel blockers can be added to the alpha blocker if BP control is not achieved. After adequate alpha blockade, a beta blocker can be added to normalize heart rate. If needed, metyrosine (catecholamine synthesis inhibitor) can be added to alpha blockade to further stabilize BP for a short period of time before surgery. Medical treatment aims to normalize BP and heart rate before surgery.[1]

A high degree of clinical suspicion is required for early case detection of pheochromocytomas. Impaired glucose tolerance or overt diabetes can be the initial presentation in such patients. Resolution of diabetes or impaired glucose tolerance has been described in the literature in several cases after pheocromocytoma resection. The combination of hypertension and diabetes should be considered a clinical clue for the diagnosis of pheochromocytoma.

References

1. Lenders JW, Duh QY, Eisenhofer G, Gimenez-Roqueplo, AP, Grebe SK, et al. Pheochromocytoma and paraganglioma: an Endocrine Society clinical practice guideline. *J Clin Endocrinol Metab* 2014;99:1915–1942

2. Wiesner TD, Bluher M, Windgassen M, Paschke R. Improvement of insulin sensitivity after adrenalectomy in patients with pheochromocytoma. *J Clin Endocrinol Metab* 2003;88:3632–3636

3. Cases A, Bono M, Gaya J, Jimenez W, Calls J, Esforzado N, et al. Reversible decrease of surface beta 2-adrenoceptor number and response in lymphocytes of patients with pheochromocytoma. *Clin Exp Hypertens* 1995;17:537–549

4. Jones CT, Ritchie JW. The metabolic and endocrine effects of circulating catecholamines in fetal sheep. *J Physiol* 1978;285:395–408

5. Okamura T, Nakajima Y, Satoh T, Hashimoto K, Sapkota S, Yamada E, et al. Changes in visceral and subcutaneous fat mass in patients with pheochromocytoma. *Metabolism* 2015;64:706–712

Case 48:
Pheochromocytoma and Preexisting Diabetes

Padmaja Akkireddy, MD;[1] and Andjela Drincic, MD[1]

Case

A 65-year-old male presented with intermittent episodes of nausea, vomiting, and dizziness over a period of 6 months. Patient has history of hypertension for more than 20 years, with worsening blood pressure control over the last 5 years resulting in multiple admissions for hypertensive urgency. He was on five different antihypertensive medications including carvedilol, spironolactone, amlodipine, lisinopril, and hydrochlorothiazide. He was diagnosed with type 2 diabetes five years ago, which was managed with oral agents initially but over the last two years his hyperglycemia worsened, necessitating insulin use. At the time of admission his diabetes regimen included insulin glargine 30 units daily, insulin aspart 5 units with meals, and metformin 1,000 mg twice daily. Patient reported adherence to his therapy and diet but his HbA$_{1c}$ was 10.1%.

His other medical history includes coronary artery disease, gastroesophageal reflux disease, and dyslipidemia. Family history was positive for hypertension in his father and his siblings, but negative for diabetes. He denied any tobacco, alcohol, or illicit drug use. Review of systems was positive for palpitations, fatigue, and sweating episodes. He weighed 95 kg with a body mass index of 34.3 kg/m^2; physical examination was remarkable for mild epigastric and left upper quadrant tenderness without any

[1]Division of Diabetes, Endocrinology, and Metabolism, University of Nebraska Medical Center, Omaha, NE

rebound tenderness. Computed tomography (CT) imaging of abdomen was done as part of evaluation, which showed heterogeneously enhancing left adrenal mass measuring 5.2 x 5.2 cm with unenhanced attenuation of 54 Hounsfield units and contrast enhancement washout of 56% (Figure C48.1).

Hormonal evaluation showed normal renin-aldosterone ratio, normal 24-hour urine free cortisol, and his 8 A.M. cortisol appropriately suppressed to 1.4 mcg/dL following overnight low-dose dexamethasone. Plasma meta-nephrines were elevated at 12.51 nmol/L (reference range 0–0.49), and plasma normetanephrines were elevated at 2.52 nmol/L (reference range 0–0.89). He was diagnosed with pheochromocytoma arising from left adrenal gland.

After adequate alpha and beta adrenergic blockade, patient underwent laparoscopic left adrenalectomy; surgery was uneventful without any compli-cations. Postoperative pathology showed tumor consisting of a nested and insular pattern of cells with neuroendocrine-like nuclear features consistent with pheochromocytoma. Postoperatively patient's insulin requirements

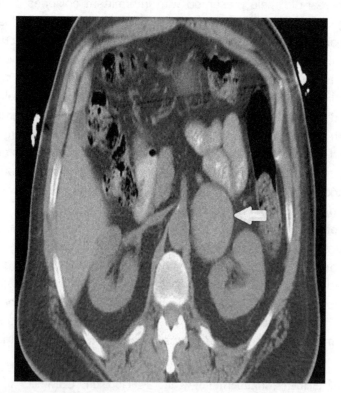

Figure C48.1—CT imaging of patient's abdomen.

decreased significantly. He did not need any insulin during his postoperative period; hence patient was discharged on metformin alone. At his two-month follow-up, patient reported improved appetite with the resolution of his nausea and vomiting. Repeat plasma and urinary metanephrines were within normal range and his HbA_{1c} came down to 7.0%, despite increase in his appetite and carbohydrate intake.

Discussion

Pheochromocytoma is a rare tumor arising from the intra- or extra-adrenal chromaffin cells that synthesize and secrete excessive catecholamines. Several metabolic derangements could result from the excess catecholamines, impaired glucose tolerance being one of them. Impaired glucose tolerance is seen in about 50% of the patients with pheochromocytoma, and 33% of patients with pheochromocytoma have diabetes.[1] New-onset hyperglycemia or worsening of preexisting diabetes may be the presenting feature in some patients with pheochromocytoma.

Glucose metabolism is affected by catecholamines at various tissue and organ levels (Figure C48.2). Glucose intolerance in pheochromocytoma is mainly due to decrease in insulin secretion related to α_2-mediated inhibitory effects of excess catecholamines on β-cells of pancreas.[2] Catecholamines stimulate hepatic glucose output by promoting gluconeogenesis and glycogenolysis, and inhibit peripheral glucose utilization through beta adrenergic mechanisms. Catecholamines also stimulate lipolysis in adipose tissue and glycolysis in skeletal muscles, thereby producing increased substrates for gluconeogenesis.[3] Elevated plasma free fatty acid from lipolysis in turn decreases insulin sensitivity in the liver and peripheral tissues.

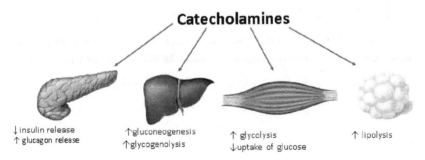

Catecholamines

↓ insulin release
↑ glucagon release

↑gluconeogenesis
↑glycogenolysis

↑ glycolysis
↓uptake of glucose

↑ lipolysis

Figure C48.2—Catecholamine and glucose metabolism.

The severity of hyperglycemia associated with pheochromocytoma is variable. Patients without preexisting diabetes may have mild hyperglycemia, which can be managed by oral medications. Patients with preexisting diabetes often need insulin for management. Diabetic ketoacidosis as a presenting feature is rare, and there are very few cases reported in the literature. In a retrospective study of 191 patients with pheochromocytoma, diabetes was present in 36% of the patients; age at presentation, duration of hypertension, and plasma catecholamine concentration were significantly and independently associated with diabetes.[4]

Management of diabetes in pheochromocytoma patients is no different than in patients without pheochromocytoma. There may be mild improvement in hyperglycemia with alpha blockade but not complete resolution. Impaired glucose tolerance will improve and often resolves following successful surgical resection of pheochromocytoma. Postoperative hypoglycemia is commonly encountered, owing to rebound hyperinsulinemia as the β-cells are no longer under the α_2-inhibitory effect caused by high catecholamines.[5] The risk of postoperative hypoglycemia is associated with larger tumor size, longer operative time, and higher concentrations of urinary metanephrines.[6] Therefore, it is important to closely monitor and follow these patients and make necessary adjustments to insulin doses.

Our case illustrates the importance of recognizing that pheochromocytoma can worsen glycemic control in patients with preexisting diabetes and the need for closely monitoring these patients in the postoperative period. In addition, secondary causes of diabetes ought to be considered in patients, especially if there is no family history of this disease.

References

1. Adlan MA, Bondugulapati LN, Premawardhana LD. Glucose intolerance and diabetes mellitus in endocrine disorders - two case reports and a review. *Curr Diabetes Rev* 2010;6:266–273

2. Isles CG, Johnson JK. Pheochromocytoma and diabetes mellitus. Further evidence that α_2 receptors inhibit insulin release in man. *Clin Endocrinol* 1983;18:37–41

3. Spergel G, Bleicher SJ, Ertel NH. Carbohydrate and fat metabolism in patients with pheochromocytoma. *N Engl J Med* 1968;278:803–809

4. La Batide-Alanore A, Chattellier G, Plouin P. Diabetes as a marker of pheochromocytoma in hypertensive patients. *J Hypertens* 2003;21:1703–1707

5. Wiesner TD, Buher M, Windgassen M, Paschke R. Improvement of insulin sensitivity after adrenalectomy in patients with pheochromocytoma. *J Clin Endocrinol Metab* 2003;88:3632–3636

6. Chen Y, Hodin RA, Pandolfi C, Ruan DT, McKenzie TJ. Hypoglycemia after resection of pheochromocytoma. *Surgery* 2014;156:1404–1408

Case 49:
Glucagonoma as a Cause of Diabetes

Henning Beck-Nielsen, MD[1,2]

Case

This patient was diagnosed with type 2 diabetes in 2001 (at the age of 50) and treated initially by diet alone. Later, sulfonylureas were added, and, lastly, insulin treatment became necessary eight years after the initial diagnosis.

In the years before and after the diagnosis of diabetes, the patient suffered from abdominal pain and from regular vomiting, often daily and often in the morning. She was diagnosed with reflux esophagitis, but gastroscopy, colonoscopy, and ultrasound of the abdomen were found to be normal.

The symptoms worsened and she developed necrolytic migratory erythema. The patient was finally referred to the hospital with severe vomiting, abdominal pain, diarrhea, and anemia. The investigations mentioned above were repeated and an abdominal computed tomography (CT) scan was carried out due to suspicion of an abdominal tumor. The scan showed a large vascular tumor with central necrosis localized between the cauda pancreatis and the upper pole of the left kidney (Figure C49.1). The tumor was removed, and the tissue staining showed positive results for gluca-

[1]Department of Endocrinology, Odense University Hospital, Odense, Denmark
[2]Department of Clinical Research, University of Southern Denmark, Odense, Denmark

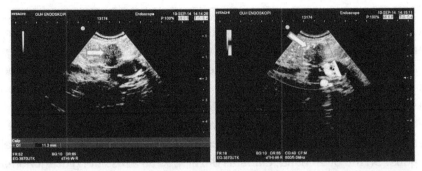

Figure C49.1—Hypervascular tumor in the tail of the pancreas with metastases in segment V of the liver. Adapted with permission from Al-Faouri et al.[1]

gon in alpha cells, but not insulin. Fasting plasma glucagon was severely increased (115 pmol/L compared with a reference value of 5–20 pmol/L), but also pancreatic polypeptide was increased threefold (gastrin was not measured). The patient was also examined for multiple endocrine neoplasia syndrome 1 (MEN1), but no mutation in the MEN1 gene was found.

After removal of the tumor and cauda pancreatis, plasma glucagon normalized, but the diabetic phenotype did not disappear. The tumor metastasized later on and plasma glucagon increased again.

At the time of diagnosis of diabetes, fasting plasma C-peptide was found to be 1,200 pmol/L (three times the normal values). The diabetes was, however, mild and easy to treat. Initially, the patient was treated with diet only and finally with 10 units of Insulatard (intermediate-acting insulin, Novo-Nordisk) daily. The patient developed no diabetic microvascular complications or thromboembolic diseases, and hypoglycemia was never detected.

Discussion

Type 2 diabetes is a heterogeneous disease with several causes of hyperglycemia, but in most type 2 diabetes patients, hyperglycemia is due to an imbalance between insulin secretion and insulin action. Moreover, the second pancreatic hormone, glucagon, may occasionally influence this balance. For example, in patients with glucagonoma where glucagon secretion is significantly increased, the ratio of insulin to glucagon changes in favor of glucagon and may induce hyperglycemia.

Glucagonoma is one of the most uncommon causes of diabetes, since only 1 in 20 million people develop this disease. Glucagonoma is a very rare disease (only a few percentages of pancreatic tumors are glucagonomas) and is therefore often overlooked in patients with newly diagnosed diabetes.[2] However, the diagnosis of glucagonoma should be considered in newly diagnosed diabetes patients with specific signs of this tumor. A failure of identifying glucagonoma in patients with newly diagnosed diabetes may have a deleterious effect since they may metastasize to other vital organs. On the other hand, diabetes developed as a result of glucagonoma is usually mild and easy to treat. To help clinicians in diagnosing glucagonoma, the foregoing case is presented.

The diagnosis should be considered in newly diagnosed diabetes patients presenting gastrointestinal symptoms such as diarrhea, vomiting, abdominal pain, nausea, anemia, and specifically necrolytic migratory erythema. A CT scan of the abdomen and staining of the removed tumors for glucagon could be used as tools for diagnosing glucagonoma. Plasma glucagon is increased initially and should be followed during treatment.

Diabetes that develops due to glucagonoma is mild and can be treated with insulin secretagogues alone or insulin in low doses.

The cause of hyperglycemia is an increase in the insulin/glucagon ratio, specifically with increased gluconeogenesis and glycogenolysis in the liver, and thereby an increase of fasting blood glucose. Therefore, measurement of fasting plasma glucose values in the clinical diagnostic situation is of specific value.

These patients rarely develop diabetic complications, and hypoglycemia does not occur due to the increased glucagon values. Early diagnosis and surgical removal of the tumor may cure the patient, and therefore glucagonoma should be considered in patients with mild diabetes even though the disease is rare.[2]

References

1. Al-Faouri A, Ajarma K, Alghazawi S, Al-Rawabdeh S, Zayadeen A. Glucagonoma and glucagonoma syndrome: a case report with review of recent advances in management. *Case Rep Surg* 2016;2016:1484–1489

2. John AM, Schwartz RA. Glucagonoma syndrome: a review and update on treatment. *J Eur Acad dermatol Venereol* 2016;30:2016–2022

Case 50:
Type 1 or Type 2 Diabetes vs. LADA

Ifrah Jamil, MD;[1] and Janice L. Gilden, MS, MD[1]

Case

A 39-year-old African-American male was evaluated for diabetes diagnosed at age 36. He was asymptomatic at the time. The diagnosis was made
after bloodwork done for evaluation after a knee injury. He was told he had
prediabetes and metformin 1,000 mg extended release daily was recommended. However, the patient could not tolerate this dose due to diarrhea,
and it was changed to 500 mg nightly. He reported a history of elevated
creatinine phosphokinase (CPK) levels initially thought to be secondary to
statin therapy for hyperlipidemia. His statin was discontinued. Despite this
measure, CPK level remained high, and metformin was discontinued.

Medical history is significant for an episode of rhabdomyolysis secondary to intense physical activity occurring approximately seven years
prior to diagnosis of diabetes. Renal function recovered. He continued to
undergo intense daily physical activity without any further complications.
He also reported drinking six cases of beer a week for many years until
two years ago, when he decreased his intake to minimal amounts. Family
history is significant for diabetes in mother, maternal uncle, and maternal
grandmother. Age of diabetes onset and treatment regimen for the mother
were unknown. Physical examination was significant for BMI of 31, muscular body habitus, and perioral vitiligo, but otherwise unremarkable.

---

[1]Rosalind Franklin University of Medicine and Science/Chicago Medical School and
Captain James A. Lovell Federal Health Care Center, North Chicago, IL

Upon initial evaluation, the patient presented with fasting blood sugars between 82–134 mg/dL (4.6–7.4 mmol/L). Glycosylated hemoglobin (HbA$_{1c}$) was 6.5% (4.0–6.0). The patient participated in diabetic education, and the decision was made not to restart metformin. A follow-up evaluation soon thereafter revealed excellent blood glucose control.

Approximately six months after initial evaluation, the patient was admitted to the critical care unit for polyuria, polydipsia, fatigue, and blood glucose levels over 450 mg/dL (25 mmol/L), without evidence of ketonemia or hyperosmolar state. He was hydrated and treated with intravenous insulin, then transitioned by the primary care team to detemir 10 units nightly and sitagliptin 10 mg daily. HbA$_{1c}$ was 8.9%.

Upon return to Endocrinology, he continued to have fatigue, polyuria, and polydipsia with hyperglycemia. Thus, sitagliptin was discontinued and insulin aspart 2 units with meals was prescribed. Islet cell antibodies were negative, and glutamic acid decarboxylase antibody level was <1.0 unit/mL (<1.0). Although glycemic control was improved, he continued to have symptomatic hyperglycemia. Insulin was further titrated upward to detemir 20 units nightly and aspart 10 units with meals, along with correction insulin. Symptoms of polyuria and polydipsia resolved with improvement in blood glucose levels. Metformin was started and slowly increased. However, the patient could not tolerate the medication. He stopped taking metformin on his own accord.

After titrating the diabetic therapy over a two-month period, the patient began having episodes of hypoglycemia fluctuating with hyperglycemia. Continuous blood glucose monitoring was performed over a four-day period, and the patient's blood glucose patterns were slightly above normal, without any evidence of hypoglycemia. However, given his hypoglycemic symptoms at euglycemia, his insulin doses slowly were decreased. HbA$_{1c}$ was 9.6%. He began more physical activity and controlled his diet more effectively. Thereafter, he had frequent episodes of symptomatic hypoglycemia. Over a ten-week period, insulin doses were slowly decreased to levemir 18 units nightly and aspart 3 units with meals. He stopped taking insulin on his own accord and continued to have slightly above-normal blood sugar readings. A random serum glucose level of 161 mg/dL (8.9 mmol/L) corresponded to C-peptide level of 3.04 (0.81–3.85). Thus, insulin was not restarted.

HbA$_{1c}$ decreased to 7.8%. Another attempt was made to start low-dose metformin. However, the patient could not tolerate minimal doses and eventually it was discontinued. The patient was then administered a trial of sitagliptin. His blood sugars became normal. Fifteen months after initial evaluation, HbA_{1c} was 6.4%. He remains euglycemic with therapy.

Discussion

With features of both type 1 and type 2 diabetes, this patient was suspected of having latent autoimmune diabetes of adults (LADA), also known as diabetes type 1.5. The current definition of LADA includes patients with markers of immunity similar to type 1 diabetes (TID) who can usually be managed on oral therapy initially, but they eventually require insulin.[1] LADA is prevalent in 8–22% of newly diagnosed diabetes according to some European studies. However, the prevalence in the United States, particularly in minorities, is less defined.[2]

Although the delayed destruction of β-cell function of patients with LADA is a distinguishing feature compared to T1D, the pathogenesis of this phenomenon is unknown. Studies suggest protective genetic factors, regeneration of β-cells, and environmental factors all may play a role in the time course of LADA.[3,4]

Our patient's age and neutral weight, like those of other minorities with LADA, is similar to the phenotypic pattern of T1D. These similarities make the distinction between T1D and LADA unclear.[5] Antibodies in our patient were negative; however, his clinical presentation was characterized by features of both T1D and type 2 diabetes (T2D). It took several months to appropriately titrate his medications. He currently requires no insulin. Our future management will include monitoring of antibody status, as patients with LADA and positive immune markers are more likely to require insulin long term.

There are no established pharmacological treatments specifically for LADA. At onset, patients are treated T2D. Our patient could not tolerate metformin and is prone to hypoglycemia. Therefore, sulfonylureas were not used. Insulin has also been studied in LADA patients and shows promising results in maintaining β-cell function over a longer period of time. However, the spectrum of patients studied has been small. In addition, patients are hesitant to begin insulin injections if blood sugars are well controlled without therapy.[2]

This case demonstrates the perplexity associated with the distinction between T1D and T2D, and LADA. Certainly, control of diabetes improves insulin resistance and prevents complications. However, the concomitant β-cell destruction is yet to be understood. Ultimately, the clinician's awareness of the complexity of diabetes is crucial to prescribing and monitoring proper care of the patient.

This research was supported in part by the Captain James A. Lovell Federal Health Care Center.

References

1. Palmer J, Hirsch I. What's in a name: latent autoimmune diabetes of adults, type 1.5, adult-onset, and type 1 diabetes. *Diabetes Care* 2003;26:536–538

2. Pozzilli P, Di Mario U. Autoimmune diabetes not requiring insulin at diagnosis (latent autoimmune diabetes of the adult). *Diabetes Care* 2001;24:1460–1467

3. Brahmkshatriya P, Mehta A, Saboo B, Goyal R. Characteristics and prevalence of latent autoimmune diabetes in adults (LADA). *ISRN Pharmacol* 2012; 2012:580202

4. Weyer C, Bogardus C, Mott D, Pratley R. The natural history of insulin secretory dysfunction and insulin resistance in the pathogenesis of type 2 diabetes mellitus. *J Clin Invest* 1999;104:787–794

5. Djekic K, Mouzeyan A, Ipp E. Latent autoimmune diabetes of adults is phenotypically similar to type 1 diabetes in a minority population. *J Clin Endocrinol Metab* 2012;97:E409–E413

Case 51:
LADA Masquerading as Type 2 Diabetes

Negin Misaghian-Xanthos, MD;[1] and Laura Young, MD, PhD[1]

Introduction

Autoantibodies to glutamic acid decarboxylase (GAD-Ab) have a well-established link to type 1 diabetes (T1D) and latent autoimmune diabetes of adults (LADA).[1] While a rare disease, stiff person syndrome (SPS) has also been linked in literature to GAD-Ab.[2] A lesser-known neurologic phenomenon, cerebellar ataxia, appears to also have a link between autoimmune diabetes but has been infrequently described, particularly in the endocrinology literature.[3,4] Here we report a case of a patient diagnosed initially with type 2 diabetes (T2D) and soon after with cerebellar ataxia. However, with further investigation, she was determined to have LADA associated with cerebellar ataxia.

Case Report

A 67-year-old African-American female was referred to our clinic in 2015 for presumed T2D management. She had been diagnosed about 8 years prior after noted polydipsia and had been initially placed on metformin, but due to gastrointestinal intolerance, she was switched to subcutaneous insulin within 6 months of diagnosis. Approximately 1 year after

[1]University of North Carolina School of Medicine, Division of Endocrinology and Metabolism, Chapel Hill, NC

her diabetes diagnosis, she had developed symptoms of dysarthria and weakness with ultimate workup by neurology consistent with autoimmune cerebellar ataxia. At that time, workup for paraneoplastic syndrome by neurology had been negative. Her workup was also notable for elevation of serum glutamic acid decarboxylase antibodies (GAD 65-Ab) to 330 nmol/L (reference range <0.02 nmol/L). This had been attributed to her underlying neurologic disease, for which she received treatment with both cellcept and intravenous immunoglobulin with some improvement in symptoms. Interestingly, treatment for her underlying cerebellar ataxia did not correspond to improvements in her glycemic control.

On our initial evaluation, we had concern for underlying autoimmune-mediated diabetes given her elevated serum GAD 65-Ab in 2015, along with interim history of hypothyroidism. For this reason, a C-peptide was obtained, which was abnormally low at 0.8 in the setting of hyperglycemia (venous blood glucose = 194 mg/dL or 10.8 mmol/L). No other autoimmune testing was done including anti-islet cell antibodies or thyroid-peroxidase antibodies. However, given that our patient had GAD-Abs, a history of autoimmune disease, and an inappropriately low C-peptide, we felt her diagnosis of T2D was inaccurate and instead LADA was a more apt classification.

Discussion

LADA has been more thoroughly characterized in recent years and its association with other autoimmune diseases, particularly thyroid and celiac disease, is well established. While it has been characterized as a disease in which time from diagnosis to insulin treatment is delayed, a hallmark of the disease is the presence of islet cell autoimmunity, particularly GAD-Ab.[1] GAD, which is the enzyme that is responsible for the ultimate production of gamma-amino butyric acid, is narrowly expressed, primarily in the central and peripheral nervous systems, fallopian tubes, and β-cells of the pancreas.

In the neurology and endocrinology literature, in addition to clinical signs and symptoms, GAD-Ab positivity in either serum or CSF is well documented with SPS being reported in over 80% of cases in some literature.[3,4] With this, over 50% of patients with SPS have documented autoimmune diabetes, ranging from T1D to LADA.[3] More recently but infrequently reported is cerebellar ataxia and its association with autoimmune diabetes, with over 50% of patients having documented autoimmune diabetes in the few case series available. In what has been reported, it appears that the diabetes precedes the development of symptoms and diagnosis of cerebellar ataxia in the majority of patients who ultimately develop diabetes, which is similar to our patient.[3,4] Additionally, the majority of cases are women >50 years old at onset of neurologic symptoms, as was our patient.[3]

While the diagnosis of cerebellar ataxia makes this case a part of only a handful of patients reported in literature, her concurrent diagnosis of autoimmune diabetes is not unique in this population. It does, however, raise the question: are LADA cases being underdetected and underreported in this population, as was initially the case in our patient? On the whole, there is emerging evidence that LADA is universally underdiagnosed, currently being reported in up to 14% of cases initially classified as having T2D.[1] Universal screening is not routinely recommended for LADA in patients with T2D. However, given that the majority of patients with cerebellar ataxia have concurrent LADA, this case highlights the need to specifically screen patients with cerebellar ataxia and diabetes for LADA. Furthermore, while there is a scarcity of evidence regarding if and how we should treat LADA patients differently, the potential rapidity of loss of β-cell function in this patient population may provide us with the impetus to treat these patients more aggressively and quickly with insulin to potentially prevent episodes of metabolic decompensation.

References

1. Fourlanos S, Dotta F, Greenbaum CJ, Palmer JP, Rolandsson O, Colman PG, Harrison LC. Latent autoimmune diabetes in adults (LADA) should be less latent. *Diabetologia* 2005;48:2206–2012

2. Kono S, Miyajima H, Sugimoto M, Suzuki Y, Takahashi Y, Hishida A. Stiff-person syndrome associated with cerebellar ataxia and high glutamic acid decarboxylase antibody titer. *Intern Med* 2001;40:968–971

3. Saiz A, Blanco Y, Sabater L, Gonzalez F, Bataller L, Casamitjana R, et al. Spectrum of neurological syndromes associated with glutamic acid decarboxylase antibodies: diagnostic clues for this association. *Brain* 2008;131:2553–2563

4. Honnorat J, Saiz A, Giometto B, Vincent A, Brieva L, Andres CD, et al. Cerebellar ataxia with anti–glutamic acid decarboxylase antibodies. *Arch Neurol* 2001;58:225–230

Case 52:
LADA during the Obesity Epidemic

Lavanya Viswanathan, MD;[1] and Cherie Vaz, MD[1]

Case

A 32-year-old obese Caucasian male was referred to Endocrinology for management of uncontrolled type 2 diabetes (T2D). He was diagnosed with T2D at the age of 29 on routine blood tests. He had no previous episodes of diabetic ketoacidosis or hospitalizations for diabetes. He denied a family history of type 1 diabetes and autoimmune diseases. He did report history of T2D in his grandmother and aunt. He had no other medical problems other than diabetes.

The patient was diagnosed with diabetes when he was morbidly obese at 100 lb over his current weight of 210 lb. His BMI then was 43.2 mg/k². He was initially started on metformin twice a day and titrated up to maximum dose. He followed appropriate lifestyle changes and achieved weight loss of approximately 100 lb over 4 years. He was doing well until recently when he noticed increasing glucose levels. Over a period of 12 months a sulfonylurea - glimepiride 4 mg twice daily, and dipeptidyl peptidase 4 (DPP4) inhibitor, sitagliptin 100 mg daily, were added. Lastly, a sodium-glucose co-transporter 2 (SGLT2) inhibitor - canagliflozin 100 mg daily was started. Metformin 2,000 mg daily was continued through all these

---

[1]Temple University, Section of Endocrinology, Diabetes and Metabolism, Philadelphia, PA

Table C52.1—Antibody and C-peptide Panel

Test	3/21/2016
Insulin antibodies uIU/mL (<5)	<5
Anti-GAD 65 units/mL (<5)	21.3
IA-2 antibodies units/mL (<1)	4.8
C peptide ng/mL (1.1–4.4)	0.6
Glucose mg/dL	144

therapeutic steps. However, his diabetes was still uncontrolled on the four-drug regimen and Endocrinology was consulted.

His physical exam was unremarkable except for loose folds of skin on the abdomen presumably from the significant weight loss. He weighed 210 lb and BMI was 31. Although he was obese by BMI criteria, we suspected autoimmune diabetes based on his history and presentation. In addition, there is inherent inaccuracy in using BMI for diagnosing obesity in a young male due to higher percentage of muscle mass.

Laboratory evaluation showed HbA$_{1c}$ was 8.7%, C peptide was 0.6 ng/mL (1.1–4.4), Insulin was 2.1 uIU/mL (2.6–24.9), glutamic acid decarboxylase (GAD)-65 antibody was 21.3 units/mL (reference range <5), islet antigen (IA)-2 antibody was 4.8 units/mL (reference range <1), insulin antibody was <5 uIU/mL (reference range <5), and glucose was 144 mg/dL (8 mmol/L) (Table C52.1). The low insulin and C-peptide levels confirmed low endogenous insulin production. The positive antibodies were consistent with latent autoimmune diabetes of adults (LADA) as was suspected.

The sulfonylurea was discontinued and the patient was started on basal insulin in addition to his existing regimen. This patient is being cautiously managed with an SGLT2 inhibitor after understanding the possible risk of ketoacidosis and need for daily insulin on board to avoid this complication. His glucose is currently being controlled on metformin 2,000 mg daily, sitagliptin 100 mg daily, canagliflozin 100 mg daily, and glargine insulin 14 units daily. While on this current regimen, he has been following our lifestyle intervention program incorporating a low–glycemic index, low-carbohydrate diet. He has since shown an improvement in HbA$_{1c}$ to 7.8% and remains off prandial insulin (Figure C52.1).

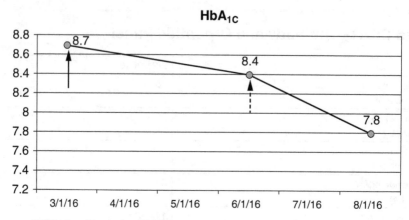

Figure C52.1 — Trend of HbA_{1c}.

Solid arrow indicates when long-acting basal insulin (glargine) was initiated and sulfonylurea was discontinued.

Dashed arrow indicates increase in basal insulin (glargine) dosing by 4 units to control fasting hyperglycemia.

Discussion

LADA is defined as an autoimmune type of diabetes diagnosed at age greater or equal to 30 years with positive antibodies in a patient not requiring insulin for at least 6 months after diagnosis. It was first reported by Groop et al.[1] in 1986 and later labelled as LADA following two other studies by Tuomi et al.[2] and Zimmet et al.[3] Cases with LADA typically manifest with a type 2 phenotype. In this type of diabetes, there is preserved β-cell function at diagnosis and slow progressive β-cell failure despite the presence of antibodies. Hence, these patients may not require insulin for the initial 6 months after diagnosis. We present here a case of LADA in a young male who was presumed to have T2D as a complication of obesity. Unfortunately, his glycemic control progressively worsened despite adequate pharmacotherapy for type 2 diabetes and lifestyle changes.

Studies have shown that among patients with T2D, LADA occurs in 10% of those above age 35 years and in 25% below that age.[4] In this case, it is possible that the patient did in fact have diabetes as a result of his morbid obesity three years ago and went on to develop LADA at a later point. It is also plausible that he had mild autoimmune diabetes with preserved β-cell reserve at diagnosis, which has gradually progressed over the past three years. Since it was first reported, there have been many studies to identify risk factors for progression of this atypical form of diabetes. High concentrations of islet antibodies predict future β-cell failure. Prospective studies of β-cell function have shown that patients with multiple islet antibodies develop failure within 5 years whereas it may take as long as 12 years in those with only one type of antibody. Though not requiring insulin at the time of diagnosis, these patients have been shown to have impaired β-cell function compared to controls without diabetes. This case highlights that not all patients with LADA are lean. With obesity reaching epidemic proportions worldwide, it may be worthwhile to revisit the etiology of diabetes in younger overweight or obese individuals. Restricting calories in obese patients with LADA along with treatment with metformin and appropriate physical activity has shown benefit in previous trials.[5] As such, our patient is able to remain off prandial insulin while following a low–glycemic index, low-carbohydrate diet along with the current oral regimen.

In cases of LADA, treatment with sulfonylureas may cause faster progression of β-cell failure compared to treating with insulin alone. This is particularly true if antibody levels were high at the time of diagnosis.[6] The hypothesis is that sulfonylureas facilitated the autoimmune process. Alternatively, insulin at the time of diagnosis seems to help by combating glucose toxicity and thereby helping with β-cell recovery. This patient was justifiably taken off the glimepiride considering the low C-peptide level.

References

1. Groop LC, Bottazzo GF, Doniac D. Islet cell antibodies identify latent type 1 diabetes in patients aged 35-75 years at diagnosis. *Diabetes* 1986;35:237–241

2. Tuomi T, Carlsson A, Li H, Isomaa B, Miettinen A, et al. Clinical and genetic characteristics of type 2 diabetes with and without GAD antibodies. *Diabetes* 1999;48:150–157

3. Zimmet PZ, Tuomi T, Mackay IR, Rowley MJ, Knowles W, Cohen M, Lang DA. Latent autoimmune diabetes mellitus in adults (LADA): the role of antibodies to glutamic acid decarboxylase in diagnosis and prediction of insulin dependency. *Diabet Med* 1994;11:299–303

4. Turner R, Stratton I, Horton V, Manley S, Zimmet P, Mackay IR, Shattock M, Botazzo GF, Holman R; UK Prospective Diabetes Study (UKPDS) Group. UKPDS 25 autoantibodies to islet-cell cytoplasm and glutamic acid decarboxylase for prediction of insulin requirement in type 2 diabetes. *Lancet* 1997;350:1288–1293

5.　Lóriz Peralta O, Campos Bonilla B, Granada Ybern ML, Sanmartí Sala A, Arroyo Bros J; Investigadores Asociados del Catalonian Overweight and Diabetes Study Group. [Detection of LADA-type diabetes in overweight diabetic patients. Is treatment with metformin suitable?]. *Aten Primaria* 2007;39:133–137

6.　Alvarsson M, Sundkvist G, Lager I, Henricsson M, Berntop K, Fernqvist-Forbes E, Steen I, Westermark G, Westermark P, Orn T, Grill V. Beneficial effects of insulin versus sulphonylurea on insulin secretion and metabolic control in recently diagnosed type 2 diabetic patients. *Diabetes Care* 2003;26:2231–2237

Case 53:
LADA in Older Adults

Lavanya Viswanathan, MD;[1] and Cherie Vaz, MD[1]

Case

A 67-year-old female with a past medical history of type 2 diabetes (T2D), osteoporosis, dyslipidemia, and mitral valve prolapse was referred to Endocrinology for management of uncontrolled diabetes. She was initially diagnosed at 61 years of age with symptoms of increased thirst, polyuria, fatigue, and progressive weight loss. She denied any previous episodes of ketoacidosis or family history of diabetes.

At the time of the initial consultation, she was on oral antidiabetic agents including pioglitazone 15 mg twice a day, metformin 850 mg twice a day, glimepiride 2 mg twice a day, and sitagliptin 100 mg daily, which were progressively added to her diabetes regimen over a period of 4 years. Despite the escalation of therapy, she continued to have rising HbA$_{1c}$ levels. HbA$_{1c}$ checked at the time of initial consult with Endocrinology was 9.6%.

Based on her disease course and thin body habitus, autoimmune diabetes was suspected. The patient was phenotypically very similar to a person with type 1 diabetes (T1D). She weighed 125 lb with BMI of 21.46. Laboratory workup revealed C-peptide was 0.2 ng/mL (1.1–4.4), insulin antibodies were 179 uIU/mL (reference range <5), glutamic acid decarboxylase (GAD) antibodies were 1,495 units/mL (reference range <5),

[1]Temple University, Section of Endocrinology, Diabetes and Metabolism, Philadelphia, PA

glucose was 113 mg/dL (6.3 mMol/L). She was diagnosed with latent auto-immune diabetes of adults (LADA). A diagnosis of autoimmune diabetes in the sixth decade of life is very rare. Some of the risk factors for developing autoimmune diabetes are family history and presence of certain HLA alleles, exposure to certain viruses, and living in northern climates. Coexistence of other autoimmune diseases such as Graves' disease, pernicious anemia, and multiple sclerosis increases the chance of developing autoimmune diabetes.

The patient was started on treatment with basal insulin, glargine 10 units, and glimepiride, pioglitazone, and metformin were discontinued. She had labile blood glucose readings with frequent hypoglycemia with even small changes in diet or exercise patterns. Some patients with "mild" or early stages of LADA may behave similar to patients with T2D and can be managed similarly. However, this patient's glycemic pattern that included labile blood glucose readings and increased insulin sensitivity was akin to a more advanced case of T1D. A few months later she was started on mealtime insulin (lispro) 3 units three times a day with meals. Her HbA_{1c} improved to 7.8% on this regimen (Figure C53.1). She is currently requiring only 18–20 units of insulin in total daily (divided into multiple daily injections with glargine 11 units and lispro 2–3 units with meals) along with metformin. She is on a separate regimen of lispro insulin on days that she goes to the gym to avoid hypoglycemia. She is requiring coverage for small snacks in between meals with 2 units of lispro. Thus, this patient of LADA exhibits insulin sensitivity and glycemic patterns very similar to a patient with T1D. As she was experiencing frequent hypoglycemia, we are targeting a slightly relaxed HbA_{1c} goal for her. The further plan for this patient is an insulin pump with continuous glucose monitoring.

Discussion

LADA is an atypical form of diabetes with a prevalence rate of 2.8–10% in patients with T2D.[1,2] Presence of detectable levels of autoantibodies in non–insulin-requiring diabetes at the time of diagnosis defines this subgroup of diabetic patients as LADA. In 1997, the U.K. Prospective Diabetes Study (UKPDS — a study of individuals with T2D) showed that 12% of subjects thought to have T2D tested positive for antibodies. These positive islet cell antibodies and GAD antibodies detected in a significant number of patients in the UKPDS database who were originally thought to have T2D prompted further studies to understand the pathogenesis of LADA and risk factors for it in these individuals. It was then discovered that higher antibody titers and presence of multiple antibodies were associated with lower β-cell function.[1] The same subset of patients also tended to have a lower BMI and higher glycosylated hemoglobin (HbA$_{1c}$) at diagnosis. This subset of patients with LADA also progressed more rapidly to insulin requirement and had lower C-peptide secretion (Tables C53.1 and C53.2).[3] Though initially identified by Groop et al. in patients aged 35–75 years at diagnosis, the average age at diagnosis is usually around the fourth and fifth decades. Here we present a case of LADA diagnosed in the sixth decade of life and currently being managed as an individual with T1D.

This patient developed autoimmune diabetes in the sixth decade of life, which is very rarely seen. She also became completely insulin dependent due to the severity of autoimmunity. With disease progression, she now has more labile glycemia as is seen in T1D. The diagnosis of autoimmune diabetes had been missed for several years. However, routine testing of antibodies in clinical practice has been debated extensively and there is no consensus as to when to test for antibodies in patients

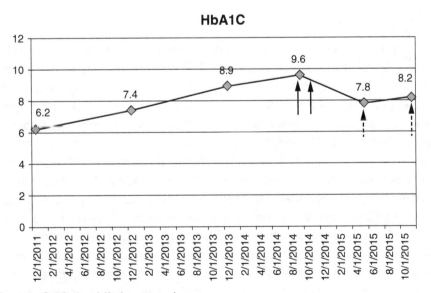

Figure C53.1—HbA$_{1c}$ trend.

Table C53.1—Antibody and C-peptide Panel

Date	C-Peptide ng/mL (1.1-4.4)	Glucose (mg/dL)	Insulin Antibodies uIU/mL (<5)	Anti-GAD 65 units/mL (<5)
9/26/2014	0.2	113	179	1495
5/22/2015	0.4	198		
3/15/2016	0.2	229		

Table C53.2—Lipid and Renal Panels

Date	LDL mg/dL	TG mg/dL	Total Chol mg/dL	Creatinine mg/dL	eGFR mL/min/1.73
9/26/2014	112	66	196	0.61	95
3/15/2016	84	57	175	0.71	88

without T1D. Antibodies to islet autoantigens are very reproducible and currently the best validated predictive markers for autoimmune diabetes, particularly GAD 65, islet antigen (IA)-2, and insulin antibodies through radiobinding assays.[4] Despite the ease of access, high sensitivity, and specificity of these assays, it must be remembered that cutoffs are arbitrary and represent a spectrum. Therefore, a higher antibody titer is of more value in predicting future insulin requirement as was seen in the Botnia study.[5]

As is illustrated in this case, the treatment of LADA can vary at different times of the disease course. While oral agents may be sufficient initially, these patients eventually require insulin. We prefer to manage our patients with LADA on a combination of both insulin and oral agents. We successfully use metformin as well, given its effects on reducing hepatic gluconeogenesis. We prefer not to use sulfonylureas in the management of LADA even in patients with relatively higher β-cell reserve. Maruyuma et al.[2] compared treatment with insulin and sulfonylurea in 60 subjects with LADA. They followed their progression to a fully insulin-dependent state over 4 years. They found that C-peptide secretion decreased less rapidly with insulin treatment than with sulfonylurea use in antibody positive individuals, particularly those with preserved C-peptide level at baseline.[2] However, due to its small sample size and no difference in comparison with high or low antibody titers, the implications of their findings have been debated.

References

1. Turner R, Stratton I, Horton V, Manley S, Zimmet P, Mackay IR, Shattock M, Botazzo GF, Holman R; UK Prospective Diabetes Study (UKPDS) Group. UKPDS 25: autoantibodies to islet-cell cytoplasm and glutamic acid decarboxylase for prediction of insulin requirement in type 2 diabetes. *Lancet* 1997;350:1288–1293

2. Maruyama T, Tanaka S, Shimada A, Funae O, Kasuga A, Kanatsuka A, Takei I, Yamada S, Harii N, Shimura H, Kobayashi T. Insulin interventions in slowly progressive insulin–dependent (type 1) diabetes mellitus. *J Clin Endocrinol Metab* 2008;93:2115–2121

3. Irvine WJ, McCallum CJ, Gray RS, Duncan LJ. Clinical and pathogenic significance of pancreatic-islet-cell antibodies in diabetics treated with oral hypoglycemic agents. *Lancet* 1977;1:1025–1027

4. Törn C, Mueller PW, Schlosser M, Bonifacio E, Bingley PJ. Diabetes Antibody Standardization Program: evaluation of assays for autoantibodies to glutamic acid decarboxylase and islet antigen-2. *Diabetologia* 2008;51:846–852

5. Lundgren VM, Isomaa B, Lyssenko V, Laurila E, Korhonen P, Groop LC, Tuomi T; Botnia Study Group. GAD antibody positivity predicts type 2 diabetes in an adult population. *Diabetes* 2010;59:416–422

Case 54:
Stiff Person Syndrome

Han Na Kim, MD;[1] and Nestoras Mathioudakis, MD, MHS[1]

Case

The patient is a 31-year-old man with uncontrolled type 1 diabetes (T1D) diagnosed at age 8 and complicated by diabetic retinopathy, Hashimoto's thyroiditis, and vitiligo, who was seen for management of his diabetes. He had been on an insulin pump since age 10 with historically poor glycemic control (average HbA$_{1c}$ 8.5–9% range). Three years after the initial visit, he experienced ascending severe right calf pain and spasm lasting for more than a week. The cramping and discomfort spread to involve all extremities, abdomen, lower back, and at times his face. Two months later, he developed diffuse body tightening, spasm, and excruciating pain with movement during a stressful situation at work. He received symptomatic treatment at a local hospital and was discharged with clonazepam. Outpatient evaluation revealed a normal brain magnetic resonance imaging and an elevated anti-glutamic acid decarboxylase (GAD) antibody titer at 90 (reference range 0-1.5 units/mL), raising suspicion for stiff person syndrome (SPS).

He was referred to our neurology department, and on initial visit he endorsed ongoing symptoms of muscle spasms and pain worsened by stress and loud noises, although symptoms improved with clonazepam. He sustained several falls and had gait instability from stiffness. Physical exam revealed increased tone and spasticity on all extremities and torso

[1]Division of Endocrinology, Diabetes, & Metabolism, Johns Hopkins University School of Medicine, Baltimore, MD

rigidity. His initial gait was normal but timed 25-foot walk performed unassisted in 5 seconds resulted in intense pain and spasms in his feet.

Extensive laboratory and imaging evaluations ruled out other neurologic conditions and repeat anti-GAD antibody was 148.5 U/mL (normal ≤1.0). Electromyogram (EMG) was normal.

His clinical picture was consistent with SPS and he received intravenous immunoglobulin (IVIg) therapy for 6 months without improvement. He was then treated with five sessions of plasmapheresis followed by rituximab. He showed significant positive response and is now maintained on regular rituximab treatment.

Discussion

SPS, previously known as stiff man syndrome, is a rare autoimmune neurologic disorder characterized by presence of anti-GAD65 antibody and association with autoimmune conditions, most commonly T1D. In one SPS case series, of the 79 patients with anti-GAD65 antibody positivity, T1D was seen in 43% of patients either preceding or following the diagnosis of SPS during median follow-up period of 5 years (range 0–23 years).[1] In contrast, however, incidence of SPS in T1D is low at 1:10,000 and overall prevalence of SPS has been estimated to be 1 case per million.[2] SPS is also seen in non-autoimmune context, and paraneoplastic and idiopathic cases have been described.

In SPS, there is axial muscle stiffness and rigidity from simultaneous contracture of opposing muscle groups and intermittent spasms. These result in hyperlordosis, torso rigidity, and wide and slow gait to compensate for imbalance. Spasms are triggered by unanticipated sounds, touch, visual stimuli, or emotional disturbance.[3]

GAD is an important presynaptic rate-limiting enzyme needed for synthesis of GABA, the main inhibitory neurotransmitter in the central nervous system (CNS). GAD exists in two isoforms, GAD65 and GAD67, and antibodies against them have been detected up to 80% and <50% of SPS cases respectively.[4] Unlike T1D, anti-GAD65 antibody titers in SPS are elevated to at least 50 times above the baseline, and in SPS, antibody recognizes linear epitopes whereas in T1D, conformational epitope is recognized.[3] Although anti-GAD65 antibodies are good disease biomarkers, whether they have a pathogenic role is questionable as there has been no correlation between anti-GAD65 antibody titers and severity or duration of SPS or treatment response.[4] Additional autoantigens have been identified (amphiphysin, gephyrin, GABA receptor-associated protein), but their pathogenicity also remains unclear.

SPS is a debilitating condition that leads to significant pain, falls, inability to perform daily activities, and immobility. It is an underdiagnosed disorder and early recognition and initiation of treatment are crucial to prevent chronic disability. SPS can be categorized into several different forms (classic, partial, paraneoplastic, and progressive encephalomyelitis with rigidity and myoclonus) based on clinical presentation, antibody status, and presence of malignancy. The majority of cases are classic SPS form, which is characterized by axial muscle stiffness, diffuse rigidity, intermittent spasms, and awkward gait. Common nonneurologic symptoms of SPS are anxiety and "task-specific phobias" that stem from true functional disability and not from underlying primary psychiatric condition.[3]

Partial SPS is characterized by focal stiffness, particularly one lower limb (Stiff Limb syndrome) or trunk (Stiff Trunk syndrome) and only 15% of cases have positive anti-GAD antibodies.[5] SPS as part of a paraneoplastic phenomenon is seen in 5% of patients, and anti-GAD antibodies are usually absent but antibodies against amphiphysin and gephyrin can be present. [3]

There are no standardized diagnostic criteria, but in general, the following features are considered necessary for the diagnosis of SPS:

- Rigidity of truncal and limb muscles, particularly of the abdominal and thoracolumbar paraspinal muscles (involvement of one limb or trunk is partial SPS)
- evidence of simultaneous agonist and antagonist muscle contraction on physical exam or EMG
- intermittent muscle spasms triggered by auditory, tactile, or emotional stimuli
- exclusion of other neurologic conditions that could explain symptomatology
- anti-GAD65 antibody positivity[3]

However, absence of anti-GAD65 antibody does not rule out SPS, and positive response to a trial of diazepam treatment has also been used to support the diagnosis without the need for EMG.

Paraneoplastic SPS, however, can be difficult to diagnose. Anti-GAD antibody is typically negative, and thus a high level of suspicion is required with search for occult malignancy if clinical symptoms otherwise fit SPS.

Treatment of SPS consists of symptomatic treatment with use of GABA-enhancing drugs and immunomodulators in severe cases. Benzodiazepines, particularly diazepam, are first-line treatment. The drug is started at a low dose and gradually increased to reach a dose that allows for maximal mobility without excessive sedation, which is often the major adverse effect limiting titration. Daily dose of diazepam required for symptom relief varies among patients and can range from 5–100 mg/d in divided doses.[3] Antiepileptics that enhance GABAergic transmission (vigabatrin, tiagabine, levetiracetam) are effective and can be used either as the sole treatment agent or adjunctive to benzodiazepine. Baclofen, an antispasticity agent, has been shown to improve symptoms and is the second most beneficial drug, but its use is also limited by CNS side effects.[3]

Immunomodulators are used when GABA-enhancing drugs are ineffective or in patients with severe disease. Corticosteroids, immunosuppressants, rituximab, plasmapheresis, and IVIg have been used to treat SPS. Immunomodulator selection is based on experience and expert opinions. IVIg is the only therapy that has been studied in a randomized controlled trial (crossover design), albeit small, and has shown symptom improvement.[3] Thus IVIg is the initial preferred immunomodulator, and in patients resistant to IVIg, alternative treatments with plasmapheresis, rituximab, or other immunosuppressants can be attempted but evidence is limited and outcomes are highly variable.

References

1. McKeon A, Robinson MT, McEvoy KM, et al. Stiff-man syndrome and variants: clinical course, treatments, and outcomes. *Arch Neurol* 2012;69:230–238

2. Dalakas MC, Fujii M, Li M, McElroy B. The clinical spectrum of anti-GAD antibody-positive patients with stiff-person syndrome. *Neurology* 2000;55:1531–1535

3. Dalakas MC. Advances in the pathogenesis and treatment of patients with stiff person syndrome. *Curr Neurol Neurosci Rep* 2008;8:48–55

4. Alexopoulos H, Dalakas MC. A critical update on the immunopathogenesis of stiff person syndrome. *Eur J Clin Invest* 2010;40:1018–1025

5. Sarva H, Deik A, Ullah A, Severt WL. Clinical spectrum of stiff person syndrome: a review of recent reports. *Tremor Other Hyperkinet Mov (N Y)* 2016;6:340

Case 55: Polyglandular Failure and Diabetes

Bushra Z. Osmani, MD;[1] Janice L. Gilden, MS, MD;[1] Alvia Moid, DO;[1] and Degaulle Dai[1]

Case

A 46-year-old female was referred to the Endocrine Clinic for the management of hypothyroidism (5–6 years' duration) and recent patchy hair loss of a few months' duration. TSH was 6.22 µIU/mL (normal = 0.34–4.82), free T4 0.88 ng/dL (normal = 0.59–1.61), thyroglobulin antibody level was 80.9 units/mL (normal = 0–60), thyroid peroxidase antibody level 474.3 units/mL (normal = 0–60). Therefore, levothyroxine dose was increased from 0.1 mg to 0.125 mg.

Laboratory testing: Elevated random blood glucose of 163 mg/dL (9.05 mmol/L). History was significant for gestational diabetes, but no treatment was required and the child was born of normal weight without fetal abnormalities. She also had fatty liver disease, obesity, and hyperlipidemia. Family history was significant for obesity, diabetes, psoriasis, rheumatoid arthritis, systemic lupus erythematosus, and alopecia.

At this point, our patient demonstrated the presence of at least one autoimmune condition: autoimmune thyroiditis. There was also a possibility that alopecia was of autoimmune origin. She was referred to dermatology and a scalp biopsy was done.

[1]Rosalind Franklin University of Medicine and Science/Chicago Medical School and Captain James A. Lovell Federal Health Care Center, North Chicago, IL

During the next visit, glycosylated hemoglobin (HbA$_{1c}$) was 6.0%. Since there were other autoimmune conditions, the question was raised as to whether she had also developed autoimmune type 1 diabetes (T1D). 65 glutamic acid decarboxylase (GAD) antibodies were negative.

She began a calorie-controlled low-carbohydrate diet and exercise program and lost five pounds. However, HbA$_{1c}$ increased to 6.6%. She was then lost to follow-up. Three years later, she returned with the diagnosis of type 2 diabetes (T2D). Pharmacotherapy included metformin 1,000 mg twice a day and glipizide 5 mg twice a day.

Three years later, she was admitted to hospital with 3 days of recurrent episodes of hypoglycemia, mainly during the night with the lowest reading of 45 mg/dL (2.5 mmol/L). Oral medications were discontinued. HbA$_{1c}$ was 7.2%. GAD, adrenal, and insulin antibodies were negative. ACTH and cortisol levels were also normal, which ruled out autoimmune hypoglycemia and adrenal insufficiency.

The patient was seen in the clinic one month later. Metformin therapy was restarted. Due to continued high suspicion of increasing autoimmune disorders, GAD antibodies were reevaluated and were positive (2.4 units/mL, normal = <1.0 unit/mL). To eliminate the possibility of a laboratory error, this level was re-checked six weeks later and was found to be even higher (26 IU/mL) (Table C55.1).

At this point the positive GAD antibodies now suggested autoimmune T1D.

Table C55.1—Patient's Laboratory Results over Time

	01/2005	05/2011	08/2015	04/2016	05/2016
HbA$_{1c}$ (normal: 4.0-6.0%)	5.5%	6.0%	7.2%		6.1%
GAD-65 Antibodies (normal: <1.25IU/mL)	<0.2		<1.0	2.4	26
Islet Cell Antibody (normal: negative)					Negative
Insulin Antibodies (normal: negative)			<0.4		
Adrenal Antibodies (normal: negative)			Negative		Negative
C-peptide (normal 0.81–3.85 ng/mL)			4.51		2.66
Glucose			126		103

Table C55.2—Polyglandular Autoimmune Syndromes

	PAS I	PAS II	PAS III	PAS IV
Age of Onset	Infancy or childhood or early adolescence	Peak incidence at ages 20–60 years	Peak incidence at ages 20–60 years	
Inheritance	Monogenic, autosomal recessive	Polygenic, autosomal dominant	Polygenic, autosomal dominant	
Clinical Manifestations	Mucocutaneous candidiasis Acquired hypoparathyroid Addison's disease Hypothyroidism Hypogonadism Malabsorption syndromes Pernicious anemia Alopecia Vitiligo T1D Hypopituitary diabetes insipidus	Adrenal insufficiency T1D Autoimmune thyroid disease Hypoparathyroidism Hypogonadism Alopecia Pernicious anemia	T1D Autoimmune thyroid disease Hypoparathyroidism Hypogonadism Alopecia Pernicious anemia	Any combination of autoimmune conditions that does not fulfill the criteria of PAS I–III

T1D, type 1 diabetes

The diagnosis of polyglandular autoimmune syndrome (PAS) was considered in our patient. PAS is a group of endocrine disorders characterized by the presence of at least two glandular autoimmune diseases.[1,2] PAS can be classified into four types, PAS I–IV (Table 55.2).[3]

PAS I is a rare autosomal recessive disease that usually presents in infancy or early childhood. It is a monogenic disease with mutation in autoimmune regulator (AIRE) gene on chromosome 21. Mutations in this gene affect central tolerance and can cause production of defective AIRE proteins, causing autoimmune destruction of target organs.[4] PAS I is generally found in populations with a high degree of consanguinity as in Iranian Jews (1:600-9,000) and Finns (1:25,000). It typically first presents as chronic mucocutaneous candidiasis and then Addison's disease and acquired hypoparathyroidism. Affected individuals may have at least two out of three of these conditions.[1]

PAS II is more common, and typically occurs in adults, with peak incidence at ages 20–60 years of age. This syndrome is more common in women as compared to men with a male-to-female ratio of 1:3. There is usually familial clustering, and multiple generations of the same family may be affected.[5] This syndrome is characterized by presence of Addison's disease with either autoimmune thyroid disease and/or T1D in addition to other endocrine and nonendocrine conditions. PAS II is a polygenic disease with autosomal dominant inheritance. It is proposed that while genetic factors play a major role in determining disease susceptibility, environmental factors may also be involved, and together they contribute to the loss of immune self-tolerance.[1]

PAS II may present initially with only one endocrinopathy, with the next one diagnosed more than 20 years later. Individuals with a single autoimmune disease are at higher risk to develop a second disease compared to the general population. Therefore, it is important to screen these individuals periodically to diagnose autoimmune conditions earlier.

PAS III presents similarly to PAS II, but without involvement of the adrenal glands. PAS IV should be considered in patients with autoimmune endocrine gland disorders who do not fulfill the criteria of PAS I–III.[3]

In our patient, we can consider the diagnosis of PAS III. She presented in her forties (consistent with PAS II and III) with autoimmune thyroid disease and negative GAD antibodies. Over the course of the next few years, she developed positive GAD antibodies, which is consistent again with PAS II and PAS III. Adrenal antibodies were negative, which makes the diagnosis of PAS III more likely for her than PAS II. However, she will need to be followed closely and monitored for the development of adrenal antibodies, as these may develop years later.

Our patient was counseled regarding the diagnosis of T1D since the risk was higher considering she has other autoimmune conditions (Hashimoto's thyroiditis and alopecia, and strong family history for multiple autoimmune disorders). She was started with low-dose insulin therapy and is currently doing well. Her blood sugar levels are in the range of 108–198 mg/dL (6 –11 mmol/L). She will be monitored closely in the Endocrine Clinic for development of other antibodies.

It is important to have a high index of suspicion for PAS in patients who do not fit the typical presentations for certain conditions. Screening for PAS should be directed at detection of organ-specific antibodies. Our case illustrates a patient who fit the description for T2D but eventually developed GAD antibodies and was, therefore, reclassified as having T1D.

It is important to recognize that the initial classification of diabetes may need to change in the presence of other autoimmune disorders. Diagnosing these syndromes early has implications for management, long-term follow-up, and the need to screen family members.

This research was supported in part by the Captain James A. Lovell Federal Health Care Center.

References

1.   Kahaly GJ. Polyglandular autoimmune syndromes. *Eur J Endocrinol* 2009;161:11–20

2.   Eisenbarth GS, Gottlieb PA. Autoimmune polyendocrine syndromes. *N Engl J Med* 2004;350:2068–2079

3.   Cutolo M. Autoimmune polyendocrine syndromes. *Autoimmunity Rev* 2014;13:85–89

4.   Halonen M, Eskelin P, Myhre AG, Perheentupa J, Husebye ES, Kämpe O, Rorsman F, Peltonen L, Ulmanen I, Partanen J. AIRE mutations and human leukocyte antigen genotypes as determinants of autoimmune polyendocrinopathy-candidiasis-ectodermal dystrophy phenotype. *J Clin Endocrinol Metab* 2002;87:2568–2574

5.   Neufeld M, MacLaren N, Blizzard R. Autoimmune polyglandular syndromes. *Pediatr Ann* 1980;9:154–162

Case 56:
Type B Insulin Resistance Syndrome

Susan Ahern, DO;[1] Hoa Nguyen, MD;[1] Yung Lyou, MD;[1] Samar Singh, MD; [1] and Ping H. Wang, MD[1]

Case

Ms. PC is a 21-year-old Hispanic female with past medical history of systemic lupus erythematosus, insulin-dependent diabetes, and end-stage renal disease requiring hemodialysis, who presented to the hospital in January 2013 with cough, dyspnea, and fever. Her vitals were notable for pulse of 115, blood pressure 200/130 mmHg, and laboratory tests revealed glucose greater than 1,000 mg/dL, sodium of 119 mEq/L, and potassium of 6.4 mEq/L. Physical exam revealed skin hyperpigmentation, acanthosis nigricans, and hirsutism (Figures C56.1 and C56.2). The patient was urgently dialyzed for volume overload and electrolyte abnormalities. She was started on regular insulin infusion of 20 units per hour and subcutaneous glargine insulin 60 units twice daily. After acute issues stabilized, she still required more than 200 units of insulin per day and was eventually discharged on U-500 insulin, 100 units three times per day. She continued to have poor glycemic control at clinic follow-up appointments on U-500 insulin, reporting glucoses in the 200–300 mg/dL range. Lab workup was notable for normal TSH, testosterone, C-peptide, DHEAS, LH, FSH, and estradiol. Anti-insulin antibodies were negative. Her hemoglobin A1C (HbA$_{1c}$) level was 12%. Patient was continued on U-500 with titration instructions.

[1]Department of Internal Medicine, Division of Endocrinology, University of California Irvine Medical Center, Orange, CA

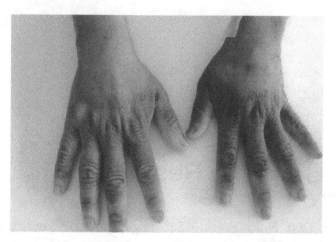

Figure C56.1—Dermatological features of type B insulin resistance syndrome—hands.

In April 2013, she was readmitted to the hospital with hyperglycemic hyperosmolar state and severe sepsis with bacteremia from arteriovenous graft. With concern for type B insulin resistance, intravenous immunoglobulin therapy was initiated for 5 days. In addition, patient was given high-dose methylprednisolone, rituximab, and mycophenolate mofetil. The patient's extreme insulin resistance led to titration of insulin up to a maximum daily dose of 38,690 units of regular insulin, which was administered at an average rate of 1,612 units an hour, and even at these doses her glucose was not controlled. Plasmapheresis was initiated and her insulin requirement decreased dramatically. By the fourth day of plasmapheresis, her insulin drip was discontinued and blood glucose levels remained in 100–200 mg/dL off insulin. She was discharged without insulin with normal glucose levels. Insulin receptor antibody results were sent; however, they returned back as negative. It was presumed that this could have been due to low titers of the antibody since the blood sample was sent after plasmapheresis.

Over the next few years, the patient began to develop episodes of hypoglycemia but was clinically asymptomatic. Hypoglycemia was demonstrated to be as low as 30–50 mg/dL on routine tests and HbA$_{1c}$ dropped to 4.4%. C-peptide levels were high despite hypoglycemia. By this point, she was still off insulin and was continued on a regimen of mycophenolate mofetil and rituximab. A cosyntropin stimulation test was done to rule out adrenal insufficiency due to prior history of steroid use; results were normal. She was started on prednisone, which did not help resolve hypoglycemia. With concern that low titers of insulin receptor antibodies were causing an agonist effect, patient received another five sessions of plasmapheresis as an outpatient in October 2015, with some improvement in severity of hypoglycemia, but not complete resolution. Her immunosuppressive regimen is being titrated up with the assistance of her rheumatologist with stabilization of glucose.

Discussion

Type B insulin resistance syndrome (IRS-B) is a rare disorder characterized by a spectrum of effects on glucose homeostasis related to autoantibodies to the insulin receptor.[1,2] The autoantibody, at high titers, can promote downregulation of insulin receptors leading to insulin resistance. Conversely, at low titers, the antibody can act as a partial agonist leading to hypoglycemia.[3] In most cases hyperglycemia and severe insulin resistance are seen; however, hypoglycemia has also been reported.[1-3] Some patients transition from severe hyperglycemia and insulin resistance to refractory hypoglycemia.[1,2] A recent review reported 25.37% of all cases had some form of hypoglycemia during the course of disease.[2]

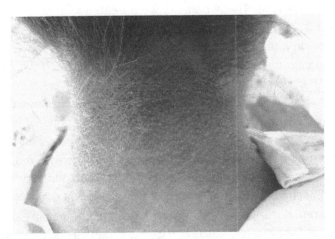

Figure C56.2—Dermatological features of type B insulin resistance syndrome—neck.

Biddinger and Kahn first described IRS-B in 1976.[4] Since then, there have been several case reports and a few case series published describing therapeutic strategies. In the largest review, done by Arioglu et al.[1] in 2002, 24 patients were studied over a 28-year period. Approximately 45% of patients carried a diagnosis of systemic lupus erythematosus (SLE), 80% presented with hyperglycemia, and 12.5% presented with hypoglycemia. SLE is the most common underlying disease state in insulin resistance syndrome. In another 2013 systematic review, the incidence of underlying SLE was as high as 62.69%.[2] Hypoglycemic manifestations have been typically associated with lower titers of insulin receptor antibodies, and those who transitioned from hyperglycemia to hypoglycemia typically had a drop in antibody titers. Our patient developed hypoglycemia after several sessions of plasmapheresis. Although the insulin receptor antibody was not quantified, it can be presumed that titers dropped with plasmapheresis and the antibody carried out partial agonist activity at the insulin receptor.

Treatment is targeted at the underlying autoimmune process, and therefore immunosuppressive agents such as glucocorticoids, cyclophosphamide, azathioprine, cyclosporine A, rituximab, leflunomide, mycophenolate mofetil, intravenous immunoglobulin, and plasmapheresis have all been used to induce remission.[2,5] In most cases, as in our case, a combination of therapies has been used, making it difficult to draw conclusions and derive a standard treatment plan. Glucocorticoids generally are the mainstay of treatment.[3] One case series included seven patients with a more standard therapeutic approach. These patients were treated with rituximab, pulse-dose steroids, and maintenance with cyclophosphamide or cyclosporine. Once remission was achieved, most patients were switched to azathioprine for maintenance for one year following remission. To achieve remission, between 1–2 cycles of rituximab were required, with 1–5 pulses of steroids, and time to remission was 2–16 months.[3] Plasmapheresis has been used in approximately one-sixth of cases with variable responses, is generally recommended for high titers of autoantibodies, and has poor long-term efficacy so may be combined with other immunosuppressive agents. For severe cases, cyclophosphamide and methylprednisolone may be recommended. Rituximab is used in patients who respond poorly to glucocorticoids and immunosuppression.[2] Intravenous immunoglobulin has shown a dramatic response in a few cases of IRS-B and can be considered first-line therapy in select cases. One case reported improvement in hyperglycemia with glucocorticoids and cyclosporine after the patient failed to improve with rituximab therapy; however, long-term remission in this case has not been evaluated.[5] Treatment must be individualized based on patient and clinical scenario; however, treatment responses seem to be highly variable. Spontaneous remission has also been reported.[6]

IRS-B is a rare but important subset of diabetes that should be recognized as highly associated with other autoimmune disorders, specifically SLE. This is a fascinating antibody-mediated disease that can be reversed with removal or suppression of antibody production. If recognized properly, it can be successfully treated and remission can be achieved. Hypoglycemia is a common and lethal manifestation of this disease as well, so long-term follow-up after remission is crucial.

References

1. Arioglu E, Andewelt A, Diabo C, Bell M, Taylor SI, Gorden P. Clinical course of the syndrome of autoantibodies to the insulin receptor (type B insulin resistance): a 28-year perspective. *Medicine* 2002;81:87–100

2. Zhang S, Wang G, Wang J. Type B insulin resistance syndrome induced by systemic lupus erythematosus and successfully treated with intravenous immunoglobulin: case report and systematic review. *Clin Rheumatol* 2013;32:181–188

3. Malek R, Chong AY, Lupsa BC, Cochran EK, Soos MA, Semple RK, Balow JE, Gorden P. Treatment of type B insulin resistance: a novel approach to reduce insulin receptor autoantibodies. *J Clin Endocrinol Metab* 2010;95:3641–3647

4. Biddinger SB, Kahn CR. From mice to men: insights into the insulin resistance syndromes. *Annu Rev Physiol* 2006;68:123–158

5. Takei M, et al. Efficacy of oral glucocorticoid and cyclosporine in a case of rituximab-refractory type B insulin resistance syndrome. *J Diabetes Investig* 2015;6:734–738.

6. Coll AP, Thomas S, Mufti GJ. Rituximab therapy for the type B syndrome of severe insulin resistance. *N Engl J Med* 2004;350:310–311

Case 57:
Remission of Type B Insulin Resistance

Jennifer Giordano, DO;[1] Maitri Shelly Kalia-Reynolds, DO;[1] Caroline Houston, MD;[1] Robert J. Tanenberg, MD;[1] Rebecca J. Brown, MD;[2] Robert K. Semple, MB, PhD;[3] Fiona J. Cook, MD[1]

Case

A 68-year-old African-American woman with a previously unremarkable medical history presented with sudden unintentional weight loss and abdominal pain. Shortly thereafter, she was diagnosed with diabetes (HbA$_{1c}$ 6.8%) and was started on metformin. During the subsequent two months, she experienced recurrent acute pancreatitis episodes and rapidly worsening symptomatic hyperglycemia (HbA$_{1c}$ 11.1%). Physical exam revealed cachexia with a reported 70-pound weight loss, patchy alopecia, facial hirsutism, acanthosis nigricans, and painful enlargement of both parotid glands (Figure C57.1).

During hospitalization for parotid surgery, her postoperative blood glucose was 507 mg/dL, requiring initiation of intravenous insulin. Hyperglycemia persisted despite administration of over 1,500 units of insulin daily.

[1]Division of Endocrinology, Brody School of Medicine at East Carolina University, Greenville, NC

[2]National Institute of Diabetes and Digestive and Kidney Diseases, National Institutes of Health, Bethesda, MD

[3]Institute of Metabolic Science, University of Cambridge, Addenbrooke's Hospital, Cambridge, U.K.

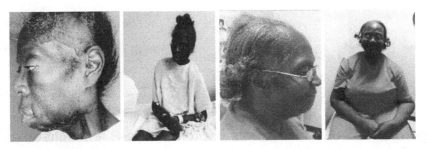

Figure C57.1—Physical exam findings upon diagnosis and after remission.

Laboratory tests were remarkable for pancytopenia, positive anti-nuclear antibodies, positive anti-Sjögren-syndrome-related antigen A (anti-SSA) antibody, low serum C3, and elevated erythrocyte sedimentation rate and C-reactive protein (Table C57.1). A diagnosis of mixed connective tissue disorder was made.

The combination of autoimmune disease, severe insulin resistance, and features of insulin deficiency raised suspicion for type B insulin resistance (TBIR). The patient's serum was sent to a research laboratory for analysis and returned positive for insulin receptor antibodies (Figure C57.2).

Table C57.1—Pertinent Laboratory Evaluation Performed within the First Week of Hospitalization

Test	Result	Reference Range
Erythrocyte Sedimentation Rate	86	0–23 mm/h
C-Reactive Protein	6.2	<2.6 mg/L
Complement C3	60	90–170 mg/dL
Anti-Nuclear Antibody Titer	1:80, Speckled Pattern	>1:40
Extractable Nuclear Antigen SSA/ Ro Antibody	Positive	Negative
Hemoglobin	7.9	10.2–17.0 g/dL
Hematocrit	27.8	30.6–49.6 %
Mean Corpuscular Volume	92	80–96 fL
White Blood Cells	3.4	2.80–10.40 k/uL
Platelets	128	117–366 k/uL
Total Cholesterol	102	<200 mg/dL
High Density Lipoprotein	60	In Females ≥ 50mg/dL
Low Density Lipoprotein	34	< 100mg/dL
Triglycerides	38	< 150mg/dL

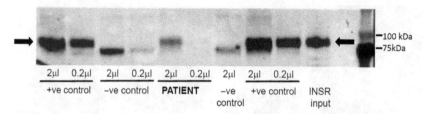

| 2μl | 0.2μl | 2μl | 0.2μl | 2μl | 0.2μl | 2μl | 2μl | 0.2μl | |
| +ve control | | −ve control | | **PATIENT** | | −ve control | +ve control | | INSR input |

Figure C57.2—Gel electrophoresis for anti-INSR autoantibodies.

The semi-quantitative antibody assay is based upon the ability of patient serum to immunoprecipitate a human insulin receptor antibody.

Impaired insulin receptor function was evidenced by a combination of severe hyperinsulinemia with an insulin level of 6,120 uIU/mL (normal 5–65), low serum triglycerides (38 mg/dL), and a high adiponectin of 30.3 ug/mL (normal 3–21.1). A high molar ratio of insulin to C-peptide (9:1) reflected the impaired clearance of insulin.

The patient was treated at our institution according to the protocol published from the National Institute of Diabetes and Digestive and Kidney Diseases (Malek R, et al.)[1] (Study Protocol 76-DK-0006). Cycles 1 and 2 consisted of a two-dose pulse of intravenous rituximab 750 mg/meter body surface area, given 2 weeks apart, and a four-day pulse of oral dexamethasone 40 mg given with each rituximab dose (Figure C57.3). The protocol also includes cyclophosphamide 100 mg by mouth daily, starting on Day 1 of the first cycle, until remission.

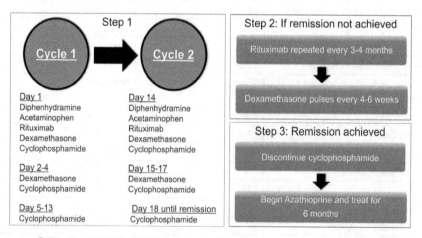

Figure C57.3—NIH/NIDDK Study Protocol 76-DK-0006 (Malek et al.)[1].

As per the protocol published by Malek et al., criteria for remission include the following: euglycemia off insulin, and fasting insulin <30 uIU/mL. Additional treatment may be given if remission is not achieved and CD-19 B lymphocyte levels remain detectable. Adjunctive therapy includes rituximab every 3–4 months and dexamethasone pulses every 4–6 weeks. Once remission is achieved, cyclophosphamide is discontinued and azathioprine is given for 6–12 months.[1]

After two cycles of treatment, our patient's insulin requirement dissipated (Figure C57.4), and mild hyperglycemia was managed with metformin 500 mg twice daily. She continued cyclophosphamide 100 mg daily. The CD-19 lymphocyte count was <1% and her insulin level was 112.1 uIU/mL.

After two months of therapy, her HbA$_{1c}$ improved to 6.1% and she experienced episodic hypoglycemia. Therefore, metformin was discontinued. She also developed cyclophosphamide-induced leukopenia, which prompted substitution with azathioprine 100 mg daily. She received two pulses of dexamethasone 40 mg per day for 4 days at 4-week intervals. Due to financial restraints, she did not receive further rituximab therapy. Ultimately, our patient achieved remission of her TBIR approximately 12 months after initial diagnosis, with a follow-up insulin level of 20.4 uIU/mL, HbA$_{1c}$ of 5.1%, and return to her prior baseline weight. She was continued on azathioprine 100 mg daily for one year following documentation of remission to suppress a rebound of insulin receptor

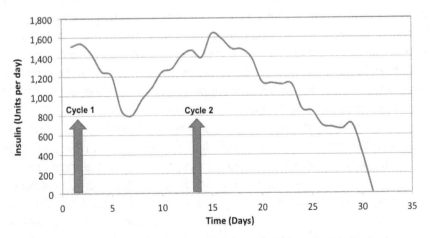

Figure C57.4—Falling insulin requirement over time during two cycles of therapy.

antibody production. She remains in remission 3 months after discontinuation of azathioprine.

Discussion

Type B insulin resistance (TBIR) is a rare syndrome in which autoantibodies act at high titers to downregulate signaling at the insulin receptor and lead to extreme insulin resistance.[1,2] Patients can present with rapidly progressive diabetes refractory to massive doses of insulin, weight loss, acanthosis nigricans, and hyperandrogenism. This syndrome occurs most often in reproductive-aged women with concomitant rheumatologic disease or as a paraneoplastic manifestation.[2]

Multiple experimental therapies for TBIR have been attempted, including plasmapheresis, intravenous immunoglobulin, and various immunosuppressive agents.[1-3] Malek et al. conducted the only prospective clinical trial to date, using a combination of rituximab, cyclophosphamide, and steroids to induce disease remission.[1] In this report, we describe the clinical course of a female patient with TBIR and mixed connective tissue disease, who was successfully treated with this protocol at our institution.

TBIR is caused by an autoantibody to a cell surface receptor (as is also observed in Graves' disease and myasthenia gravis[2]). This concept of antibodies that impair insulin receptor binding was first reported in 1975.[3] Disparate clinical manifestations can result from variation in the antibody titer, with hypoglycemia occurring when low antibody titers act as a partial agonist to the receptor. Conversely, severe hyperglycemia develops when high antibody titers block the response to insulin.[1] Unlike the more common insulin-resistant patient, patients with TBIR tend to have low triglyceride levels and a normal or high adiponectin level.[1] Prior to the use of immunosuppressive therapy, the original 2002 NIH case series indicated a mortality rate of 54% in <10 years after diagnosis.[2] The rarity of this syndrome has precluded randomized controlled trials, and therapy has not been standardized. However, in 2010 the NIH described seven patients treated prospectively with the protocol, all of whom achieved remission.[1] Rituximab is used to target antibody-producing B lymphocytes, while pulse steroids are used to suppress the activity of preexisting plasma cells. Adjunctive immunosuppressants (e.g., cyclophosphamide) are used to suppress B and T cell function. Reported time to remission from TBIR is variable with a range of

6–27 months, but with the NIH protocol remission was achieved in 2.5–9 months, with a mean of 5 months.[1,3] However, the rarity and variable natural history of the disease prohibits firm conclusions. Our report is currently the third to describe a patient treated with this regimen outside of the NIH[4] and lends further credence to the use of combined rituximab/cyclophosphamide/steroids in the treatment of TBIR syndrome. This treatment is now considered a standard of care and will likely become increasingly accessible to patients outside the NIH.

References

1. Malek R, Chong AY, Lupsa BC, et al. Treatment of type B insulin resistance: a novel approach to reduce insulin receptor autoantibodies. *J Clin Endocrinol Metab* 2010;95:3641–3647

2. Arioglu E, Andewelt A, Diabo C, Bell M, Taylor SI, Gorden P. Clinical course of the syndrome of autoantibodies to the insulin receptor (type B insulin resistance): a 28-year perspective. *Medicine (Baltimore)* 2002;81:87–100

3. Willard D, Stevenson M, Steenkamp D. Type B insulin resistance syndrome. *Curr Opin Endocrinol Diabetes Obes* 2016;23:318–323

4. Manikas ED, Isaac I, Semple RK, Malek R, Fuhrer D, Moeller L. Successful treatment of type B insulin resistance with rituximab. *J Clin Endocrinol Metab* 2015;100:1719–1722

Case 58:
Ketosis-Prone Type 2 Diabetes

Jignesh Patel, MD;[1] and Colette M. Knight, MD[1,2]

Case

A 49-year-old man with no significant past medical history presented to the emergency room with complaints of weakness, increased thirst, frequent urination, dizziness, loss of appetite, and unintentional weight loss over three weeks. Initial laboratory tests were suggestive of diabetic ketoacidosis (DKA): glucose 529 mg/dL (29.4 mmol/L), serum HCO3 12 m eq/L, arterial pH: 7.20, and elevated urine and serum acetone. Additional studies revealed a low C-peptide, 0.9 ng/mL, and anti-GAD (glutamic acid decarboxylase) >30 u/mL (Table C58.1). The patient was treated with continuous IV insulin infusion and then transitioned to a basal-bolus regimen: insulin detemir 25 units nightly and insulin lispro 6 units with meals. Insulin therapy was tapered and eventually discontinued after three months. The patient was subsequently treated with metformin 500 mg twice daily and has had normalization of glucose. Repeat laboratory tests showed an increase in fasting C-peptide to 2.3 ng/mL.

Discussion

Ketosis-prone type 2 diabetes (KPDM) is a subtype of type 2 diabetes (T2D) that is associated with severe hyperglycemia and ketoacidosis

[1]Montefiore Medical Center, Department of Pediatrics, Bronx, NY
[2]Montefiore Medical Center, Department of Medicine, Division of Endocrinology, Bronx, NY

Table C58.1—Lab Data at Diagnosis and after Treatment

Test	Initial Labs	Labs after 3 Months
Plasma glucose (mg/dL)	529	139
A1C (%)	16.3	6.7
HCO3 (meq/L)	12	22
pH, arterial	7.20	N/A
Anion Gap	32	14
Serum Acetone	Moderate	N/A
Urine Ketone (mg/dL)	>80	
BUN (mg/dL)	14	20
Cr (mg/dL)	1.12	1.3
C-peptide (1.3–4.2 ng/mL)	0.9	2.3
GAD Ab (n < 1 unit/mL)	>30.0	

on presentation followed by remission after intensive insulin therapy. This form of diabetes has been called several names including atypical diabetes, idiopathic type 1 diabetes, Flatbush diabetes, and diabetes type 1.5. Patients with KPDM have markedly impaired insulin secretion and insulin action but more than half of them with unprecipitated DKA experience significant improvement in β-cell function and insulin sensitivity sufficient to allow discontinuation of insulin therapy within a few months after initiation.[1-3] Upon discontinuation of insulin, the period of near-normoglycemic remission may last months to several years. KPD is most commonly seen in Africans, African Americans, or Afro-Caribbean blacks but has been seen in other ethnic groups such as Latinos and Asians. It is more often seen in adults in the fourth or fifth decade of life but there is increasing incidence in children as well. There is also a gender disparity as the incidence in men is almost threefold higher compared to women.[3]

The typical presentation of patients with new-onset KPD is polyuria, polydipsia, and unintentional weight loss. The majority of these patients are overweight or obese at baseline but usually report significant weight loss at the time of diagnosis. On presentation they may have nausea, vomiting, and abdominal pain. Lab abnormalities are significant for marked hyperglycemia associated with ketonuria/ketonemia and high anion gap metabolic acidosis. Patients may also have cutaneous manifestations of insulin resistance such as acanthosis nigricans and abdominal obesity. Among the African diaspora, sub-Saharan African individuals with KPD are often thin/lean compared to patients with KPD in the U.S. who are obese.[4] The patients can usually be grouped into two different phenotypes: those with no identifiable precipitating factor who are more likely to discontinue insulin therapy and those with a clear precipitant and who may require long-term insulin therapy. The patient in the case report had no prior illnesses and there were no known triggers for his onset of hyperglycemic crisis.

The pathogenesis of KPDM is complex and includes many factors such as genetic predisposition, attenuation of β-cell function, glucotoxicity, and lipotoxicity (Figure C58.1). Sustained hyperglycemia has been associated with decreased β-cell function. Similarly, prolonged exposure to free fatty acids has been shown to induce insulin resistance. However, recent studies were unable to show an impairment in insulin secretion in subjects with KPDM after short-term infusion of glucose or lipids suggesting that longer exposure is required.[3] Impaired insulin signaling via the Akt-pathway may also account for decreased insulin action as insulin-stimulated expression

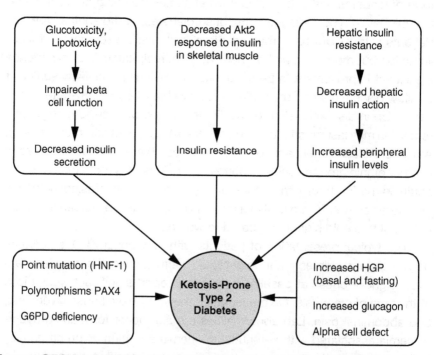

Figure C58.1—Pathogenesis of ketosis-prone type 2 diabetes. HGP, hepatic glucose production; Akt2, protein kinase B.

and phosphorylation of Akt-2 in skeletal muscle was decreased in subjects with KPD but improved after remission of the hyperglycemic state.[3,5] In most patients with KPD there is generally a lack of autoantibodies to the β-cells. HLA associations also seem to be rare, but one study showed increased frequency of HLA-DR3 and HLA-DR4.[1] There is significant interest to identify and characterize associated putative genes. G6PD deficiency seems to be more prevalent in individuals with KPD compared to controls with T2D. Point mutation in HNF-1 or high polymorphisms in PAX4 was associated with KPD in select patients of African ethnicity. Overall it seems that there may be a confluence of multiple factors that may promote and accelerate the progression to KPD.[3,5]

Acute management of DKA in KPD is the same as that of any DKA patient. Insulin is required to achieve near-normoglycemic remission after presentation. Over the course of 10–12 weeks, most patients can completely discontinue insulin. In clinical practice a target A1C of <7.0% and FBS <130 mg/dL are used while lowering insulin dose or to guide complete discontinuation of insulin. Patients with negative GAD antibody and positive C-peptide response a few weeks after diagnosis are likely to maintain euglycemia with oral antidiabetic drugs. However, patients with positive GAD antibody and insufficient C-peptide response will likely need insulin or will require close follow-up if a decision is made to discontinue insulin as was the case with the patient in this report.

Recurrence of hyperglycemia or ketosis after the discontinuation of insulin occurs within 12–24 months in nearly 60% of patients who are on diet alone. These findings led to studies to evaluate the effects of oral hypoglycemic agents on maintaining insulin-free remission and β-cell function that can prevent or delay hyperglycemic relapse after the discontinuation of insulin. It was found that use of glipizide compared with placebo significantly prolonged remission. Low-dose secretagogues such as glipizide (0.625–2.5 mg/day) and glyburide (1.25–2.5 mg/day) and the insulin sensitizer pioglitazone (30 mg/day) were found to be beneficial in some studies.[3] Other drugs like metformin, DPP4 inhibitors, and incretin mimetic are currently being investigated. Another treatment strategy to prevent relapse is to continue to use insulin even during remission.

In summary, KPD is a subtype of T2D where the initial presentation is one of hyperglycemic crisis with ketoacidosis. These patients improve significantly after intensive insulin therapy. However, unlike T2D patients, >50% of KPD patients present with recurring episodes of relapse-remission within 2 years of diagnosis, and with each relapse, there is a risk of becoming chronically insulin dependent. The most common subtype of KPD is antibody negative with preservation of β-cell. However, other subtypes with islet antibody positivity and some preservation of β-cell as described in the clinical case have been documented. These patients should be monitored very carefully to determine the best options for long-term management. More research needs to be done to better identify the mechanisms that are involved in the pathogenesis of KPD and to determine the optimal pharmacological treatment approach in affected patients.

References

1. Banerji MA, Chaiken RL, Huey H, Tuomi T, Norin AJ, Mackay IR, Rowley MJ, Zimmet PZ, Lebovitz HE. GAD antibody negative NIDDM in adult black subjects with diabetic ketoacidosis and increased frequency of human leukocyte antigen DR3 and DR4. Flatbush diabetes. *Diabetes* 1994;43:741–745

2. Mauvais-Jarvis F, Sobngwi E, Porcher R, Riveline JP, Kevorkian JP, Vaisse C, Charpentier G, Guillausseau PJ, Vexiau P, Gautier JF. Ketosis-prone type 2 diabetes in patients of sub-Saharan African origin: clinical pathophysiology and natural history of beta-cell dysfunction and insulin resistance. *Diabetes* 2004;53:645–653

3. Smiley D, Chandra P, Umpierrez GE. Update on diagnosis, pathogenesis and management of ketosis-prone type 2 diabetes mellitus. *Diabetes Manag (Lond)* 2011;1:589–600

4. Gaillard TR, Osei K. Racial disparities in the pathogenesis of type 2 diabetes and its subtypes in the African diaspora: a new paradigm. *J Racial Ethn Health Disparities* 2016;3:117–128

5. Nyenwe EA, Kitabchi AE. The evolution of diabetic ketoacidosis: an update of its etiology, pathogenesis and management. *Metabolism* 2016;65:507–521

Case 59:
Ketosis-Prone Type 2 Diabetes: Case Report

Anna Milanesi, MD, PhD;[1] and Jane E. Weinreb, MD[1]

Case

A 57-year-old African-American male with no previous history of diabetes presented in May of 2008 with 3 weeks of polyuria, polydipsia, and blurred vision and was diagnosed with new-onset diabetes with ketoacidosis (DKA). He had a history of hypertension treated on a multidrug regimen (metoprolol, lisinopril, spironolactone, and nifedipine), chronic obstructive pulmonary disease, and strong family history of type 2 diabetes. On examination, he was morbidly obese (BMI 41 kg/m²), afebrile, and hemodynamically stable. Examination was otherwise unremarkable. Laboratory testing on admission revealed significant hyperglycemia (plasma glucose 654 mg/dL or 36.3 mmol/L), with anion gap of 21.7 mEq/L (3–11 mEq/L), acidemia with arterial pH 7.27 (7.35–7.45) and bicarbonate of 12.8 mmol/L (22-26 mmol/L), and positive ketonemia and ketonuria, confirming DKA. Creatinine was 2.2 mg/dL (0.5–1.4 mg/dL), but it quickly improved to normal after aggressive intravenous hydration, confirming reversible acute kidney injury secondary to dehydration. There were no apparent precipitant factors. Workup for possible secondary hypertension was negative. The hemoglobin A1C (HbA$_{1c}$) was 12% at admission, increased from 6.5% three months before admission and was always below 6% previously (Figure C59.1A).

[1]Division of Endocrinology, VA; Greater Los Angeles Healthcare System, Los Angeles, CA; Department of Internal Medicine, David Geffen School of Medicine at UCLA, Los Angeles, CA

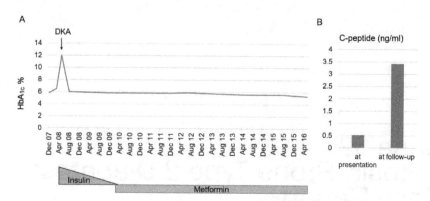

Figure C59.1—Hemoglobin A1C trend from 2007 to date (A). Time on insulin and metformin therapy. Fasting C-peptide level (ng/mL) at presentation and 3 months after DKA (at follow-up) (B).

The C-peptide, measured on day 3 during admission, was 0.42 mg/mL (0.8-3.9 mg/mL) (Figure C59.1B) with concurrent plasma glucose of 151 mg/dL (8.4 mmol/L). Anti-glutamic acid decarboxylases and anti-islet cell antibodies were negative.

He received standard treatment for DKA with hydration and an intravenous insulin drip and was discharged home on multiple daily insulin injections (total 0.7 units per kg body weight). At 3 months follow-up, his HbA$_{1c}$ was 6% (Figure C59.1A) and fasting C-peptide was 3.4 mg/ml with concurrent plasma glucose 113 mg/dL (Figure C59.1B). For almost 2 years he was kept on insulin therapy. However, the dose of insulin was down-titrated to about 0.2 unit/kg due to recurrent symptomatic hypoglycemia, and ultimately, because of persistent hypoglycemia, insulin was completely discontinued and he was started on metformin 1 gram daily. He remains to date in optimal glucose control on metformin monotherapy (Figure C59.1A). During the 8-year follow-up since diabetes diagnosis, there has been no change in weight, and he remains morbidly obese (BMI 40 kg/m^2).

Discussion

Over the course of the past two decades, ketosis-prone type 2 diabetes (KPD2) has emerged as a new clinical entity. Despite growing interest and recent studies dedicated to improve current understanding of KPD2, the pathophysiologic mechanism behind this "atypical diabetes" remains unknown. Although these individuals present with severe hyperglycemia and ketosis similar to type 1 diabetes, they have clinical and biochemical features typical of type 2 diabetes and can discontinue insulin and maintain acceptable glycemic control on diet and/or oral agents.[1] Most adults with KPD2 are African American or Hispanic, overweight or obese, middle-aged, have a strong family history of type 2 diabetes, and present with new onset of diabetes with unprovoked ketosis.[2] Our patient meets the clinical and biochemical criteria for KPD2. He is middle-aged, African American, obese, with no previous history of diabetes and presented for the first time with an unprovoked episode of DKA. He regained β-cell function following a few weeks on multiple daily insulin injections and eventually was able to completely discontinue insulin therapy with good glucose control on metformin alone for more than 6 years now. After treatment of the acute episode, 40 to 70% of the patients with KPD2 are able to sustain near- normoglycemic remission after insulin discontinuation.[2] However, even during near-normoglycemic remission, these patients have impaired glucose response to intravenous insulin, as well as impaired glucagon suppression.[5] Early identification of KPD2 patients is important to predict viable candidates for insulin therapy discontinuation in outpatient follow-up. The main reason why our patient was kept on insulin for 2 years after discharge was the perception that he had type 1 diabetes because of his clinical presentation with DKA. This could have potentially led to life-threatening hypoglycemia. There is not a clear consensus about the prediction of recovery after the first presentation with new-onset DKA. The presence of β-cell autoantibodies has been linked to latent autoimmune diabetes, and it has been suggested that patients with ketosis-prone diabetes and positive autoantibodies are more likely to become insulin dependent.[2] We recently reviewed the database at a single large Veterans Affairs Medical Center and found that over a ten-year period, more than half of patients with new-onset diabetes presenting with DKA had KPD2. Further, higher fasting C-peptide levels at follow-up (1 month after DKA resolution) were strongly predictive of recovery.[3] This has been previously reported and was not surprising, as high C-peptide levels have been directly correlated to successful insulin therapy discontinuation in multiple studies and is compatible with the theory that KPD2 may be the result of an innately higher β-cell propensity toward glucose toxicity.[2] It is well known that insulin secretion can be dramatically improved after insulin treatment with associated improved glycemic control in both animal and human studies.[4] Because C-peptide and pancreatic islet autoantibodies are not routinely measured in the clinical setting, these should be checked in all patients hospitalized with new onset of DKA in order to clarify what type of diabetes a patient has and therefore optimize long-term management.

Another important challenge in KPD2 is outpatient follow-up after insulin discontinuation. Patients with KPD2 tend to relapse and have recurrent episodes of DKA. For this reason, patient education and close follow-up are important to avoid hospitalization. In addition, it has been reported that sulfonylurea treatment during the near-normoglycemic remission prevents recurrence of hyperglycemia.[4]

Clearly, KPD2 presents in a manner that challenges traditional beliefs about how type 2 diabetes is expected to behave in the clinical setting and represents a unique entity that often is unrecognized. Early recognition of this peculiar clinical presentation of diabetes is important to guide appropriate management and follow-up with the aim to avoid potentially life-threatening hypoglycemia and recurrent hospitalization.

References:

1. Umpierrez GE, Smiley D, Kitabchi AE. Narrative review: ketosis-prone type 2 diabetes mellitus. *Ann Intern Med* 2006;144:350–357

2. Mauvais-Jarvis F, Sobngwi E, Porcher R, Riveline JP, Kevorkian JP, Vaisse C, Charpentier G, Guillausseau PJ, Vexiau P, Gautier JF. Ketosis-prone type 2 diabetes in patients of sub-Saharan African origin: clinical pathophysiology and natural history of beta-cell dysfunction and insulin resistance. *Diabetes* 2004;53:645–653

3. Goodstein G, Milanesi A, Weinreb J. Ketosis-prone type 2 diabetes in a veteran population. *Diabetes Care* 2014;37:e74–e75

4. Umpierrez GE, Clark WS, Steen MT. Sulfonylurea treatment prevents recurrence of hyperglycemia in obese African-American patients with a history of hyperglycemic crises. *Diabetes Care* 1997;20:479–483

5. Choukem SP, Sobngwi E, Boudou P, Fetita LS, Porcher R, Ibrahim F, Blondeau B, Vexiau P, Mauvais-Jarvis F, Calvo F, Gautier JF. β- and α-cell dysfunctions in Africans with ketosis-prone atypical diabetes during near-normoglycemic remission. *Diabetes Care* 2013;36:118–123

Case 60:
Ketosis-Prone Diabetes

Sumera Ahmed, MD;[1] and Robert J. Tanenberg, MD, FACP[1]

Case

A 17-year-old African-American male with no past medical history presented to the emergency department of an outside hospital with vomiting and worsening fatigue. He had a 1–2-week history of polyuria, nocturia, polydipsia, and fatigue. He was found to be in diabetic ketoacidosis (DKA) with initial glucose 1,228 mg/dL (68 mmol/L), pH 7.22, and bicarb 14 and transferred to our tertiary care hospital. Physical exam revealed obesity (weight 106 kg, BMI 30 mg/k²) with acanthosis nigricans. He was newly diagnosed with diabetes (HbA$_{1c}$ 12.2%) with initial presentation in DKA and treated with IV insulin and fluids. DKA resolved uneventfully.

Labs sent for GAD-65, insulin, and islet cell antibodies were negative, ruling out autoimmune diabetes (Table C60.1).

Formal diabetes education was completed. By the time of discharge, he tolerated appropriate oral intake. Patient and his family demonstrated proficiency in checking fingerstick blood glucose, counting carbohydrates, calculating insulin doses, treatment of hypo- and hyperglycemia, and sick day rules. He was discharged on insulin glargine 53 units at bedtime every night; carbohydrate coverage with insulin aspart 2 units per 5 grams of carbs; and correctional scale 2 units aspart for every 50 mg/dL and metformin-XR 500 mg daily. When seen in endocrine clinic 6 weeks later,

[1]Division of Endocrinology Brody School of Medicine, East Carolina University, Greenville, NC

Table C60.1—Pertinent Labs during Hospitalization

TEST	RESULT
β-hydroxybutyrate	77.20 mg/dL
A1C	12.2%
C-peptide	1.06 ng/ml (corresponding blood glucose 754)
Fructosamine	794 umol/L
Free T4	0.9 ng/dL
TSH	0.24 uIU/ml
Insulin Ab	<0.4
GAD 65	<1.0 unit/ml
Islet cell Ab screen	negative
Ig A	negative
Anti-thyroid peroxidase Ab	negative
Thyroglobulin Ab	negative
Transglutaminase IgG	negative

fingerstick blood glucose levels were noted to be below 90 mg/dL with occasional hypoglycemia. No reported severe hypoglycemia and HbA$_{1c}$ was 5.0%. Insulin doses were reduced by half and metformin dose was increased. Six months after initial presentation, HbA$_{1c}$ was 4.5% and insulin was discontinued with maximization of metformin dose.

On subsequent follow-up 3 months later, HbA$_{1c}$ was 4.4% off insulin and on metformin 2,000 mg daily. At that time, a 90-minute post–mixed meal stimulated C-peptide was 9.45 ng/ml with a corresponding glucose level of 122 mg/dL (6.8 mmol/L).

Discussion

Ketosis-prone diabetes (KPD) is a form of atypical type 2 diabetes mellitus in which patients under certain circumstances can develop a near-complete but mostly reversible β-cell failure causing life-threatening DKA. Aggressive medical intervention usually promotes restoration of β-cell function. It is a rare form of type 2 diabetes characterized by sudden, severe, and phasic insulin dependence, but lacking markers of autoimmunity observed in type 1 diabetes. KPD has been found primarily in nonwhite populations, especially those of sub-Saharan African descent (particularly West Africa), although Native Americans, Hispanics, Asians,

Table C60.2—Classification Scheme for Ketosis-Prone Diabetes

Classification system

ADA	Type 1a: + autoantibodies Type 1b: – autoantibodies
Modified ADA classification	Type 1a: + autoantibodies Type 1b: – autoantibodies • Insulin-dependent (KPD-ID) • Non-insulin-dependent (KPD-NID)
BMI	Lean: BMI <28 kg/m^2 Obese: BMI 28 kg/m^2
Aβ	A+β–: autoantibodies +, β-cell function – A+β+: autoantibodies +, β-cell function + A–β–: autoantibodies –, β-cell function – A–β+: autoantibodies –, β-cell function +

Aβ – most accurate in terms of sensitivity (99.4%), NPV, - LR and has high degree of specificity (95.9%), + LR, PPV [2]

Table C60.3—Subtypes of Diabetes Based on Antibodies and β-cell Function

Subtype	Autoantibodies	Beta-cell Function
A+β+	+	+
A+β–	+	–
A–β+	–	+
A–β–	–	–

Source: Balasubramanyam A et al.[4]

and some Caucasians have been diagnosed with it.[1,2] In the U.S, prevalence has been estimated to be between 20% and 50% in African-American and Hispanic patients with new diagnoses of DKA.[1]

This variant of type 2 diabetes has been referred to in the literature as diabetes type 1B, idiopathic type 1 diabetes, atypical diabetes, Flatbush diabetes, type 1.5 diabetes, Type J diabetes, and more recently, ketosis-prone type 2 diabetes.

A published classification system of patients presenting with DKA has been noted to predict which patients will have preserved β-cell function and thus long-term insulin independence.[3] Absent or preserved β-cell function is a strong determinant of long-term insulin dependence and clinical phenotype (Table C60.2; Table C60.3).

Recommend Treatment Protocol

The literature supports the following treatment protocol:[1]

Initial Management of DKA

Start an initial intravenous bolus at 0.1 unit/kg of body weight, followed by continuous infusion at 0.1 unit/kg per hour. When blood glucose levels <250 mg/dL, change IV fluids to 5% dextrose and 0.45% saline, and reduce the insulin infusion rate to 0.05 unit/kg per h to keep glucose levels at approximately 200 mg/dL (11.1 mmol/L) until resolution of DKA.

After Resolution of DKA

Start basal/bolus insulin at a dose of 0.8 unit/Kg of body weight. Adjust insulin dose to achieve target fasting and premeal glucose levels <120 mg/dL (6.7 mmol/L). Monitor patients every 2 weeks for first 2 months to adjust insulin therapy. Depending on glycemic control, subsequently monitor every 2 or 3 months. To achieve target blood glucose level, the mean insulin requirement is usually 1–1.2 units/kg of body weight. Begin tapering insulin dose once fasting blood glucose levels are <6.7 mmol/L (<120 mg/dL) for 2 weeks or if hypoglycemia. Decrease total insulin dose by 25–50% at each visit.

Measure GAD antibodies and β–cell function (fasting C-peptide or glucagon-stimulated C-peptide test) after resolution of DKA. If β-cell function is absent, irrespective of presence or absence of autoantibodies, lifelong insulin therapy is indicated.

If β–cell function is present, irrespective of presence or absence of autoantibodies, and if blood glucose level is above goal, continue/intensify insulin therapy. Reassess β-cell function every 6 months. If blood glucose is at goal, reduce insulin dose as mentioned earlier. Reassess β-cell function every 6 months.

In A–β+ patients, insulin-sensitizing agents such as metformin are recommended. If blood glucose levels do not achieve therapeutic targets within eight weeks, addition of low doses of a sulfonylurea, thiazolidinedione, meglitinide, or alpha-glucosidase inhibitor should be considered. Patients with KPD2 and positive autoantibodies have considerably reduced basal and stimulated insulin secretion compared with those with negative auto-antibodies. These patients need to be watched closely and probably should be left on insulin. They act more like slow-onset type 1 or LADA patients. When this protocol is followed, approximately 70% of obese patients with new diagnoses of DKA are able to discontinue insulin therapy after a mean follow-up of 9 weeks.[2]

Summary

A ketosis-prone form of diabetes has emerged as a new clinical entity. This syndrome of episodic DKA without autoimmune markers of type 1 diabetes is characterized by severe impairment of insulin secretion and action at presentation, but followed by absence of insulin requirements for years. The KPD syndrome includes one major subgroup with preserved insulin secretion and negative autoantibodies (A-β+). Most patients are obese, middle-aged men with a strong family history of type 2 diabetes.[1] Aggressive diabetic management results in marked improvement in β-cell function and insulin sensitivity (generally to allow discontinuation of insulin treatment within a few months). Remission phase is usually less than 2 years when patients are treated with diet alone. Low-dose sulfonylureas and metformin have been found to delay the recurrence of hyperglycemia. Use of the newer incretin agents has not been studied but their mechanism of action, safety profile, and anecdotal evidence lend support to their use after diabetes has been stabilized with subcutaneous insulin.

References

1. Umpierrez GE, Smiley D, Kitabchi AE. Narrative review: ketosis-prone type 2 diabetes mellitus *Ann Intern Med* 2006;144:350–357

2. Umpierrez GE, Kelly JP, Navarette JE, Casals MM, Kitabchi AE. Hyperglycemic crises in urban blacks. *Arch Intern Med* 1997;157:669–675

3. Balasubramanyam A, Garza G, Rodriguez L, et al. Accuracy and predictive value of classification schemes for ketosis-prone diabetes. *Diabetes Care* 2006;29:2575–2579

4. Balasubramanyam A, Nalini R, Hampe C, Maldonado M. Syndromes of ketosis-prone diabetes mellitus. *Endocr Rev* 2008;29:292–302

Case 61:
Prader-Willi Syndrome

Janice L. Gilden, MS, MD;[1,2] and Bushra Z. Osmani, MD[1]

Case

A 30-year-old Latino male with approximately one year duration of type 2 diabetes (T2D), taking glipizide XL 5 mg and metformin 1,000 mg, both twice daily, was admitted to the hospital for a week of very high blood glucose levels, reportedly in the 400–500 mg/dL range (22.2–27.8 mmol/L), with cellulitis of his hands and legs. He was known to have self-mutilating behavior, and these subcutaneous areas became infected. An endocrine consult was requested for glycemic control.

History was obtained from his mother, with whom he now lives. She stated that he was known to have the Prader-Willi syndrome (PWS) and uncontrollable hyperphagia. However, she refused genetic testing and photographs at this time for protective emotional reasons. Complications included: morbid obesity (BMI 67.6 kg/m²), sleep apnea with episodes of respiratory failure, atherosclerosis, umbilical hernia, an episode of paralytic ileus, hypogonadism, seizure disorder with episodes of "collapse," a mood disorder, episodic uncontrollable behavior and cognitive deficits, gastroesophageal reflux disease, and intermittent rectal bleeding. Physical examination was limited due to his inability to cooperate but showed

[1]Rosalind Franklin University of Medicine and Science/Chicago Medical School, Captain James A. Lovell Federal Health Care Center, North Chicago, IL
[2]Presence Saints Mary and Elizabeth Medical Center, Chicago, IL

a shy morbidly obese male, 4 feet 5 inches tall (134.6 cm), with a very fair complexion, rosy cheeks, and characteristic facial features of almond-shaped eyes with esotropia, a child-like appearance with large fatty body composition, lack of facial and chest hair, bilateral gynecomastia, small gonads, and child-like speech with an impediment and childlike mentation (although he was bilingual). Extremities showed deep scarring and exudates with cellulitis on multiple areas of his arms and legs from the chronic skin-picking behavior.

While an inpatient, he received intravenous antibiotics and insulin therapy. Despite increasing doses of insulin, blood glucose levels remained elevated, and he continued to demand food with tantrums. A DPP-4 inhibitor was then administered, in addition to the insulin therapy, and blood glucose levels began to decrease, although they did not normalize (Table C61.1).

The plan was to administer a trial of a glucagon-like polypeptide (GLP)-1 receptor agonist, which has been suggested as an adjunctive treatment for T2D in PWS, due to its effect of decreasing appetite in the short term.[1] However, he was discharged to a home for mentally challenged and disabled adults, due to the difficulty with behavioral and other care issues, despite many years of attempted interventions, and lost to follow-up.

PWS is the most common cause of obesity as a syndrome and has a birth incidence of approximately 1:15,000 to 1:30,000 and a population prevalence of about 1 in 50,000.[2] It is a genomic disorder, caused by the absence of expression of the `active genes on the long arm of chromosome 15 (15q11.3-q13.3 region) and can be due to deletions from the paternal chromosome, maternal disomy, or defects in the imprinting center.[3] PWS can present clinically with neonatal hypotonia, short stature, developmental delay, childhood obesity, hypogonadism, and characteristic facial features.[2]

The clinical diagnostic consensus criteria for PWS were proposed in 1993 and include major and minor criteria (Table C61.2).[4] A diagnosis of PWS is highly likely in children, aged 0–36 months, with a score of five (four of major criteria), and in children aged 3 years to adults, if the score is at least eight points, with five or more from the major criteria. Our patient had a score of ≥9. The severe hyperphagia and lack of satiety are thought to be partly due to a dysregulation of the hypothalamic-pituitary axis. If PWS is clinically suspected, the diagnosis should be confirmed by genetic testing (Table C61.3).[3]

Table C61.1—Laboratory Data

	Blood Glucose Values	Other Lab tests
Hospital Admission	578 mg/dL (32.1 mmol/L	No ketosis
		Hemoglobin A1C: 12.0%
Day 4	243 mg/dL (13.5 mmol/L)	C-peptide: 2.91 ng/mL
		Negative GAD *
		TSH: 2.391 mIU/L
		Serum Albumin: 3.3 g/dL

*GAD, 65 Glutamic Acid Decarboxylase

Table C61.2—Clinical Diagnostic Criteria for Prader-Willi Syndrome[4]

		Points
Major Criteria:	• Neonatal and infantile hypotonia	1
	• Feeding problems during infancy	1
	• Excessive weight gain after infancy	1
	• Characteristic facial features	1
	• Global developmental delay or mild to moderate intellectual disability	1
		1
	• Hyperphagia	1
	• Hypogonadism	
Minor Criteria	• Decreased fetal movement	½
	• Characteristic behavior problems	½
	• Sleep disturbance or sleep apnea	½
	• Short stature	½
	• Hypopigmentation	½
	• Small hands and/or feet	½
	• Narrow hands with straight ulnar border	½
	• Eye abnormalities (esotropia, myopia)	½
	• Thick viscous saliva with crusting at the corners of the mouth	½
	• Speech articulation defects	½
	• Skin picking	½

Various studies of individuals with PWS have observed impaired glucose metabolism (impaired fasting glucose, impaired glucose tolerance, and T2D) in 7–40% of patients. This abnormal glucose metabolism often occurs after puberty and is more commonly seen in obese subjects with a mean age of 20 years.[4] Although the relationship between obesity and T2D is not clear, children and adults with PWS have been noted to have relative hypoinsulinemia and high insulin sensitivity. The high insulin sensitivity is thought to be explained by lower growth hormone levels, with generalized obesity, as opposed to visceral obesity, and higher relative ghrelin levels for the degree of obesity.

A recent Italian multicenter study of PWS observed that the prevalence of altered glucose metabolism correlated with age, BMI, and HOMA-IR (a measure of insulin resistance). These investigators suggested that the main reason for individual metabolic risk clustering in PWS was obesity and recommended that the most important goal for any PWS treatment program was weight control. This study also confirmed that routine screening for altered glucose metabolism should be performed in all PWS patients, especially in those with obesity.[5] Therefore, it is important to identify and treat the T2D, as well as the obesity, which can lead to increased risks for premature death, cardiovascular disease, and respiratory insufficiency.

Therefore, the most important goal for effective management of PWS is to control obesity through limiting food intake. Individuals with PWS should be placed on low-calorie diets, and often require supplementation of vitamins and minerals, with calcium in order to meet daily requirements. Behavior modification techniques are helpful and may require strict limitation

Table C61.3 — Summary of Testing Used in Prader-Willi Syndrome

Genetic Mechanism	Test Method Used to Detect Defect
Deletions	• DNA methylation • MS-MLPA • FISH • CMA • CMA-SNP array
Uniparental Disomy	• DNA Methylation • MS-MLPA • CMA-SNP array • DNA polymorphisms
Imprinting Defect	• DNA methylation • MS-MLPA • DNA polymorphisms • DNA sequence
Imprinting Center Deletions	• DNA sequence

FISH, fluorescence in situ hybridization; MS-MLPA, Methylation-specific multiplex ligation-dependent probe amplification; CMA, chromosomal microarray; CMA-SNP, chromosomal microarray - small nucleotide polymorphisms

Table C61.4—Pharmacotherapy for Management of Obesity in Prader-Willi Syndrome

Pharmacotherapy	Effect
Phentermine Fenfluramine	• Anorectic • Not been shown to be effective in controlling appetite in patients with PWS
Selective serotonin reuptake inhibitors (SSRIs)	• Effective for behavioral symptoms • Little evidence that they affect binge eating or weight gain
Topiramate	• Not shown to decrease appetite, food intake, or weight status • May decrease self-injurious behaviors
Somatostatin Octreotide	• Predicted to suppress ghrelin and its orexigenic properties • Not been shown to be beneficial in patients with PWS
Exenatide	• Shown to significantly decrease appetite • No effect on weight, BMI, or adiposity when used without diet or lifestyle modifications[5] • Significant decrease in HbA_{1c}[5]

to access of food, such as using physical barriers. Pharmacotherapy has shown to be effective in reducing appetite and weight in some cases but has shown to be more effective if combined with diet and other lifestyle modifications (Table C61.4).

Our patient demonstrates the typical features of PWS with hyperphagia; survival into adulthood is somewhat unusual. Glycemic management of patients who also have T2D presents further challenges and is problematic. Therefore, further research is needed to develop effective pharmacologic, behavioral, and other lifestyle interventions.

References

1.   Salehi P, Hsu I, Azen CG, Mittelman SD, Geffner ME, Jeandron D. Effects of exenatide on weight and appetite in overweight adolescents and young adults with Prader-Willi syndrome. *Pediatr Obes* 2017;12:221–228

2.   Basheer R, Jalal MJ, Gomez R. An unusual case of adolescent type 2 diabetes mellitus: Prader-Willi syndrome. *J Family Med Prim Care* 2016;5:181–183

3.   Driscoll DJ, Miller JL, Schwartz S, Cassidy SB. Prader-Willi syndrome. In *GeneReviews* [Internet]. Pagon RA, Adam MP, Ardinger HH, et al., Eds. Seattle, WA, University of Washington, Seattle, 1993–2016

4. Holm VA, Cassidy SB, Butler MG, Hanchett JM, Greenswag LR, Whitman BY, Greenberg F. Prader-Willi syndrome: consensus diagnostic criteria. *Pediatrics* 1993;91:398–402

5. Fintini D, Grugni G, Bocchini S, Brufani C, Di Candia S, Corrias A, Delvecchio M, Salvatoni A, Ragusa L, Greggio N, Franzese A, Scarano E, Trifirò G, Mazzanti L, Chiumello G, Cappa M, Crinò A. Disorders of glucose metabolism in Prader-Willi syndrome: results of a multicenter Italian cohort study. *Nutr Metab Cardiovasc Dis* 2016;26:842–847

Case 62:
Bardet-Biedl Syndrome

Jennifer J. Iyengar, MD;[1] Roma Y. Gianchandani, MD;[1] and Jennifer Wyckoff, MD[1]

Case

A 56-year-old woman presents with previously diagnosed Bardet-Biedl syndrome (BBS). She originally presented in infancy with postaxial polydactyly, specifically a sixth digit on her hands bilaterally, and webbing between her 2nd and 3rd toes bilaterally. At age 4, visual difficulty led to a diagnosis of cone-rod retinal dystrophy. When she was 10 years old, her older brothers were diagnosed with BBS, prompting an evaluation that led to her diagnosis. She has one sister without manifestations of BBS. Her pedigree was extensively traced without finding evidence of other affected family members. There is no known consanguinity. The diagnosis was made on a clinical basis and neither she nor her brothers underwent genetic testing.

Her primary manifestations of BBS are polydactyly, obesity, cone-rod dystrophy, and renal defects. She denies any neurocognitive delay. She attended regular elementary school until second grade. Then, due to progressive visual impairment, she transferred to a school for the blind where she completed high school. She was completely blind by age 32. She had recurrent urinary tract infections and at the age of 20 underwent a partial nephrectomy for urinary obstruction due to congenital anomaly. Her renal

---

[1]Department of Metabolism, Endocrinology, & Diabetes, University of Michigan, Ann Arbor, MI

history also includes nephrolithiasis and contrast-induced nephropathy with progression to renal insufficiency and dialysis at the age of 55. Radiology showed atrophic, lobular kidneys with minimal cystic changes.

Secondary manifestations include poor balance, premature menopause, and type 2 diabetes with severe insulin resistance. She has no congenital heart defects. Poor balance led to frequent falls in her 40s which resulted in her being wheelchair bound. Menarche was at age 14 and oligomenorrhea started in her 20s. She did have one pregnancy resulting in therapeutic abortion due to medical comorbidities. She developed premature menopause at age 35.

Obesity began in early childhood with peak weight of 309 pounds at the age of 39 (BMI 62m/kg^2). She was diagnosed with type 2 diabetes at age 28. She was treated with oral agents initially but progressed to basal-bolus insulin within 6 months due to poor control. Total daily insulin requirements during this period were 250–300 units. More recently her insulin requirements had declined in the setting of end-stage renal disease and weight loss. Due to visual impairment, she uses insulin pens.

Discussion

BBS is autosomal recessive syndrome. Prevalence has been reported to be 1 per 3,700 in the Faroe Islands, 1 per 13,500 in Bedouin communities, 1 per 17,500 in Newfoundland, and 1 per 160,000 in Switzerland.[1,2]

The diagnosis of BBS is made clinically. Various diagnostic criteria have been proposed.[3-5] Generally, four of the primary features listed in Table C62.1 should be present to make a clinical diagnosis. The average age at diagnosis is 9 years old.[4] Early diagnosis can be difficult because although polydactyly is present at birth, other manifestations often become evident later in life and there is considerable phenotypic variability both between and within families.

BBS is similar to Laurence-Moon syndrome (LMS) and controversy exists as to whether they represent distinct syndromes or a single clinical entity. Both syndromes are characterized by rod-cone dystrophy, cognitive impairment, and hypogonadism but polydactyly is common in BBS whereas spastic paraplegia is more common in LMS.[5] More recently, families who were diagnosed with LMS have been found to have pathogenic variants in BBS-related genes, which suggests that these two syndromes may really be one and the same.[2,6]

Table C62.1—Primary and Secondary Features of Bardet-Biedl syndrome

Primary Features	Secondary Features
• Rod-cone dystrophy • Polydactyly • Truncal obesity • Genital abnormalities • Renal defects • Developmental delay	• Brachydactyly or syndactyly • Dental crowding • Ataxia/poor coordination/spasticity/dysdiadochokinesia • Type 2 diabetes • Congenital heart disease • Olfactory defects • Nephrogenic diabetes insipidus • Male hypogonadism • Hepatic involvement • Craniofacial dysmorphism (wide spaced eyes, down-slanted palpebral fissures, depressed nasal bridge, retrognathia) • Hirschsprung disease

Source: Suspitsin EN, Imyanitov EN,[1] Forsythe E, Beales OL,[2] Green et al.,[3] Beales P et al.,[4] Schachat AP, Maumenee IH[5]

More than 20 genes have been associated with BBS, most commonly BBS1 and BBS10, which code for cilia proteins in the BBSome and chaperonin complex, respectively.[1,7] All genes associated to date with BBS are important for the development and maintenance of immotile cilia, but the genotype–phenotype correlation is poor. While disease states such as cystic fibrosis and maturity-onset diabetes of the young type 5 are associated with ciliary dysfunction and diabetes, the exact mechanism by which BBS genes produce the pleiotropic effects seen in BBS, including diabetes, remains unclear.

Obesity and type 2 diabetes are both commonly found in patients with BBS. Rates of obesity vary depending on cohort and the definition used. However, in the Moore cohort,[6] all patients with BMI data were overweight and 25% had BMI >40 kg/m^2. Early studies likely underestimated rates of diabetes because A1C testing was not commonly available and glucose tolerance testing was not performed in all patients. Table C62.2 gives the estimated frequency of diabetes in different cohorts. The severity of obesity and insulin resistance is higher in patients with BBS10 variants compared to BBS1.[2]

There are no trials comparing diabetes treatment options in BBS. However, weight negative/neutral agents such as metformin, dipeptidyl peptidase-4 (DPP-4) inhibitors, glucagon-like peptide-1 (GLP-1) receptor agonists, or sodium-glucose co-transporter 2 (SGLT2) inhibitors are most

Table C62.2—Estimated Prevalence of Diabetes in Patients with Bardet-Biedl Syndrome[3-6]

Cohort	Year	Cohort Size (Patients)	Location	Prevalence	Considerations and Limitations
Schachat and Maumenée	1982	214	Various	4% (9/214)	Based on English literature case reports from 1959–1982; not all patients tested for diabetes
Green et al.	1989	28	Newfoundland, Canada	45% (9/20)	3 patients with known diabetes on study entry; 6/17 tested positive for diabetes with OGTT
Beales et al.	1999	109	United Kingdom	6% (7/109)	A minority of patients underwent testing for diabetes
Moore et al.	2005	46	Newfoundland, Canada	48% (22/46)	Diabetes screened by either glucose tolerance or A1C

Source: Green et al.,[3] Beales P et al.,[4] Schachat AP, Maumenee IH,[5] Moore SJ et al.[6]

appropriate. Renal dysfunction and unrecognized nephrogenic diabetes insipidus should be considered. Insulin-requiring patients may have visual impairment and need talking glucose meters and insulin pens. More research is needed to identify the underlying mechanisms of diabetes in BBS and to identify optimal diabetes and obesity management in BBS.

References

1. Suspitsin EN, Imyanitov EN. Bardet-Biedl syndrome. *Mol Syndromol* 2016;7:62–71

2. Forsythe E, Beales PL. Bardet-Biedl syndrome. In *GeneReviews* [Internet]. Pagon RA, Adam MP, Ardinger HH, et al., Eds. Seattle, WA, University of Washington, Seattle, 1993–2016

3. Green JS, Parfrey PS, Harnett JD, et al. The cardinal manifestations of Bardet–Biedl Syndrome, a form of Laurence-Moon-Biedl syndrome. *N Engl J Med* 1989;321:1002–1009

4. Beales P, Elcioglu N, Woolf A, Parker D, Flinter F. New criteria for improved diagnosis of Bardet-Biedl syndrome: results of a population survey. *J Med Genet* 1999;36:437–446

5.   Schachat AP, Maumenee IH. Bardet-Biedl syndrome and related disorders. *Arch Ophthalmol* 1982;100:285–288

6.   Moore SJ, Green JS, Fan Y, et al. Clinical and genetic epidemiology of Bardet-Biedl syndrome in Newfoundland: a 22-year prospective, population-based, cohort study. *Am J Med Genet A* 2005;132A:352–360

7.   Forsythe E, Beales PL. Bardet-Biedl syndrome. *Eur J Hum Genet* 2013;21:8–13

Case 63:
Williams-Beuren Syndrome and Diabetes

Meghan Gaule, MD;[1] and Andjela Drincic, MD[1]

Case

A 44-year-old male, with a history of Williams-Beuren syndrome, was seen for routine follow-up of diabetes. He was diagnosed with diabetes 9 years prior to this visit and was well controlled for years with HbA_{1c} <7% on pioglitazone 30 mg daily, metformin ER 500 mg twice daily, and glimepiride 1 mg twice daily. He had no diabetes complications. His fasting blood glucose ranged from 118 to 143 mg/dL (6.5 to 7.9 mmol/L); and his premeal glycemia was in the 92–144 mg/dL (5.1–8 mmol/L) range. He was feeling quite well, without any reported hypoglycemia.

His history was significant for Williams-Beuren syndrome, complicated by supravalvular aortic stenosis and mild mental retardation, hypertension, recurrent urinary tract infections (UTIs), and hyperlipidemia. In addition to the aforementioned medications for diabetes, he was also taking diltiazem, nitrofurantoin, atorvastatin, uroxatral, aspirin, vitamin D3, and lisinopril. He had no family history of Williams-Beuren syndrome, diabetes, hyperlipidemia, or thyroid disease.

On physical exam, he weighed 54.6 kg with a BMI of 22 kg/m², had a blood pressure of 102/64 mmHg, and pulse of 70. He was noted to be quiet and pleasant, with facial features consistent with Williams-Beuren syndrome such as upturned nose, long philtrum, and a wide mouth.

[1]Division of Diabetes, Endocrinology, and Metabolism, University of Nebraska Medical Center, Omaha, NE

Cardiopulmonary exam was notable for a systolic murmur and loud S2 over the right upper sternal border. Feet were without any ulcerations or calluses. Monofilament examination was intact.

Laboratory evaluation showed a HbA_{1c} of 7.0%, TSH 2.36 mcIU/mL (0.4-5.0 mcIU/mL) with FreeT4 of 0.9 ng/dL (0.6–1.5 ng/dL). Calcium level, obtained 3 months after starting 1,000 IU vitamin D3 daily, was elevated at 10.4 mg/dL with an albumin of 4.3 g/dL; 25-OH-vitamin D level was 45 ng/mL. His calcium prior to starting vitamin D supplementation was 9.3 mg/dL and it returned the baseline after stopping his vitamin D supplementation. He later had a bone density scan which showed decreased bone mineral density in the lumbar region of 0.816 g/cm^2, indicating a T-score of –2.5 SD, and at the femoral neck of 0.711 g/cm^2, indicating a T-score of –1.6 standard deviations. As a result of his DEXA scan, his pioglitazone was stopped, and he was continued on only metformin and glimepiride and maintained his HbA_{1c} at ~7 %.

Discussion

Williams-Beuren syndrome (also known as Williams syndrome) was initially described as a syndrome with "peculiar" facies, a distinctive cardiovascular lesion, and "mental retardation." However, it is now known to be a disorder that can affect nearly all organ systems. The features of Williams syndrome are due to deletion of 26–28 genes within a 1.5–1.8 million basepair Williams-Beuren syndrome chromosome region on chromosome 7q11.23.[1] Its prevalence is estimated at 1 in 10,000 persons. Diagnosis is made by fluorescence in situ hybridization (FISH) of ELN (elastin gene). FISH using ELN-specific probes shows the presence of a single ELN allele, rather than two alleles. A number of organ systems can be affected. In particular, cardiovascular manifestations are common and include supravalvular aortic stenosis in 70% of patients and hypertension in 50% of patients. They also have global cognitive impairment but display characteristically a very friendly personality.[2] In addition, patients with Williams-Beuren syndrome suffer from many endocrine abnormalities, including hypercalcemia, osteopenia or osteoporosis, diabetes, subclinical hypothyroidism, and early onset of puberty. We will focus our discussion on the endocrine abnormalities as they relate to our patient.

There is a high prevalence of impaired glucose tolerance in patients with Williams-Beuren syndrome. In one study, a standard oral glucose tolerance test (OGTT) was given to 28 adults with Williams syndrome, and three-fourths of these patients showed abnormal glucose curves and met diagnostic criteria for either diabetes or prediabetes.[1] OGTT was used because HbA$_{1c}$ levels were not as reliable as OGTT in diagnosing diabetes. In fact, only using the HbA$_{1c}$ levels would have missed diabetes diagnosis in half of the cohort. Adults with Williams syndrome should thus be screened for diabetes. It is thought that deletion of a gene in the Williams-Beuren syndrome critical region is the major risk factor for abnormal glucose metabolism, in combination with some environmental factors. Syntaxin-1A is considered to be a possible gene responsible for the high frequency of diabetes in these patients due to its location in the Williams syndrome chromosome region and its role in insulin release. Mouse models with abnormal expression of STx-1a have abnormal glucose metabolism. Another gene, MLXIPL, may also contribute to abnormal glucose metabolism. Environmental factors that may have contributed to abnormal glucose metabolism in this cohort (and generalized to all those with Williams syndrome) include hypertension, prescription medications (such as beta blockers, antipsychotics), and limited physical activity in these patients.[1]

In terms of treatment of diabetes in patients with Williams syndrome, there are no clear guidelines for pharmacotherapy. In our patient, there were multiple considerations to take into account. As mentioned, he was initially on metformin, pioglitazone, and glimepiride. His metformin dose could not be optimized to maximum dose because he had a tendency for weight loss with increasing doses, which was a problem given his BMI. Population studies have identified that about 40% of adults with Williams syndrome have normal weight, while 25% are obese and 30% are overweight. Certainly, glimepiride carries a risk of hypoglycemia, and there are no recommendations for or against this medication in patients with Williams syndrome. Thiazolidinediones may not be a good option due to increased risk of bone loss in these patients who are already at an increased risk, as outlined below. In addition, our patient had a history of recurrent UTIs, typical for William's syndrome, so DPP-4 inhibitors and SGLT-2 inhibitors could possibly further increase UTI risk. Insulin is always an option, but certainly it carries risks of hypoglycemia and difficulty of administering. Pharmacotherapy for diabetes in patients with Williams-Beuren syndrome remains an area where more research is needed.

Our patient exhibited a few other commonly seen endocrinopathies in patients with Williams syndrome, including osteoporosis as mentioned above and hypercalcemia. This patient's elevated calcium level was felt to be a result of vitamin D supplementation. Hypercalcemia is common in Williams-Beuren syndrome, and it has been reported that 5–50% of patients have at least one episode of hypercalcemia.[2] Typically, the hypercalcemia seen is mild, but can be severe, especially during infancy. Multiple mechanisms for the hypercalcemia have been posited and include heightened vitamin D sensitivity, increased 1,25-dihydroxyvitamin D levels, and defective calcitonin synthesis or release.[2,3] In our patient's case, serum calcium returned to normal after stopping vitamin D supplementation, suggesting it was related to heightened vitamin D sensitivity. His follow-up calcium was 9.2 mg/dL with an albumin of 4.2 g/dL.

In terms of his osteoporosis, it is unclear if this is related to his Williams syndrome. In one study of patients with Williams syndrome, nearly half (9/20) of adult subjects had decreased bone mineral density at multiple sites on DEXA (dual-energy x-ray absorptiometry), and all but one had normal calcium levels.[4] However, it is felt that this may be a nonspecific finding, as low bone density is more common among adults with developmental disabilities. One possibility in our patient is that his low bone density could be at least partially attributable to the pioglitazone he had been taking. Thiazolidinediones (TZDs) are a cause of secondary osteoporosis. PPARγ activation with TZDs leads to unbalanced bone remodeling: bone resorption increases and bone formation decreases.[5] Notably, our patient has not exhibited evidence of subclinical hypothyroidism, which is common in patients with Williams but continues to be monitored for this.

Our patient exhibited diabetes, hypercalcemia, and osteoporosis. Specifically, in our patient, treatment of diabetes was altered because of his osteoporosis on DEXA scan. His pioglitazone was stopped out of concern for his osteoporosis. It is also important to be aware of the need for cautious vitamin D repletion as in this patient, who developed hypercalcemia on only 1,000 IU of vitamin D3. Thus, in diabetes treatment in patients with Williams syndrome, it is important to know about the various associated endocrinopathies.

References

1.   Pober BR, Wang E, Caprio S, Petersen KF, Brandt C, et al. High prevalence of diabetes and pre-diabetes in adults with Williams syndrome. *Am J Med Genet* 2010;154C:291–298

2.   Pober BR. Williams-Beuren syndrome. *N Engl J Med* 2010;362:239–252

3. Garabedian M, Jacqz E, Guillozo H, et al. Elevated plasma 1,25-dihydroxyvitamin D concentrations in infants with hypercalcemia and an elfin facies. *N Engl J Med* 1985;312:948–952

4. Cherniske EM, Carpenter TO, Klaiman C, et al. Multisystem study of 20 older adults with Williams syndrome. *Am J Med Genet A* 2004;131:255–264

5. Lecka-Czernik B. Bone loss in diabetes: use of antidiabetic thiazolidinediones and secondary osteoporosis. *Curr Osteoporosis Rep* 2010;8:178–184

Case 64:
Spinal and Bulbar Muscular Atrophy and Diabetes

Sarena Ravi, MD;[1] Janice L. Gilden, MS, MD;[1] Alvia Moid, DO;[1] Boby G. Theckedath, MD;[1] and Jennifer Afranie-Sakyi, BS, MS[1]

Case

A 65-year-old Japanese-American male was diagnosed with type 2 diabetes mellitus in 1995, and spinal and bulbar muscular atrophy (SBMA), also known as Kennedy's Disease, in 2000. Two of his brothers also have SBMA. For control of blood glucose, initial pharmacologic therapy included metformin and nataglinide, which was eventually changed to glipizide, and then glyburide, due to insurance restrictions. Metformin therapy was continued until 2003, then stopped due to the concern of elevated liver enzymes. Liver biopsy showed fatty infiltration. Metformin was eventually restarted and is continued through the current time with close monitoring of liver function tests.

Glutamic acid decarboxylase antibodies and islet cell antibodies were negative. (C-peptide 2.03 ng/mL [0.80–3.10] with blood glucose 125 mg/dL [7.0 mmol/L]). By the year 2003, he began to experience muscle weakness in the upper and lower extremities, muscle cramps with chewing, dysphagia, hand tremors, and facial muscle twitching. He also developed sleep apnea, gastroparesis, and erectile dysfunction. Creatine phosphokinase (CPK) test results were >1,300 u/L (35–232) and echocardiogram showed mild to concentric left ventricular hypertrophy and diastolic dysfunction (EF 69%).

[1]Rosalind Franklin University of Medicine and Sciences/Chicago Medical School and Captain James A. Lovell Federal Health Center, North Chicago, IL

By 2005, he required insulin therapy due to increasing blood glucose levels, and later transitioned to insulin pump therapy (continuous subcutaneous insulin infusion) for better glycemic control. Initial pump settings included a basal rate of 1.1–2 units/hour. By 2011, the basal rate was 1–1.5 units/hour and currently the basal rate is 0.5 unit/hour. Insulin to carbohydrate ratio (I:C) has remained about the same at 1:4–1:5.

He also has developed neuropathic pain, controlled with gabapentin therapy. Blood glucose levels have been well controlled over the years with rare hypoglycemia and HbA_{1c} averages around 7%. However, upper and lower limb proximal muscle weakness has gradually worsened. He now requires an electric wheelchair. Although he has had several episodes of upper respiratory infections and sinusitis, there have been no hospitalizations for hypo- or hyperglycemia, diabetic ketoacidosis, respiratory distress, or pneumonia. He is still able to consume an oral diet, despite dysphagia and cramping of facial muscles.

Although various neurologic complications occur in patients with diabetes, there is limited research regarding the role of neurodegenerative disorders as disease modifiers (Tables C64.1 and C64.2). SBMA is an adult-onset rare X-linked motor neuron disease caused by CAG-repeat expansion in the androgen receptor gene.[1] Hand tremors usually occur in the early 30s, followed by muscular weakness predominantly in lower limbs by age 44, with increasing proximal muscle weakness by age 49, dysarthria and dysphagia in the 50s, and need for use of a cane and wheelchair commonly occurs by late 50s and early 60s.[1] Common endocrine manifestations of SBMA include partial androgen insensitivity, gynecomastia, testicular hypotrophy, testicular exocrine dysfunction, and reduced fertility.[2]

In a review of 20 SBMA patients reported by the Mayo Clinic, half had either impaired glucose tolerance or diabetes. This study reported that diabetes is more likely to occur in SBMA and other trinucleotide repeat disorders, but the cause is unknown. The patients with more severe disease did not have a higher incidence of diabetes. However, the degree of decreased mobility and activity was not thought to be the cause of diabetes. In addition, diabetes did not influence the age of onset or rate of progression of SBMA. However, in other neurodegenerative diseases, such as amyotrophic lateral sclerosis, one study reported that patients have lower rates of glucose utilization, higher post-glucose insulin levels after an intravenous glucose tolerance test, and resistance to exogenous insulin compared to other

Table C64.1—Other Conditions Associated with Neuromuscular Issues and Diabetes

Disease	Characteristics	Genetics	Findings on Muscle Biopsy
Maternally Inherited Diabetes and Deafness (MIDD)	Diabetes, deafness, Maculopathy In one study, 43.1% of cases (22 of 51) had muscular disorders (6) Myopathy-Lower limb muscle weakness and pain with exertion	3243A>G mitochondrial point mutation Mitochondrial diabetes Maternal heritability In 2–3 generations	Muscle biopsy in 6 patients revealed ragged red fibers consistent with mitochondrial myopathy[6]
Kearns-Sayre syndrome	Opthalmoplegia, proximal myopathy, cerebellar ataxia, deafness, diabetes commonly present	Deletion of mitochondrial DNA, others m.3243A>G	Deficiency in cyclooxygenase mainly in ragged-red fibers[6]
Wolfram syndrome (DIDMOAD)	Myoclonus Ataxia Diabetes Insipidus, diabetes, optic atrophy, deafness	Autosomal recessive-mutations in WFS1 gene	
Prader-Willi syndrome	Hyptonia Hyperphagia Obesity Diabetes	Chromosome 15- loss of gene function	

neuromuscular diseases.[3] It is unclear if this is related to muscular dysfunction (Table C64.2).[3,4]

Insulin resistance and hyperinsulinemia, which eventually lead to the development of diabetes, has also been demonstrated in patients with myotonic dystrophy (MD). Although the true prevalence of diabetes in MD is unknown, the etiology is thought to be at the genetic level, leading to defects in insulin receptors. It has also been suggested that muscle wasting and low physical activity can lead to worsening of insulin resistance and further derangements in protein catabolism.[5] Unlike MD, the patients with SBMA may not have insulin resistance, nor have hyperglycemia due to their neuromuscular disease. However, it is still

Table C64.2—Various Neuromuscular Disorders and Glucose Metabolism

	Prevalence of Diabetes	Impaired Glucose Metabolism	Defective Muscle Role in Impaired Glucose Metabolism
SBMA	Suggested by one study to be increased[3]	Yes – suggested by one study to be increased[3]	Unknown
ALS	Not found or proposed in literature	Yes – suggested hyperinsulinemia post-GTT, insulin resistance, lower rates of glucose utilization[4]	Unknown
MD	Not found or proposed in literature	Yes – suggested insulin resistance, hyperinsulinemia, genetic defects in insulin receptors[5]	Genetic defect in insulin receptor Muscle wasting and low physical activity[5]

GTT, glucose tolerance test

controversial whether SBMA affects diabetes at the genetic, molecular, or muscular level. Although SBMA patients do not have the same genetic defects as MD, they also have similar muscle atrophy, progressive proximal muscle weakness, with low to minimal physical activity capabilities. This may also be the explanation for the prevalence of diabetes, rather than SBMA being a modifier of diabetes.

Patients with SBMA may require other modifications to the diabetes treatment regimen, since they may have dysphagia, limiting oral intake and/or the need for tube feedings or parenteral nutrition, with increased risk for aspiration pneumonia. Decreased mobility and inability to do physical exercise may also result in pressure ulcers and other infections that compromise glycemic control. If SBMA disease progression leads to variations in muscle utilization of glucose, it may be better to manage these patients with insulin, as this antihyperglycemic agent allows for continual rapid adjustment, thus avoiding severe hypo- and hyperglycemic events.

Our patient is currently able to consume an oral diet well at this time. However, he may develop abnormalities that can limit oral intake due to progression of his neuromuscular condition. A dietitian is monitoring him for future needs. He has also not yet developed other chronic diabetic complications, such as nephropathy, or peripheral vascular disease. Glycemic control at this time requires insulin therapy. Further, despite the fact that he has maintained good glycemic control, his SBMA has progressed.

Future treatment requirements and glycemic goals may need to change at a later time due to his progressive neuromuscular disease.

Although previous studies have suggested that there is a high prevalence of diabetes in SBMA, they have been of low power.[3] Studies of larger populations of SBMA to assess correlations and interactions with diabetes are needed, and may give a better understanding of the interaction between neuromuscular disorders and glucose metabolism. Furthermore, in the presence of a progressive neurologic disease, such as SBMA, whether there is an etiological association or not, it is important to recognize that traditional diabetic treatment recommendations may need to be modified in order to decrease the burden of care for these patients and their families.

This research was supported, in part, by the Captain James A. Lovell Federal Health Care Center.

References

1.   Atsuta N, Watanabe H, Ito M, Banno H, Suzuki K, Katsuno M, Tanaka F, Tamakoshi A, Sobue G. Natural history of spinal and bulbar muscular atrophy (SBMA): a study of 223 Japanese patients. *Brain* 2006;129:1446–1455

2.   Dejager S, Bry-Gauillard H, Bruckert E, Eymard B, Salachas F, LeGuern E, Tardieu S, Chadarevian R, Giral P, Turpin G. A comprehensive endocrine description of Kennedy's disease revealing androgen insensitivity linked to CAG repeat length. *J Clin Endocrinol Metab* 2002;87:3893–3901

3.   Sinnreich M, Sorenson EJ, Klain CJ. Neurologic course, endocrine dysfunction and triplet repeat size in spinal bulbar muscular atrophy. *Can J Neurol Sci* 2004;31:378–382

4.   Meuller PS, Quick DT. Studies of glucose, insulin, and lipid metabolism in amyotrophic lateral sclerosis and other neuromuscular disorders. *J Lab Clin Med.* 1970;76:190–201

5.   Guzman O, Garcia A, Rodriguez-Cruz M. Muscular dystrophies at different ages: metabolic and endocrine alterations. *Int J Endocrinol* 2012;2012:1–12

6.   Guillaussea PJ, Massin P, Dubois-LaForgue D, Timsit J, Virally M, Gin H, Bertin E, Blickle JF, Bouhanick B, Cahen J, Caillat-Zucman S, Charpentier G, Chedin P, Derrien C, Ducluzeau PH, Grimaldi A, Guerci B, Kaloustian E, Murat A, Olivier F, Paques M, Paquis-Flucklinger V, Porokhov B, Samuel-Lajeunesse J, Vialettes B. Maternally inherited diabetes and deafness: a multicenter study. *Ann Intern Med* 2001;134:721–728

Index

Note: Page numbers followed by *f* refer to figures. Page numbers followed by *t* refer to tables.

B

Folinic acid, fluorouracil, oxalliplatin (FOLFOX) doses, 300
Frataxin (FXN) gene, location, 404
Free fatty acids (FFAs), 331*f*
    impact, 340
Free radicals, release (enhancement), 127
Friedman, Jeffrey, 168
Friedreich ataxia (FRDA), 404–405
Friedreich's ataxia, 395
Frontal bossing, 427*f*
Fructosamine
    HbA$_{1c}$, contrast, 319
    hemoglobin A1C, contrast, 318–321
    high/low levels, 308*t*
    measurement, 307–308
    origination, 307
    usage, 306
    usefulness, 320

G
GAA repeats, 404
Galactose-restricted diet, 131–132
Gallbladder agenesis, 20
Gamma aminobutyric acid (GABA)
    activity, potentiation, 370
    depletion, 406
    GABA receptor-associated protein, 474
    synthesis, 369
Gamma glutamyl transferase, increase, 228
Gastric inhibitory polypeptide (GIP), 405
    secretion, impairment, 185
Gastrinomas, 338
Gastroesophageal reflux disease, 447, 506
Gastrointestinal (GI) autoimmunity, risk (increase), 365–366
Gastrointestinal (GI) dysmotility, 118
Gastrointestinal (GI) intolerance, 459
Gastroparesis, 250, 522

S

9 781580 406666